HEALTHIER

Healthier

FIFTY THOUGHTS ON THE FOUNDATIONS OF POPULATION HEALTH

Sandro Galea

DEAN AND ROBERT A. KNOX PROFESSOR
BOSTON UNIVERSITY SCHOOL OF PUBLIC HEALTH

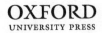

OXFORD
UNIVERSITY PRESS

Oxford University Press is a department of the University of Oxford. It furthers
the University's objective of excellence in research, scholarship, and education
by publishing worldwide. Oxford is a registered trade mark of Oxford University
Press in the UK and certain other countries.

Published in the United States of America by Oxford University Press
198 Madison Avenue, New York, NY 10016, United States of America.

© Oxford University Press 2018

Library of Congress Cataloging-in-Publication Data
Names: Galea, Sandro, author.
Title: Healthier : fifty thoughts on the foundations of population health / Sandro Galea.
Description: Oxford ; New York : Oxford University Press, [2018] |
Includes bibliographical references and index.
Identifiers: LCCN 2017000248 (print) | LCCN 2017000552 (UPDF) |
ISBN 9780190662417 (pbk. : alk. paper) | ISBN 9780190662424 (UPDF) |
ISBN 9780190662431 (EPUB)
Subjects: | MESH: Social Medicine | Health Status | Public Health Practice | Health Equity
Classification: LCC RA418 (print) | LCC RA418 (ebook) | NLM WA 31 | DDC 362.1—dc23
LC record available at https://lccn.loc.gov/2017000248

9 8 7 6 5 4
Printed by Webcom, Inc., Canada

This book is dedicated, as always, to Isabel Tess Galea,
Oliver Luke Galea, and Dr. Margaret Kruk.

Contents

Acknowledgments

THE CHAPTERS IN this book benefitted from the contributions of many, and I am grateful to all my collaborators on the book. Three sets of thanks are due in particular. First, this book would not have been possible without the work of Eric DelGizzo, whose contributions are felt on every page and on all chapters here. Thank you. Second, the following colleagues contributed to particular chapters; Salma Abdalla (Chapters 8, 31, 37, and 49), Meaghan Agnew (Chapters 11 and 29), George Annas (Chapter 1), Jennifer Beard (Chapter 45), Ulrike Boehmer (Chapter 29), Jacob Bor (Chapters 4 and 25), Lisa Chedekel (Chapter 26), Liang Chen (Chapter 10), Gregory Cohen (Chapters 6, 20, 23, 27, 33, 35, 36, 40, and 50), Harold Cox (Chapters 42 and 48), Yvette Cozier (Chapter 48), William DeJong (Chapter 45), Abdulrahman El-Sayed (Chapter 42), Catherine Ettman (Chapters 2, 7, 9, 21, 27, 28, 34, 48, and 49), Anne Fidler (Chapter 47), Lisa Fredman (Chapter 40), Bink Garrison (Chapter 46), Christopher Gill (Chapter 18), Leonard Glantz (Chapters 9 and 38), David Jones (Chapter 45), Katherine Keyes (Chapter 32), Margaret Kruk (Chapter 49), Richard Laing (Chapter 18), Revathi Penumatsa (Chapter 26), Kara Peterson (Chapter 45), Laura Sampson (Chapters 4, 8, 14, 15, 16, 17, 19, 21, 24, 28, 29, 30, 31, 37, 46, 47, 48, and 49), Michelle Samuels (Chapters 11 and 29), and Lisa Sullivan (Chapter 23). Third, these chapters originated as weekly Dean's Notes, written for the Boston University School of Public Health community. I am indebted to countless faculty, staff, students, and alumni who engaged me in conversation around the ideas put forward in those notes, sharpening my thoughts, toward the chapters included in this book. To all: Thank you.

Introduction

HEALTH MATTERS. A CONCERN with our health and well-being crosses national, partisan, and ideological divides. Our concern with health has led us to remarkable achievements that have made for a healthier world during the past century. Life expectancy worldwide is higher than it has ever been. In the past century alone, we have increased life expectancy by a mind-boggling 30 years after centuries during which life expectancy was more or less stagnant. We have dramatically reduced death from infectious disease, and large numbers of people worldwide have access to quality medical care when they need it. Yet, our health achievements leave much to be desired. Although life expectancy has increased overall, billions of people continue to die prematurely, and substantial healthy life years are lost worldwide due to disease or disability. Our collective health achievement is marred by tremendous gaps, with global life expectancy ranging from a high of 83 years in Japan to a low of 47 years in Malawi. The United States has worse health metrics than nearly all other high-income countries, even as the country spends far more on health than any other country worldwide. Population health in the United States is characterized by racial/ethnic and socioeconomic gaps, despite decades of study and effort to narrow these disparities. These successes, and failures, are all the remit of public health.

At heart, public health is concerned with the social, economic, cultural, and political conditions that shape the health of populations. The vast majority of health achievement during the past century is attributable to an improvement in these conditions: to better living conditions in cities, improved educational status for women and men, safer water and sanitation, availability of nutrient-rich food, stable housing and shelter, and reduction in violence and injury. Conversely, our shortcomings represent our failure to tackle the social divides—across countries and within countries—that become health divides. This is compounded by our mis-investment of resources in curative care and away from education, physical and social conditions of cities, social justice, and efforts at disease prevention that create the conditions for healthy populations.

These concerns have long animated my career in public health and inform this book. This collection of essays, written during a 2-year period, aims to tackle foundational concerns that I think should be of interest to anyone engaged with the work of promoting the health of populations. The book is divided into five sections. The first section is concerned with foundations, addressing some of the core principles that underlie the work of public health and that must inform how we go about improving the health of populations. The second section presents essays about the world as it is, about conditions that keep populations from being healthy, and about particular conditions that characterize unhealthy populations. The third section focuses on a topic that I consider core to any study of population health: inequities, with a particular focus on marginalized populations. The fourth section addresses some of the fundamental challenges faced by public health, ranging from methodological to conceptual issues. The final section looks ahead, toward better population health, inhabiting our aspirations toward a healthier world.

Any collection of essays such as this one is inevitably shaped by an author's experiences and perspectives. Hence, a few notes and caveats. First, I write this book from the perspective of someone who has long engaged in scholarship about the health of populations, working principally within academic schools of public health. As such, this book frequently asks the following question: What can academic public health do to tackle any particular issue? I hope that the chapters in this book are illuminating for colleagues within academic public health who may themselves be grappling with these issues. It is my hope, however, that these concerns are universal enough as to be equally interesting to anyone who is engaged in the population health enterprise in general. Reflecting this orientation, I generally use the term "public health" to refer to the discipline whose remit it is to work toward improving the health of populations, whereas I use the term "population health" to mean the subject of interest itself. Second, although this book explicitly takes a global lens, much of the focus is domestic, looking at the United States experience. This is as much a function of my engagement within a US school of public health and our peer community as it is with the challenges facing the United States at this point in time. Third, this book makes no effort at being comprehensive. There are certainly many more issues that can be raised within each of the sections in this book. The issues that I do raise reflect a combination of issues that I think are most important and ones about which I feel qualified to comment. I leave it to others to fill in the gaps. Fourth, this book is a reflection of a particular time and place, embedded within contemporary concerns. I have no doubt that some issues that I tackle will fade in importance over time, whereas other issues will rise in importance, making their omission in this book glaring.

It is my hope—as it is perhaps the hope of anyone who writes such a book—that this work provokes thought and discussion. To that end, I fully expect disagreement, both with my choice of topics and with how I handle the topics themselves. I look forward both to hearing from readers and to seeing other books and papers emerge that fill in gaps or that present alternative—perhaps better—perspectives on the topic. The study of population health is not static. As I finish this book, the United States is on the verge of a political upheaval that will undoubtedly influence the health of American populations; in addition, the global refugee crisis continues unabated, and intercountry rancor around the threat of climate change threatens continued inaction with attendant health consequences. That makes the topic of population health as interesting as it is important. I look forward to seeing where our discussion leads us in coming years, even as I hold out hope that we will be having that discussion in an ever healthier world.

SECTION 1
The Foundations of Population Health

1

The Aspirations and Strategies of Public Health[1]

DURING THE PAST century, public health has been responsible for an extraordinary number of achievements. Going forward, the field stands to make similar contributions to health in this century. Our rapidly changing world continually presents us with new challenges, including chronic diseases, increasing income disparities, the threat of bioterrorism, and climate change. In the face of these concerns, public health is well positioned to lead the way.

Yet, despite its record of achievement, organized public health appears to be on the defensive. High-profile initiatives such as the burgeoning precision medicine agenda and the continuing war on cancer have captured attention at the highest levels of politics, diverting resources into individualized efforts at disease prediction through genomic approaches, at the expense of population-based public health action geared toward the foundational drivers of health [2, 3]. Given that much public health scholarship arises from academic public health institutions that are heavily dependent on federal funding agencies, our national preference for cutting-edge technology and expensive treatment over less eye-catching prevention measures threatens to monopolize the direction of public health scholarship for decades to come. Public health is not alone in this financial uncertainty. We share funding and infrastructure deficiencies with transportation, education, and almost all other endeavors that are reliant on public funding and leadership. Investments in much of this infrastructure have been declining, or barely keeping pace with needs, for decades [4]. In this context, every extra dollar spent on medical care comes at a high opportunity cost, at the expense of public health [5].

The difficulties we face do not center on disagreements about the core goals of our field, which have always been, and remain, broad and aspirational. According to the American

---

[1] This chapter is based on an essay co-written by Professor George Annas that first appeared in *JAMA: The Journal of the American Medical Association* [1].

Public Health Association, "public health promotes and protects the health of people and the communities where they live, learn, work, and play" [6]. This statement captures public health's goal of shaping the conditions that enable healthier populations, with a key emphasis on the prevention of disease.

Rather, part of our challenge has been public health's shift toward operationalizing what we do without sufficient recognition of our aspirational, purpose-driven mission. What we as a discipline do is well-articulated by a set of "essential public health services" in three categories of function: assessment (regular surveillance of the health of communities), assurance (making services available to the public), and policy development (using scientific knowledge) [7, 8]. As a core set of foundational activities, these remain valid and reasonable today. However, simply maintaining core functions does not, in and of itself, constitute a forward-looking purpose. Instead, it suggests doing more of the same—of applying what worked in the past century to a rapidly changing environment. For example, the Director of the Centers for Disease Control and Prevention has suggested that public health should "expand its past successes to further reduce tobacco and alcohol use, control persistent infectious diseases, increase physical activity, improve nutrition, and reduce harms from injuries and other environmental risks" [9].

This agenda, although well-meaning, is too narrow. Such a focus is responsible for public health losing ground in the national conversation, with treatment-centered medical concerns dominating the debate. The bold goals implicit in the definition of public health will never be met, or even taken seriously, if we abandon or rhetorically limit them. Tension between our philosophical roots and their uncertain operational endpoint has caused public health to recede in the collective consciousness, as a burgeoning medical agenda has moved to the forefront. A lack of clarity about our purpose has further constrained our actions.

What, then, can public health do to reinvigorate itself and nudge the field into new areas of innovation? I suggest two key aspirations.

First, public health must unstintingly engage with the social, political, and economic foundations that determine population health. This has been difficult for us, likely because the conditions that make people healthy often exist outside what we have historically considered to be the remit of the health professions. For example, ample scholarship has documented the role of both income distribution and racial segregation as drivers of population health [10, 11]. A focus on the conditions that make populations healthy requires us to come to grips with such issues, reflecting as they do political and social structures. Such an engagement, however, is fraught with peril, both conceptually and operationally.

It is perhaps inevitable that our work would require us to grapple with societal conditions and political circumstances that are far less value-neutral than population health efforts such as disease surveillance. But how do we best engage with these factors? Tackling issues such as racial segregation in housing requires a clarity of advocacy by public health professionals. To be effective, these actors must work in areas such as media, business, and academia, as well as in the governmental public health infrastructure. This puts public health in the position of attempting to quarterback complex social change, motivated by an understanding that absent such change, very little is achievable that can sustain the health of populations in the long term. Actions on this front will require a boldness on the part of public health, as well as a reliance on agents of public health action, such as universities, that are less beholden to political dicta in establishing their budgets and their operating constraints. It also means that we must work with two powerful new organizational forms that have concentrated power and influence in ways that directly affect population health: the transnational corporation and the nongovernmental organization (NGO). For an example of the influence these groups wield, we need look no further than the 2014 Ebola epidemic, when NGOs, most notably Doctors Without Borders, dominated the treatment of patients, and airline corporations determined whether air transportation services would continue to be available, in what countries, and on what terms.

Our second aspiration spotlights the need for health equity. Public health must balance overall improvement of population health with the achievement of health across groups and the narrowing of health gaps. This means we must think on multiple levels. As a field, we have achieved mass legitimacy through an unstinting focus on improving the health of the aggregate. This has, perhaps not surprisingly, diminished our emphasis on the health of marginalized groups. It is not difficult to make the leap from a goal of overall health to an acceptance of health gaps as an inevitable consequence of immutable social structures. Health inequities, however, remain at the heart of why we in public health do what we do, and the drivers of these inequities are the same conditions that have animated some of the difficult national conversations that have surfaced in the past few years [12]. It is important for us to be at the forefront of this national conversation. Doing so provides us with a unique opportunity to engage with the foundational drivers of health and to shape the way people talk about health so that we might, ultimately, shape the health of populations.

What are the best strategies to meet these aspirations? I present four possible approaches.

First, we need relentless prioritization, engaging both intellectually and pragmatically with the core question of what matters most to the health of populations. As Sir Geoffrey Vickers stated in 1958, the "critical and ubiquitous question [is] what matters most *now?*" (emphasis added) [13]. This question implies a number of intellectual, practical, and operational complexities. Intellectually, our scholarship is frequently ill-suited to identify what matters most and has, for many decades, identified causes of ill health without much serious prioritization or relative weighting. To change this, we must rethink how we approach our intellectual work and how that work intersects with the actions of public health. Practically, the challenge in engaging what matters most lies in the mismatch between what we may be able to do and what will indeed have the greatest impact [14]. For too long, we have focused on smaller scale efforts—principally around engagement of lifestyles and healthy behaviors—at the expense of larger efforts that target the foundational drivers of health. Only by evaluating our actions and determining their salience toward the larger goals at hand are we likely to make progress in meeting our objectives.

Second, we must actively engage with the mechanisms whereby core foundational structures produce population health, while also maintaining our focus on these foundational drivers. Take, for example, the obesity epidemic. Although social conditions—including the widespread availability of cheap, calorie-dense, nutrient-poor food—are undoubtedly the core driver of this crisis, health behaviors such as eating patterns mediate the relationship between the corporate practices that establish food availability and obesity in populations [15]. Nonetheless, public health cannot effectively engage with eating behaviors without recognizing their place in a causal cascade. Eating behaviors do matter, but they matter only insofar as food choices represent a range of options that ill serve the ends of health promotion. It is, however, easier to tackle the mediating mechanisms than it is to address the foundational determinants, in no small part because we *think* that the former falls within the scope of public health action; while we pay definitional attention to the latter, our action on it is limited.

This challenge therefore centers on breadth of engagement, from the foundational through the mechanistic. We need to adopt a balanced perspective, as we navigate the import of understanding and intervening on mechanistic processes, without losing sight of the core foundational drivers that will determine the sustainability of our progress. This thinking also applies to our engagement with areas such as genomic medicine. It suggests that public health should by all means contribute to a conversation about the genomic research agenda and its potential while at the same time recognizing that the debate is one rather small piece of a much larger puzzle. In this puzzle, the environment, lifestyles, and even the microbiome are likely more important than genomics in determining the health of populations. Put another way, "personalized medicine" is not public health.

Third, we must embrace collaboration. The vision of public health as a government-mandated and financed activity has already been supplemented, if not replaced, by a wide recognition that public health is multisectoral. We must therefore engage actors across government, academia, industry, and not-for-profit sectors, among others, to achieve our goals. To engage these sectors, and point them toward the common cause of population health, we must create a revised narrative of the importance of public health to replace the current health narrative, centered as it is on improving clinical care. Public health must be at the forefront of generating and sustaining a broad national and global conversation around the centrality of population health. This calls for the elevation of health in the public consciousness and the recognition that individual health is glass ceilinged without an improvement in the health of the collective. Events such as the Ebola outbreak represent teachable moments—opportunities to shift the public discussion toward the foundational efforts that must be made to create a world in which similar outbreaks are prevented or quickly contained, rather than a world in which we have tertiary hospitals and new pharmaceuticals to treat people who contract Ebola when large-scale outbreaks inevitably occur.

Finally, public health needs its own ethics to help guide practice. The fact that much of public health is directed by governments suggests that human rights, as articulated in the *Universal Declaration of Human Rights*, are a solid ethical framework for public health practice [16]. Indeed, many in public health have already adopted human rights as the primary ethical guide for their work. This is perhaps to be expected. Not only do human rights proclaim a "right to health" for all people but also they provide a wide array of state obligations to "respect, protect, and fulfill" the rights of people in ways that promote population health. The World Health Organization (WHO) has adopted the "health and human rights" principles, and, like the goals of public health itself, the challenge is not so much to define these principles but to apply them. Jonathan Mann, the first head of the WHO's Global Programme for AIDS, suggested the "health and human rights" paradigm for public health at the beginning of the HIV/AIDS epidemic, when he quickly discovered that those with the disease were often severely discriminated against and lost jobs, housing, and even families as a result [17]. His legacy, as Rebecca Cook and Bernard Dickens have suggested, is "his focus on how social inequality, economic powerlessness, social exclusion, and denial of human dignity condition preventable disease, disability, and premature death" [18]. The universal scope of public health is well matched by that of human rights, with both focused on safeguarding human dignity and promoting social justice.

REFERENCES

1. Galea S, Annas G. Aspirations and strategies for public health. *JAMA: The Journal of the American Medical Association.* 2016; 315(7): 655–6. doi: 10.1001/jama.2016.0198

2. Collins FS, Varmus H. A new initiative on precision medicine. *The New England Journal of Medicine.* 2015; 372(9): 793–5. doi: 10.1056/NEJMp1500523

3. Fact sheet: President Obama's Precision Medicine Initiative. The White House web site. https://www.whitehouse.gov/the-press-office/2015/01/30/fact-sheet-president-obama-s-precision-medicine-initiative. Published January 30, 2015. Accessed August 31, 2016.

4. Public Spending on Transportation and Water Infrastructure. Congressional Budget Office web site. https://www.cbo.gov/publication/21902. Published November 17, 2010. Accessed August 31, 2016.

5. Health Crisis. Healthy People/Healthy Economy Initiative web site. http://www.tbf.org/tbf/56/hphe/Health-Crisis. Accessed August 31, 2016.

6. What Is Public Health? American Public Health Association web site. https://www.apha.org/what-is-public-health. Accessed August 31, 2016.

7. Institute of Medicine (US) Committee on Assuring the Health of the Public in the 21st Century. *The Future of the Public's Health in the 21st Century.* Washington, DC: National Academies Press; 2002.

8. Stover GN, Bassett MT. Practice is the purpose of public health. *American Journal of Public Health.* 2003; 93(11): 1799–801.

9. Frieden TR. The future of public health. *The New England Journal of Medicine.* 2015; 373: 1748–54. doi: 10.1056/NEJMsa1511248

10. Wilkinson RG, Pickett KE. Income inequality and population health: A review and explanation of the evidence. *Social Science & Medicine.* 2006; 62(7): 1768–84.

11. Williams DR, Collins C. Racial residential segregation: A fundamental cause of racial disparities in health. *Public Health Reports.* 2001; 116(5): 404–16.

12. Jee-Lyn García J, Sharif MZ. Black Lives Matter: A commentary on racism and public health. *American Journal of Public Health.* 2015; 105(8): e27–30. doi: 10.2105/AJPH.2015.302706

13. Vickers G. What sets the goals of public health? *The New England Journal of Medicine.* 1958; 258(12): 589–96.

14. Rothman KJ, Adami HO. Trichopoulos D: Should the mission of epidemiology include the eradication of poverty? *The Lancet.* 1998; 352(9130): 810–3.

15. Troy LM, Miller EA, Olson S. *Obesity and Hunger: Understanding a Food Insecurity Paradigm.* Washington, DC: National Academies Press; 2011.

16. The Universal Declaration of Human Rights. The United Nations web site. http://www.un.org/en/universal-declaration-human-rights. Accessed August 31, 2016.

17. Annas GJ, Grodin MA, Gruskin S, Mann JM, eds. *Health and Human Rights: A Reader.* New York, NY: Routledge; 1999.

18. Cook RJ, Dickens BM. The injustice of unsafe motherhood. *Developing World Bioethics Journal.* 2002; 2(1): 64–81.

2

Social Justice, Public Health

DURING THE PAST 25 years, the life expectancy of the richest quintile of 50-year-old Americans has increased, a perhaps unsurprising development. However, this improvement has not been shared by all. The life expectancy of the middle 60 percent of Americans has seen little change, and the life expectancy of the poorest 20 percent of Americans has, during this time, actually decreased [1].

These data are a core reflection of the underlying social divides that produce health divides. They are also a reminder of the concerns at the heart of public health's mission. The life expectancy gap reminds us that we will fail in our efforts if we aim to improve health without grappling with the underlying maldistribution of wealth, opportunities, and privilege within a society [2, 3, 4]. A social justice approach to population health challenges us to deal with these fundamental concerns. It forces us to recognize that problems such as racism, socioeconomic inequality, gender disparities, and hate have negative consequences for health and that we cannot improve the health of populations without tackling these foundational causes, a point made repeatedly in a large body of public health literature [5, 6, 7, 8, 9, 10].

How does a social justice approach inform action? During his imprisonment in the Birmingham, Alabama, jail in 1963, Martin Luther King Jr. had a lot of time to consider this very question. In his celebrated letter from that confinement, he said,

> I am in Birmingham because injustice is here. . . . I am cognizant of the interrelatedness of all communities and states. I cannot sit idly by in Atlanta and not be concerned about what happens in Birmingham. Injustice anywhere is a threat to justice everywhere. [11]

King's eloquence is both inspiring and direct in its implications for public health. It speaks to the urgency that informs our work, and the work of anyone who tries to help populations that are under threat. It is important to note that King took care to ground his sense of justice in an awareness of the "interrelatedness of all communities." He recognized, as we must, that inequalities are never the exclusive problem of the group they seem to most directly affect. Health, in particular, is interconnected; whenever a distinct group suffers from poor health, the burden will be shared across populations in ways both subtle and overt [12, 13].

Our pursuit of public health is therefore closely linked with how effectively we can reduce inequities between populations. The need for this approach is well captured by our country's current health expenditures. The United States spends far more on health care than any other country in the world, but it has far worse health outcomes than any of its peer countries [14]. We devote tremendous resources to delivering exceptional medical care, but we do so at the expense of correcting the underlying social, economic, and cultural structures that shape health inequities within our national population. Thus, we see troubling disparities such as the higher risk of heart trouble run by Latinos, the fact that black people die sooner than white people, or that, in 2015, the maternal mortality rate actually increased over the previous year [15, 16, 17]. Jennifer Prah Ruger has eloquently captured our skewed priorities in her work on the subject of social justice, noting, "Theories of social justice . . . have typically focused on justifying health care (medicine and public health) as a special social good. . . . In general, less attention has been paid to universal concerns of social justice with respect to health itself" [18].

In discussing the need for a public health that is centered around the creation of social justice, I realize I am saying out loud what many might consider to be implicit in our work, and so this chapter could perhaps be characterized as a statement of the obvious. I persist for three reasons.

First, we know that re-establishing first principles never comes amiss. Indeed, social justice is so central to public health that it becomes, paradoxically, easy to overlook.

Second, although we might consider the social justice component of public health to be self-evident, this is not necessarily the view taken by the wider world. Where we see disparities, for example, many may only see a need for better treatment, or perhaps reason that lopsided health outcomes are merely an unfortunate fact of life. Historically, this view has obstructed many justice-oriented change movements. At the time of King's Birmingham incarceration, the problem of Jim Crow, while clear to us now as a moral travesty, was—to many—just another aspect of normal American life [19]. Many people did not see it this way, of course, and it is in large part due to the success of these dissenters at framing the issue as a matter of social justice that we no longer have legalized segregation in this country [20]. Our own efforts would benefit from a similar, concerted emphasis.

Third, the statement and restatement of core challenges stands to nudge, to move social momentum in the direction of lasting change. History has shown us how communicating the injustice of social ills can lead to progress. Approximately 100 years ago, Upton Sinclair denounced with unprecedented fierceness the mistreatment of employees, and the inhumane conditions under which they worked, in the Chicago meatpacking industry [21]. His book, *The Jungle*, was a quintessential call to social justice, leading to legislation that regulated food production in the United States [22]. It was a notable example of the resonance of social justice as a spur to action, to the ultimate improvement of the health of the public.

Where does our sense of justice come from? What is its ethical value? In his *Nicomachean Ethics*, Aristotle deals at length with these considerations. He observes, "[J]ustice, alone of the virtues, is thought to be 'another's good,' because it is related to our neighbor; for it does what is advantageous to another" [23]. This strikes me as fitting. As we seek to improve the health of populations through our commitment to social justice, we should remember that our efforts might be motivated, at core, by a spirit of simple neighborliness.

REFERENCES

1. Committee on the Long-Run Macroeconomic Effects of the Aging US Population, Committee on Population—Phase II, Division of Behavioral and Social Sciences and Education, Board on Mathematical Sciences and Their Applications, Division on Engineering and Physical Sciences, The National Academies of Sciences, Engineering, and Medicine. *The Growing Gap in Life Expectancy By Income: Implications for Federal Programs and Policy Responses.* Washington, DC: The National Academies Press; 2015. doi: 10.17226/19015

2. Defining Economic Justice and Social Justice. Center for Economic and Social Justice Web site. http://www.cesj.org/learn/definitions/defining-economic-justice-and-social-justice. Published 2016. Accessed July 18, 2016.

3. Sidibé M. The Future We Want: Demanding Social Justice and a New Distribution of Opportunity. *The Huffington Post.* August 15, 2012. http://www.huffingtonpost.com/michel-sidib/opportunity-equality_b_1599547.html. Accessed February 11, 2017.

4. Ferguson S. Privilege 101: A Quick and Dirty Guide. Everyday Feminism Web site. http://everydayfeminism.com/2014/09/what-is-privilege. Published September 29, 2014. Accessed July 18, 2016.

5. Social Justice (definition). Dictionary.com Web site. http://www.dictionary.com/browse/social-justice. Published 2014. Accessed July 18, 2016.

6. Smedley BD. The lived experience of race and its health consequences. *American Journal of Public Health.* 2012; 102(5): 933–5. doi: 10.2105/AJPH.2011.300643

7. Pickett KE, Wilkinson RG. Income inequality and health: A causal review. *Social Science & Medicine.* 2015; 128: 316–26. doi:10.1016/j.socscimed.2014.12.031

8. Yin S. Gender Disparities in Health and Mortality. Population Reference Bureau Web site. http://www.prb.org/Publications/Articles/2007/genderdisparities.aspx. Published 2007. Accessed July 18, 2016.

9. The Health Consequences of Hate. Columbia University Mailman School of Public Health Web site. https://www.mailman.columbia.edu/public-health-now/news/health-consequences-hate. Published April 26, 2016. Accessed July 18, 2016.

10. Link BG, Phelan J. Social conditions as fundamental causes of disease. *Journal of Health and Social Behavior.* 1995; Spec No: 80–94.

11. The Atlantic Editors. Martin Luther King's "Letter from Birmingham Jail." *The Atlantic.* April 16, 2013. http://www.theatlantic.com/politics/archive/2013/04/martin-luther-kings-letter-from-birmingham-jail/274668. Accessed July 19, 2016.

12. Woodward A, Kawachi I. Why reduce health inequalities? *Journal of Epidemiology & Community Health.* 2000; 54(12): 923–9. doi:10.1136/jech.54.12.923

13. Lacapra V. Report: Racial Health Disparities Affect Everyone in St. Louis, Not Just African Americans. St. Louis Public Radio Web site. http://news.stlpublicradio.org/post/report-racial-health-disparities-affect-everyone-st-louis-not-just-african-americans#stream/0. Published May 30, 2014. Accessed July 19, 2016.

14. US Health Care from a Global Perspective. The Commonwealth Fund Web site. http://www.commonwealthfund.org/publications/issue-briefs/2015/oct/us-health-care-from-a-global-perspective. Published 2015. Accessed July 19, 2016.

15. Mehta H, et al. Burden of systolic and diastolic left ventricular dysfunction among Hispanics in the United States: Insights from the echocardiographic study of Latinos. *Circulation: Heart Failure*. 2016; 9(4). doi:10.1161/CIRCHEARTFAILURE.115.002733

16. Arias E. National Vital Statistics Report: Volume 62, Number 7. Centers for Disease Control and Prevention Web site. http://www.cdc.gov/nchs/data/nvsr/nvsr62/nvsr62_07.pdf. Published January 6, 2014. Accessed July 19, 2016.

17. Wallace K. Why Is the Maternal Mortality Rate Going Up in the United States? CNN Web site. http://www.cnn.com/2015/12/01/health/maternal-mortality-rate-u-s-increasing-why. Published December 11, 2015. Accessed July 19, 2016.

18. Ruger JP. Health and social justice. *The Lancet*. 2004; (364)9439: 1075–80.

19. Wallinger H. *Transitions: Race, Culture, and the Dynamics of Change*. LIT Verlag Münster; 2006.

20. Freedom Riders. Public Broadcasting Service Web site. http://www.pbs.org/wgbh/american-experience/freedomriders. Published 2010. Accessed July 20, 2016.

21. Sinclair U. *The Jungle* (entire text). The Literature Network Web site. http://www.online-literature.com/upton_sinclair/jungle. Novel published in 1906. Accessed online July 19, 2016.

22. Meat Inspection Act of 1906. Encyclopedia Britannica Web site. https://www.britannica.com/topic/Meat-Inspection-Act. Last updated March 28, 2016. Accessed July 19, 2016.

23. Aristotle. *Nicomachean Ethics*. Ross WD, Translator. The Internet Classics Web site. http://classics.mit.edu/Aristotle/nicomachaen.html. Accessed July 19, 2016.

3

On Mechanisms Versus Foundations

IN THIS CHAPTER, I touch on one of the primary challenges of population health, one that concerns how we might best spend our time and allocate our often limited resources. This challenge is captured in the following question: Should we, in academic public health, focus on the study of the foundational drivers of population health—on the factors that we know influence the conditions that make people healthy—or should we focus on the mechanisms whereby these foundational drivers shape the health of populations? Or, if we attempt to strike a balance between mechanisms and foundations, what relative weight should we give to each of these two areas?

There are arguments to be made for a focus on either of these approaches. Public health is concerned, foremost, with the conditions that make people healthy. It follows, then, that public health scholarship should continually seek a deeper understanding of these conditions. These foundational forces, sometimes called fundamental causes, include any number of factors, ranging from poverty to income inequality, social structures, and political policies [1]. One of my books, *Macrosocial Determinants of Population Health*, includes chapters on governance, corporate practices, taxation, culture, patent law, migration, and the mass media—all of which, among other factors, fall under the umbrella of fundamental causes [2]. In other research, my colleagues and I quantified the potential contribution of some of these foundational factors to population health. Our data suggested that approximately 245,000 deaths in the United States in 2000 were attributable to low education, 176,000 to racial segregation, 162,000 to low social support, 133,000 to individual-level poverty, 119,000 to income inequality, and 39,000 to area-level poverty [3]. It is therefore clear that a public health of consequence must be informed by an appreciation of the centrality of foundational determinants. Our scholarship should illuminate these factors, how they influence population health, and what we might do to mitigate their sometimes adverse effects.

On the other hand, there is much to agitate for a public health scholarship that focuses on more "downstream" factors—on the study of the mechanisms that explain how these foundational factors get "under the skin" [4]. Such a focus is perhaps inevitable; the relationship between large-scale social forces and population health has to be mediated by more downstream factors. Saying, for example, that poverty is associated with poor health, without acknowledging the mechanistic intermediates that bring this about, undercuts any attempt to explain this link. In fact, poverty is associated with limited access to health care resources, with greater exposure to a broad range of adversities including violence, with greater psychological burden, and with more limited and fragmented social supports, all of which are more proximally related to the production of health. Understanding these mechanisms helps us to appreciate just *how* foundational determinants influence health, and it can also provide guidance on easier ways to intervene. For example, it is perhaps easier in the short term to ensure that all populations have access to health care and better living conditions than to change the profile of poverty in this country. Aiming to inform the science in this area, we have, in our work, explored a range of biological mechanisms that explain how exogenous exposures "get under the skin" [5, 6].

But is ease of action sufficient justification for a focus on mechanisms over the foundational drivers of health? The simple answer is that surely they both matter—that we should understand both core drivers and mechanisms. However, in a world of finite resources, does an academic public health that focuses on upstream factors stand to do as much practical good as one that prioritizes downstream factors? Does it all matter equally? Let us consider one of the central public health threats currently facing the United States—the example of firearm violence. One response to the threat has been to restrict sales of firearms to individuals with mental illness. In fact, firearm-disqualifying mental health adjudications increased from 7 percent of firearm disqualifications in 2007 to 28 percent in 2013 [7]. When we compare the United States with other countries, however, we see the degree to which this intervention comes up short. Canada has a similar prevalence of psychiatric disorders compared with the United States but a much lower overall rate of gun violence and a much smaller proportion of homicides and suicides committed with guns [8]. The best evidence suggests that there is only a marginal association between mental illness and increased risk of violence [9]. This implies that among the dynamics that underlie the epidemic of firearm injury in the United States, mental health is peripheral. It is rather foundational causes—in this case, differences in firearm availability and gun culture—that likely explain the differences in firearm injury between the US and other geographic contexts [10].

Although studying the link between mechanisms and population health can indeed be interesting, and is certainly important, does such an approach in fact distract us from a focus on *what matters most* to improving the health of the public? There is much to be said about the potential distractions of an over-focus on the mechanistic drivers of heath production. Arguably, the recent surge in interest in precision medicine represents the apotheosis of this approach [11]. Francis Collins, Director of the National Institutes of Health, has suggested that "personalized medicine, also referred to as precision medicine, is a promising area for improving health outcomes" [12]. Precision medicine, of course, represents the ultimate study of "mechanisms," aiming to help us identify the causal processes that produce health. Advocates of the precision medicine juggernaut are suggesting, however, that this focus is a *si ne qua non* for the improvement of health. But is it?

At the end of the day, our choice of focus is not cost free—our energies, resources, and attention are all limited, and the areas we choose to prioritize contribute to a production of understanding that informs policy changes that impact health [13]. None of this suggests that mechanistic work is not immensely valuable for our understanding of the science behind our efforts, but it does prod us to confront why it is that we are doing what we do, and what it is we should be focusing on.

REFERENCES

1. Link BG, Phelan J. Social conditions as fundamental causes of disease. *Journal of Health and Social Behavior.* 1995; Spec No: 80–94.
2. Galea S, ed. *Macrosocial Determinants of Population Health.* New York, NY: Springer; 2007.
3. Galea S, Tracy M, Hoggatt KJ, Dimaggio C, Karpati A. Estimated deaths attributable to social factors in the United States. *American Journal of Public Health.* 2011; 101(8): 1456–65. doi:10.2105/AJPH.2010.300086
4. Taylor SE, Repetti RL, Seeman T. Health psychology: What is an unhealthy environment and how does it get under the skin? *Annual Review of Psychology.* 1997; 48: 411–47.
5. Uddin M, et al. Epigenetic and immune function profiles associated with posttraumatic stress disorder. *Proceedings of the National Academy of Sciences.* 2010; 107(20): 9470–5.
6. Toyokawa S, Uddin M, Koenen KC, Galea S. How does the social environment "get into the mind"? Epigenetics at the intersection of social and psychiatric epidemiology. *Social Science & Medicine.* 2012; 74(1): 67–74. doi:10.1016/j.socscimed.2011.09.036
7. Swanson JW, McGinty EE, Fazel S, Mays VM. Mental illness and reduction of gun violence and suicide: Bringing epidemiologic research to policy. *Annals of Epidemiology.* 2015; 25(5): 366–76. doi:10.1016/j.annepidem.2014.03.004
8. Navaneelan T. Suicide Rates: An overview. Statistics Canada Web site. http://www.statcan. gc.ca/pub/82-624-x/2012001/article/11696-eng.htm. Accessed September 20, 2016.
9. Glied S, Frank RG. Mental illness and violence: Lessons from the evidence. *American Journal of Public Health.* 2014; 104(2): e5–6. doi:10.2105/AJPH.2013.301710
10. Miller M, Azrael D, Hemenway D. Firearm availability and unintentional firearm deaths, suicide, and homicide among 5–14 year olds. *Journal of Trauma.* 2002; 52(2): 267–74; discussion 274–5.
11. Collins FS, Varmus H. A new initiative on precision medicine. *The New England Journal of Medicine.* 2015; 372(9): 793–5. doi:10.1056/NEJMp1500523
12. Collins FS. Exceptional opportunities in medical science: A view from the National Institutes of Health. *JAMA: The Journal of the American Medical Association.* 2015; 313(2): 131–2. doi:10.1001/jama.2014.16736
13. Link BG. The production of understanding. *Journal of Health and Social Behavior.* 2003; 44(4): 457–69.

4

What Health, for Whom?

WE ARE CENTRALLY concerned with the production of health. But, what health indicators are we trying to produce, and who are we trying to produce this health for? The perspective of economics—with its focus on resource allocation, models of human behavior and interaction, and the population-level consequences of political policies and other exposures [1, 2, 3, 4]—allows us a lens through which to consider this question. The concept of social welfare pushes us to consider what we are trying to achieve as we advance a population health agenda.

To avoid confusion, it is important that we first differentiate what "welfare" means in the economic sense from its other connotation of government assistance for the poor [5]. In economic terms, social welfare refers to the aggregated measure of a society's well-being and happiness [6]. "Welfare economics" is the subset of economics that concerns itself with the allocation of goods, resources, and services to optimize this allocation and promote general prosperity and satisfaction [7]. At the core of welfare economics is the concept of utility. Utility can be broadly defined as the satisfaction a person derives from the consumption of goods or from being the beneficiary of services [8]. Jeremy Bentham described utility as "that property in any object, whereby it tends to produce benefit, advantage, pleasure, good, or happiness ... or ... to prevent the happening of mischief, pain, evil, or unhappiness" [9, 10]. But utility extends beyond preferences for goods and services directly sold in the market: People may derive utility from having children, from residing in socially cohesive communities, from living without pain or activity limitations, and so on.

In economics, "social welfare" refers to the weighted sum of utility across all members of society [11]. Markets can yield many different allocations of resources across members of society that are efficient in the particular sense that no person can be made better off without making someone else worse off [12]. Social welfare analysis thus speaks to a pressing question: How can we aggregate across all members of society, to maximize utility? Given a set of weights—called a social welfare function—policies can then be compared and ranked in terms of their impact on social welfare [13].

This approach provides us with a lens through which we can view several fundamental questions of interest to populations. Given, for example, the constraints of limited resources and political intransigence, how do we value, or weigh, the welfare of different groups of people in order to maximize welfare across all groups [14, 15]? Whose utility should policy interventions seek to increase? Within the context of these questions, it seems to me that a social welfare approach has two central applications for our thinking.

First, a social welfare approach can help us formalize our thinking about our aims in population health and the values that underpin these aims. Consider the vexing problem of income inequality in the United States [16, 17]. The link between income and health is inextricable, making this issue one of central importance to public health. A social welfare view stands to deepen our understanding of inequality. It forces us to ask the question: How might a utility-focused approach be applied to maximize general prosperity? Should we advocate raising taxes on the rich and redistributing wealth and utility through social programs? Or would a cannier strategy be to promote economic efficiency by streamlining our tax code; even by redistributing income directly via a negative income tax [18, 19, 20]? Or perhaps social welfare would be better maximized through increased regulation of wages and improved bargaining power of workers?

Different types of social welfare functions—different value sets—illustrate these choices differently. A Rawlsian function measures a society by the utility of its worst-off members [21]. An intervention based on this view would reallocate resources from the best-off to the worst-off members of society until equal utility was reached. Then there is the utilitarian approach, which averages the utility of all individuals with an eye toward increasing aggregate utility for all, regardless of distribution [22]. Under this welfare function, very unequal distributions of utility may be optimal if total utility is greater than more equitable distributions. (It is worth noting that because there is decreasing marginal utility to wealth—a dollar is worth more for a poor person than for a rich person—even the utilitarian social welfare function places implicit value on equitable resource distribution.)

In public health, we, too, concern ourselves with the measurement and maximization of utility, even if we do not think about the issue in explicitly economic terms. Take, for example, the occasionally controversial practice of cost–utility analysis [23]. This approach attempts to quantify the value of a particular treatment or program, to determine its overall effect on individuals or societies. In this analysis, utility refers to general quality of life. By the metric of cost–utility analysis, a person's quality of life is measured according to a utility value scale, where the value of an intervention is determined by its translation into quality-adjusted life years (QALYs). Utility is also linked to health in other, more broadly defined ways. Longer life expectancy, for example, means a longer future utility stream; less pain has a direct utility effect; and activity limitations caused by disability or disease can influence potential utility gains from other parts of life.

A social welfare approach is centrally useful to public health in that it forces us to contend with the very "outcome" we wish to maximize and to think more deeply about the definition of "health" itself. This line of inquiry leads us to the question of how certain health states "rank" compared to others, making us ask ourselves which we may prefer if our goal is health maximization. In this sense, we share the dilemma of the economist, as she seeks to define "utility" and use her understanding to implement systems that will improve society on a large scale. Grappling with these questions—What is utility? What is health? How do we accurately measure each? —reinforces the fact that quality of life is a spectrum rather than a binary question of "sick or not sick" or "poor or not poor." Income and disease are, of course, key components that contribute to our overall well-being, but they are far from the whole story, as we well know [24, 25].

We must account for the fact that policies affecting health often have consequences that extend beyond the immediate concern of promoting health-welfare, affecting utility in different ways. Quarantine, for example, has implications for individual liberty; cigarette taxes place an economic burden on those who do not quit; and raising taxes to fund the Affordable Care Act is not free [26, 27, 28]. A social welfare view forces us to consider these factors not only as health professionals but also as citizens aspiring to behave responsibly.

In our efforts to improve population health, we must assess the overall well-being of thousands, sometimes millions, of people. The scale of our efforts means we must remain mindful of the range of factors that go into shaping health indicators within and among populations. What are the health indicators that matter? Do we judge progress by the aggregate improvement in health outcomes or by the degree to which these improvements are equally distributed within and across populations [29]? Whose health do we value? We see in social welfare function a reflection of our own engagement with these concerns.

It is important to note that I do not raise these questions with the intention of remaining neutral on them. I would argue that in public health, we ought to be firmly on the side of minimizing disparities and ensuring that no one gets left behind as we move collectively in the direction of greater health for all [30]. Doing so requires analysis, advocacy, and a willingness to engage with a range of strategies that can advance our ideas. Adopting a social welfare approach is an example of this thinking in action.

REFERENCES

1. Public Health Economics and Tools. Centers for Disease Control and Prevention Web site. http://www.cdc.gov/stltpublichealth/pheconomics. Published November 25, 2015. Accessed September 10, 2016.

2. Economics. Investopedia Web site. http://www.investopedia.com/terms/e/economics.asp. Accessed September 10, 2016.

3. Top 10 Trends of 2015. World Economic Forum. http://reports.weforum.org/outlook-global-agenda-2015/top-10-trends-of-2015. Accessed September 10, 2016.

4. Messonnier ML. Economics and public health at CDC. *Morbidity and Mortality Weekly Report (MMWR)*. 2006; 55(SUP02): 17–19.

5. US Welfare System—Help for US Citizens. US Welfare System Web site. http://www.welfareinfo.org. Accessed September 19, 2016.

6. Economics A—Z Terms Beginning with W. The Economist Web site. http://www.economist.com/economics-a-to-z/w#node-21529313. Accessed September 19, 2016.

7. Welfare Economics. Investopedia Web site. http://www.investopedia.com/terms/w/welfare_economics.asp. Accessed September 19, 2016.

8. Utility (from *International Encyclopedia of the Social Sciences*. Thomson Gale. 2008). Encyclopedia.com Web site. http://www.encyclopedia.com/topic/Utility.aspx#1-1G2: 3045001294-full. Accessed September 19, 2016.

9. Who Was Jeremy Bentham? University College London Web site. https://www.ucl.ac.uk/Bentham-Project/who. Accessed September 19, 2016.

10. Bentham J. *An Introduction to the Principles of Morals and Legislation*. Oxford: Clarendon Press; 1907 reprint of 1823 edition.

11. Weighted. Investopedia Web site. http://www.investopedia.com/terms/w/weighted.asp?layout=infini&v=5A&orig=1&adtest=5A. Accessed September 19, 2016.

12. Fundamental Theorems of Welfare Economics. Policonomics Web site. http://www.policonomics.com/fundamental-theorems-of-welfare-economics. Accessed September 19, 2016.

13. Social Welfare Functions. Statistical Consultants Ltd. Web site. http://www.statisticalconsultants.co.nz/blog/social-welfare-functions.html Published 2010.. Accessed September 19, 2016.

14. Scarcity. Investopedia Web site. http://www.investopedia.com/terms/s/scarcity.asp?layout=infini&v=5A&orig=1&adtest=5A. Accessed September 19, 2016.

15. Puzzanghera J. Political standoffs in DC could impede economic growth in '15. *Los Angeles Times*. December 31, 2014. http://www.latimes.com/business/la-fi-politics-economy-20150101-story.html. Accessed September 19, 2016.

16. Pampel FC, Krueger PM, Denney JT. Socioeconomic disparities in health behaviors. *Annual Review of Sociology*. 2010; 36: 349–70. doi:10.1146/annurev.soc.012809.102529

17. Fitz N. Economic inequality: It's far worse than you think. *Scientific American*. March 31, 2015. http://www.scientificamerican.com/article/economic-inequality-it-s-far-worse-than-you-think. Accessed September 19, 2016.

18. Economic Efficiency. Investopedia Web site. http://www.investopedia.com/terms/e/economic_efficiency.asp. Accessed September 19, 2016.

19. Taxation: Efficiency and Equity. thisMatter.com Web site. http://thismatter.com/economics/taxation.htm. Accessed September 19, 2016.

20. Allen JT. Negative Income Tax. Library of Economics and Liberty Web site. http://www.econlib.org/library/Enc1/NegativeIncomeTax.html. Accessed September 19, 2016.

21. Overview: Rawlsian Social Welfare Function. Oxford Index Web site. http://oxfordindex.oup.com/view/10.1093/oi/authority.20110803100405984. Published 2016. Accessed September 19, 2016.

22. Legal Theory Lexicon 025: Social Welfare Functions. Legal Theory Lexicon. http://lsolum.typepad.com/legal_theory_lexicon/2004/02/legal_theory_le.html Published February 29, 2004. Updated May 22, 2016. Accessed September 19, 2016.

23. World Health Organization. *Introduction to Drug Utilization Research*. Oslo, Norway: World Health Organization; 2003.

24. Diez-Roux AV, Link BG, Northridge ME. A multilevel analysis of income inequality and cardiovascular disease risk factors. *Social Science & Medicine*. 2000; 50(5): 673–87.

25. WHO Definition of Health. World Health Organization Web site. http://www.who.int/about/definition/en/print.html Published 2003. Accessed September 19, 2016.

26. Pope S, Sherry N, Webster E. Protecting civil liberties during quarantine and isolation in public health emergencies. *ABA Law Practice Today*. April 2011. https://www.americanbar.org/publications/law_practice_today_home/law_practice_today_archive/april11/protecting_

6

Producing Health over a Lifetime

AN APPROACH TO population health that prioritizes the central drivers of health must lean on organizing frameworks that help us determine where, and how best, to intervene toward healthier populations. These frameworks help us to wrap our arms around the factors that drive health and disease within and among groups, lending focus to our efforts to influence these foundational conditions. To this end, public health frequently borrows theoretical perspectives from other disciplines to guide specific aspects of our work; there are several constructive examples of our efforts in this regard [1, 2]. In this chapter, I comment on two simple frameworks that I find immensely useful in my own work: life course and multilevel frameworks, each of which aims to help organize our thinking in population health science.

A life course approach to health is based on the understanding that multiple factors influence health throughout the length of a human life. These factors include biological, social, psychological, geographic, and economic conditions that shape health over the life course through risk mechanisms that are independent, cumulative, and constantly interacting over time [3]. As John Lynch and George Davey Smith succinctly put it,

> A life course approach to chronic disease epidemiology explicitly recognizes the importance of time and timing in understanding causal links between exposures and outcomes within an individual life course, across generations, and on population level disease trends. [4]

The scope of specific factors covered within this approach is broad. They include physical growth, social mobility, behavior changes, physical environment, life role transitions, and the central, overarching influence of time. Life course approaches attempt to assess how we make sense of interconnected temporal processes and how exposures arise and produce health throughout life. Life course approaches are also not limited to the life of the individual. Rather, they seek connections in health across generations. Within the context of trauma, for example, a life course approach guides us to the question: How does childhood exposure to a traumatic event change the risk of poor mental health in adulthood? Importantly, a life course perspective suggests that we cannot ignore this question. It challenges us to understand the traumatic event experienced during one's childhood or risk limiting our understanding of poor mental health later in life.

This raises the conceptual and analytic bar, suggesting that we must take into account factors throughout life, and across generations, to better understand the health of populations at any given moment. Such an approach may indeed make our job more difficult, but it may also yield compelling answers, helping us move beyond the welter of contradictory findings that unfortunately characterize much of population health science literature [5].

The advent of formal thinking about life course approaches in population health science is relatively recent. It emerged principally in the realm of chronic disease, although further work has shown its potential to enhance the study of psychiatric and substance use disorders, infectious disease, and oral health [6, 7, 8]. The most recent precursor to the formalization of a life course approach in population health science came via David Barker and colleagues, who found a link between birth weight and lifetime risk for coronary heart disease [9]. Known as the "fetal origins hypothesis," this work focused on how prenatal programming may influence later health. Prior to this work, it was not entirely clear whether prenatal exposure mechanisms were linked to adult disease only through their correlation with later life exposures or whether these early exposures mattered entirely on their own [4]. The work of Barker and colleagues established that these early life exposures did matter on their own, above and beyond any measured confounding variables [10]. Barker's example opened the door for the formal introduction of life course thinking in the field and its continued adoption in the coming decades.

As our thinking about life course exposures has evolved, several authors have articulated key mechanistic models that may explain how exposures over the life course shape subsequent health. Key models in this regard are the critical period, sensitive period, accumulation of risk, and chains-of-risk models. The critical period model concerns itself with the timing of an exposure during specific periods of unalterable biological development, with the understanding that the exposure can affect development during this period. One example of this is fetal exposure to teratogens, which links directly to our understanding of human embryonic development. A life course approach therefore illustrates how fetal exposure to a particular event or agent can result in subsequent alterations to normal human development [11].

The sensitive periods hypothesis posits that there are sensitive periods throughout the life course that are not temporally fixed, when an exposure can wield a more potent influence than it may have at another time. An example is the effect of poverty on mental health during a period of social transition such as divorce [12].

In an accumulation of risk model, the total amount of exposure is what matters, rather than specific exposure time points. Nutrition and cancer risk provides an illustrative example (Figure 6.1) [13].

Finally, the chains-of-risk model emphasizes the sequence of exposures. It assumes that one exposure increases the risk of, or triggers, another exposure, as in the case of nicotine exposure potentiating cocaine addiction [14].

Perhaps the greatest challenge in adopting a life course approach is that of application. How can we best operationalize this approach to achieve our analytic ends? One possibility

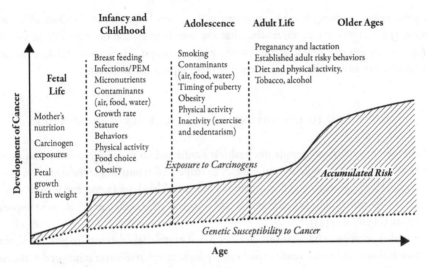

FIGURE 6.1 Accumulation of risk model, based on total cancer exposures throughout the life course. Uauy R, Solomons N. Diet, nutrition, and the life-course approach to cancer prevention. *Journal of Nutrition*. 2005; 135(Suppl 12): 2934S–2945S [13].

rests on thinking about discrete life course stages in order to consider how each stage can represent causes of later disease, manifesting the consequences of prior exposure.

By way of example, consider substance use. We can apply a life course epidemiology of substance use through an analysis of five life course stages: in utero, infancy, childhood, adolescence, and adulthood.

We know that in utero exposure to smoking is a cause of increased risk of lifetime tobacco dependence [15]. We also know that low family socioeconomic status and marital status changes during infancy predict early onset of smoking, while exposure to parental smoking during infancy is associated with sudden infant death syndrome [16, 17]. Childhood neglect and abuse are associated with binge drinking in adolescence, while maternal drug use during childhood can predict an early onset of the same drug use in children [16, 18]. Drinking in adolescence is associated with alcohol dependence later in life, while multiple substance use can be a consequence of prior physical and sexual abuse [19, 20]. Finally, in adulthood, low income has been positively associated with increased risk of substance use disorders, while injuries can be a consequence of alcohol intoxication [21, 22].

As these illustrations demonstrate, a life course perspective suggests links across, perhaps unsurprisingly, phases of life. Without an understanding of these links, it will be difficult to understand any particular "one-point-in-time snapshot" of population health. These illustrations also make it clear that this approach, while helping us better understand the determination of population health, raises substantial methodological and conceptual questions that might open up new scientific vistas and challenge dominant paradigms. At the simplest level, for example, we are compelled to ask—Why should an exposure in childhood influence health in adulthood? Clearly some process, perhaps biological, perhaps social, must link these life stages. Even more provocatively, we encounter the question of why should exposures for one generation influence the health of a subsequent generation? The recent emergence of epigenetics has evinced some promise in answering these questions while also, in some respects, raising as many questions as it answers [23, 24]. Methodologically, a life course perspective calls for approaches that rise above our typical deterministic paradigm. They must be able to take into account both long-term temporal influences and the dynamic, discontinuous, and nonlinear influences that these approaches likely suggest.

MOVING ON TO THE POTENTIAL OF A MULTILEVEL FRAMEWORK

A multilevel approach to population health is predicated on the understanding that exposures at many levels of organization interact to shape health outcomes. These exposures are positioned both upstream and downstream of individual-level risk factors and include determinants of population health that are social, biological, geographic, political, and temporal in nature (Figure 6.2) [25].

A multilevel approach leads us to the question of how social relationships produce health behaviors that may, in turn, result in pathophysiologic manifestations of injury or disease. An inquiry along these lines might ask what effect lifting a law requiring motorcycle helmet use will have on head injuries in a particular state. This, of course, is in contrast to a "single-level" question that concerns itself with individual associations and would ask, rather, what the relationship is between an individual wearing her helmet and her risk of head injury.

Through the adoption of a multilevel framework, we have an opportunity to ask questions that broaden our analytic scope beyond individual experience, toward a fuller appreciation of the levels of influence that plausibly shape the health of populations. This serves to deepen our appreciation of what matters most within the context of public health and to suggest ways we might best engage with these priorities to improve the collective well-being.

To illustrate this approach, let us use the example of coronary heart disease (CHD), the leading cause of death in the United States (610,000 per year), responsible for approximately one-fourth of all annual deaths [26]. CHD has largely been studied in relation to diet, physical activity, and smoking. These are all critical and modifiable factors that are indeed associated

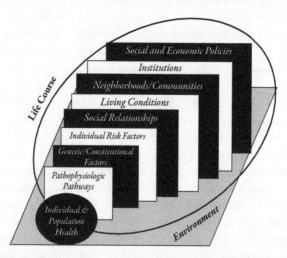

FIGURE 6.2 Upstream and downstream determinants of population health. Kaplan GA. What's wrong with social epidemiology, and how can we make it better? *Epidemiologic Reviews*. 2004; 26: 124–135 [25].

with CHD [27, 28, 29]. Yet, if we limit our perspective to these exposures, we risk confining our inquiry to the proximate prison of risk-factor epidemiology, thereby missing the upstream determinants of public health impact that lie at "higher" levels of organization [30]. In the past two decades, we have seen this broader focus at work, as the study of CHD has extended to neighborhood-level social environment [31]. As a result of this research, socio-economic environment is now associated with CHD incidence, with greater neighborhood disadvantage predicting higher incidence among both blacks and whites, beyond the influence of individual risk factors. In particular, neighborhood median housing value is inversely related to hypertension (a risk factor for CHD) among black women—again, independent of individual-level risk factors [32]. Similarly, neighborhood-level social capital is a predictor of CHD mortality [31]. Therefore, the drivers of CHD exist at both the individual level and the group level. This reality reflects the need for a multilevel perspective.

Importantly, multilevel perspectives do not simply "add" isolated "risk factors" at other levels of influence to our prediction models. Rather, multilevel frameworks lead us to examine the interface between levels and to quantify interactions across levels. To this effect, there is an established literature on theoretic and statistical considerations in appropriately modeling clustered or nested observations (e.g., people within neighborhoods) [33, 34].

Extending the CHD example, from 1979 through 2009, CHD mortality declined by 66 percent among men and 67 percent among women [35]. However, these general gains mask differences by race [35]. Despite the overall reduction in CHD mortality, the rates for African American men and women remain disproportionately high relative to other race/gender groupings [35].

WHY IS THIS?

Informed by a multilevel perspective, one could approach this question in several ways. Can genomic differences explain racial disparities in CHD? Ample evidence suggests that genomic factors do not appear to explain racial disparities in population-level CHD burden [36]. Could this difference, then, be the product of disparities in access to and quality of care [37]? Such a link is possible, although the best available evidence suggests that disparities in access to, and quality of, care explain relatively few of these observed racial differences.

Widening a multilevel lens, an exploration of the geographic differences in disparities in CHD by race shows that while mortality is higher for blacks than whites at any level of urbanization, there are substantial regional differences by race [38]. Among blacks in the United States in 2009, for example, the highest rate of CHD mortality was found in Midwestern rural areas (231 per 100,000), whereas the lowest rate was found in Northeastern rural areas (147 per 100,000). In contrast, among whites, the highest rate of CHD mortality was found among large metro areas in the Northeast (192 per 100,000), whereas the lowest rate was found in medium metro areas in the West (134 per 100,000). This begs the question: Could "higher-level" group determinants of CHD better explain racial differences in CHD? A geographically weighted regression approach demonstrated that geographic heterogeneity in black–white differences in CHD mortality was attributable both to poverty and to segregation [39]. After controlling for poverty, segregation was positively associated with CHD for blacks in some counties and negatively associated with CHD in others. This suggests that the significance of segregation varies by place. Variation in features of the built environment, including walkability and air pollution, are also jointly associated with CHD mortality [40]. Thus, in addition to mitigating racial disparities in CHD by promoting equal access to quality health care, we should also view economic deprivation and segregation as key targets for study and intervention. Encouragingly, a recent commentary by New York City Health Commissioner Mary Bassett, "#BlackLivesMatter—A Challenge to the Medical and Public Health Communities," advocates for just such an approach, calling on clinicians and researchers to contribute to the reduction of interpersonal and institutional discrimination, factors at multiple "levels" that will likely continue to contribute to substantial racial disparities in health [41].

The example of CHD demonstrates how an exploration of influences at multiple levels can illuminate the determinants of population health far more comprehensively than a focus on single levels alone. Just staying within the realm of CHD, we can see how this approach is rapidly gaining currency and broader acceptance, with the 2010 Institute of Medicine report, *Promoting Cardiovascular Health in the Developing World*, emphasizing the need for a multilevel approach to CHD promotion [42].

Taken together, the life course and multilevel perspectives both provide organizing principles that can guide our analytic and conceptual work in public health. Both can help us to better frame the questions we ask and, it is hoped, guide us toward more accurate, actionable answers. Finally, both demonstrate the complexity of population health—a complexity that extends well beyond a deterministic approach that suggests a particular health behavior is the central factor responsible for health outcomes in populations. This clearly has implications for our scholarship, our educational programs, and the practice of public health as a whole.

REFERENCES

1. Krieger N. *Epidemiology and the People's Health*. New York, NY: Oxford University Press; 2011.

2. DiClemente R, Salazar L, Crosby R. *Health Behavior Theory for Public Health: Principles, Foundations, and Applications*. Burlington, MA: Jones & Bartlett Learning; 2013.

3. Ben-Shlomo Y, Kuh D. A life course approach to chronic disease epidemiology: Conceptual models, empirical challenges and interdisciplinary perspectives. *International Journal of Epidemiology*. 2002; 31(2): 285–93.

4. Lynch J, Smith GD. A life course approach to chronic disease epidemiology. *Annual Review of Public Health*. 2005; 26:1–35.

5. Reynolds G. A handy guide to longer living through science! *The New York Times*. October 23, 2014. http://www.nytimes.com/interactive/2014/10/26/magazine/mag-26aging-ai2html.html?_r=1. Accessed September 23, 2016.

6. Koenen K, Rudenstine S, Susser E, Galea S, eds. *A Life Course Approach to Mental Disorders*. New York, NY: Oxford University Press; 2014.

7. Hall AJ, Yee LJ, Thomas SL. Life course epidemiology and infectious diseases. *International Journal of Epidemiology*. 2002; 31(2): 300–301.

8. Nicolau B, Thomson WM, Steele JG, Allison PJ. Life-course epidemiology: Concepts and theoretical models and its relevance to chronic oral conditions. *Community Dentistry and Oral Epidemiology*. 2007; 35(4): 241–9.

9. Barker DJ, Winter PD, Osmond C, Margetts B, Simmonds SJ. Weight in infancy and death from ischaemic heart disease. *The Lancet.* 1989; 2(8663): 577–80.

10. Barker DJ. Fetal origins of coronary heart disease. *The BMJ.* 1995; 311(6998): 171–4.

11. Cardonick E, Iacobucci A. Use of chemotherapy during human pregnancy. *The Lancet Oncology.* 2004; 5(5): 283–91.

12. Aseltine RH Jr. Pathways linking parental divorce with adolescent depression. *Journal of Health and Social Behavior.* 1996; 37(2): 133–48.

13. Uauy R, Solomons N. Diet, nutrition, and the life-course approach to cancer prevention. *Journal of Nutrition.* 2005; 135(Suppl 12): 2934S–2945S.

14. Kandel ER, Kandel DB. Shattuck Lecture: A molecular basis for nicotine as a gateway drug. *The New England Journal of Medicine.* 2014; 371(10): 932–43. doi:10.1056/NEJMsa1405092

15. Buka SL, Shenassa ED, Niaura R. Elevated risk of tobacco dependence among offspring of mothers who smoked during pregnancy: A 30-year prospective study. *American Journal of Psychiatry.* 2003; 160(11): 1978–84.

16. Hayatbakhsh MR, et al. Early childhood predictors of early substance use and substance use disorders: Prospective study. *Australian & New Zealand Journal of Psychiatry.* 2008; 42(8): 720–31. doi:10.1080/00048670802206346

17. US National Cancer Institute. *Health Effects of Exposure to Environmental Tobacco Smoke. Smoking and Tobacco Control Monograph No. 10.* Bethesda, MD: National Cancer Institute; 1999.

18. Shin SH, Edwards EM, Heeren T. Child abuse and neglect: Relations to adolescent binge drinking in the national longitudinal study of Adolescent Health (AddHealth) study. *Addictive Behaviors.* 2009; 34(3): 277–80. doi:10.1016/j.addbeh.2008.10.023

19. Hingson RW, Heeren T, Winter MR. Age at drinking onset and alcohol dependence, age at onset, duration, and severity. *JAMA Pediatrics.* 2006; 160(7): 739–46. doi:10.1001/archpedi.160.7.739

20. Harrison PA, Fulkerson JA, Beebe TJ. Multiple substance use among adolescent physical and sexual abuse victims. *Child Abuse & Neglect.* 1997; 21(6): 529–39.

21. Bassuk EL, Buckner JC, Perloff JN, Bassuk SS. Prevalence of mental health and substance use disorders among homeless and low-income housed mothers. *American Journal of Psychiatry.* 1998; 155(11): 1561–4.

22. Zautcke JL, Coker SB Jr, Morris RW, Stein-Spencer L. Geriatric trauma in the State of Illinois: Substance use and injury patterns. *American Journal of Emergency Medicine.* 2002; 20(1): 14–7.

23. Waterland RA, Michels KB. Epigenetic epidemiology of the developmental origins hypothesis. *Annual Review of Nutrition.* 2007; 27: 363–88.

24. El-Sayed AM, Koenen KC, Galea S. Putting the "epi" into epigenetics research in psychiatry. *Journal of Epidemiology and Community Health.* 2013; 67(7): 610–6. doi:10.1136/jech-2013-202430

25. Kaplan GA. What's wrong with social epidemiology, and how can we make it better? *Epidemiologic Reviews.* 2004; 26: 124–35.

26. Heart Disease Facts. Centers for Disease Control and Prevention Web site. http://www.cdc.gov/heartdisease/facts.htm. Updated August 10, 2015. Accessed September 23, 2016.

27. Mente A, de Koning L, Shannon HS, Anand SS. A systematic review of the evidence supporting a causal link between dietary factors and coronary heart disease. *Archives of Internal Medicine.* 2009; 169(7): 659–69. doi:10.1001/archinternmed.2009.38

28. Li J, Siegrist J. Physical activity and risk of cardiovascular disease—A meta-analysis of prospective cohort studies. *International Journal of Environmental Research and Public Health.* 2012; 9(2):391–407. doi:10.3390/ijerph9020391

29. Huxley RR, Woodward M. Cigarette smoking as a risk factor for coronary heart disease in women compared with men: A systematic review and meta-analysis of prospective cohort studies. *The Lancet.* 2011; 378(9799): 1297–305. doi:10.1016/S0140-6736(11)60781-2

30. McMichael AJ. Prisoners of the proximate: Loosening the constraints on epidemiology in an age of change. *American Journal of Epidemiology.* 1999; 149(10): 887–97.

31. Chaix B. Geographic life environments and coronary heart disease: A literature review, theoretical contributions, methodological updates, and a research agenda. *Annual Review of Public Health.* 2009; 30: 81–105. doi:10.1146/annurev.publhealth.031308.100158

32. Diez Roux AV, et al. Neighborhood of residence and incidence of coronary heart disease. *The New England Journal of Medicine.* 2001; 345(2): 99–106.

33. Diez-Roux AV. Multilevel analysis in public health research. *Annual Review of Public Health.* 2000; 21: 171–92.

34. Gelman A, Hill J. *Data Analysis Using Regression and Multilevel/Hierarchical Models.* New York, NY: Cambridge University Press; 2007.

35. Ford ES, Roger VL, Dunlay SM, Go AS, Rosamond WD. Challenges of ascertaining national trends in the incidence of coronary heart disease in the United States. *Journal of the American Heart Association.* 2014; 3(6): e001097. doi:10.1161/JAHA.114.001097

36. Kaufman JS, Dolman L, Rushani D, Cooper RS. The contribution of genomic research to explaining racial disparities in cardiovascular disease: A systematic review. *American Journal of Epidemiology.* 2015; 181(7): 464–72. doi:10.1093/aje/kwu319

37. Graham G. Population-based approaches to understanding disparities in cardiovascular disease risk in the United States. *International Journal of General Medicine.* 2014; 7: 393–400. doi:10.2147/IJGM.S65528

38. Kulshreshtha A, Goyal A, Dabhadkar K, Veledar E, Vaccarino V. Urban–rural differences in coronary heart disease mortality in the United States: 1999–2009. *Public Health Reports.* 2014; 129(1): 19–29.

39. Gebreab SY, Diez Roux AV. Exploring racial disparities in CHD mortality between blacks and whites across the United States: A geographically weighted regression approach. *Health & Place.* 2012; 18(5): 1006–14. doi:10.1016/j.healthplace.2012.06.006

40. Hankey S, Marshall JD, Brauer M. Health impacts of the built environment: Within-urban variability in physical inactivity, air pollution, and ischemic heart disease mortality. *Environmental Health Perspectives.* 2012; 120(2): 247–53. doi:10.1289/ehp.1103806

41. Bassett MT. #BlackLivesMatter—A challenge to the medical and public health communities. *The New England Journal of Medicine.* 2015; 372(12): 1085–7. doi:10.1056/NEJMp1500529

42. Fuster V, Kelly BB, eds, Committee on Preventing the Global Epidemic of Cardiovascular Disease: Meeting the Challenges in Developing Countries, Board on Global Health, Institute of Medicine. *Promoting Cardiovascular Health in the Developing World: A Critical Challenge to Achieve Global Health.* Washington, DC: The National Academies Press; 2010.

7

Shaping Values, Elevating Health

I HAVE LONG admired the work of the epidemiologist Sir Geoffrey Rose, who wrote the seminal book, *The Strategy of Preventive Medicine* [1]. Writing as a physician who was interested in disease prevention, Rose explained more clearly than anyone before him the differences between identifying the causes of individual cases and identifying the causes of disease incidence in populations. His work in this regard provided us with a framework for thinking about population health, and the perspective he expressed continues to inform much of what we do. As a proponent of the analytic capacity and responsibilities of the quantitative public health scientist, Rose attempted to capture how he saw the role of such practitioners, writing,

> [Our task] is not to tell people what they should do. That is a matter for societies and their individual members to decide. [Rather, our task is] to analyze the options, so that such important choices can be based on a clearer understanding of the issues. [1]

Rose was cautioning here that we must be clear in our understanding of what matters to population health so that this clarity might inform our scholarship and action. I have tried to echo this point under the rubric of "what matters most" in some of my own writing [2].

This perspective seems to suggest the desirability of dispassion in our work, implying that we should be value-neutral arbiters of data analysis, presenting causes of disease that are amenable to intervention, then leaving it to society to decide whether to act on them or not.

This brings us to a core question: How does society decide on these actions?

I would argue that, at a basic level, societal decisions are informed by societal values—sometimes spoken, sometimes not—and that an understanding of the role these values play in shaping decisions central to the promotion of public health should inform how we, as an academic public health community, carry out our work.

Values help us decide the worth, the usefulness of any particular construct, and the extent to which that construct is important to us in life. A fairly clear-cut explanation of values comes to us by way of economics. Economics, as a discipline, is predicated on the monetization of value and on the attribution of monetary value to all aspects of life—some readily transactional, some less so. This is why, for example, we value a car more than we value a laptop. We also, of course, place a value on all aspects of medical care provision in this country; for an enlightening look at the mechanics of monetizing medical procedures, see Steven Brill's book, *America's Bitter Pill* [3].

Values also help us determine the ideas, concerns, and characteristics that we elevate as a society. In this way, values inform our national identity. The United States, for example, clearly values freedom—of the press, of assembly, of religion—and a range of other constructs, many of which are enshrined in unifying national documents such as the Constitution or the Bill of Rights. On the global stage, international documents, such as the Universal Declaration of Human Rights, articulate standards of group and individual behavior, with the goal of establishing common values, to be shared by all nations [4]. Toward this objective, the International Bill of Human Rights—which includes components such as the International Covenant on Economic, Social, and Cultural Rights (ICESCR)—sets agreed upon standards that should hold governments to account in multiple areas, including the right to health. It is worth noting that these standards are, at least theoretically, legally binding.

There is little question that Americans value their health. An abundance of data show that health is one of the principal concerns voiced by Americans when asked [5]. This concern is reinforced by our spending—indeed, we spend more on health than any other country. Insofar as monetary investment is an expression of value, this further suggests the degree to which we prioritize health [6]. Specifically, we value the attainment of individual health—that is, my capacity to be as healthy as I can be and to spend as much money as I want to optimize my health. This is, of course, consistent with an American adherence to the notion of individual capacity for limitless achievement above all else. Our society has chosen, within the context of available options, to prioritize the health of the individual over the health of the group. This, unfortunately, stands the health of the public in poor stead.

We are therefore faced with a choice. If we, as analysts, present, as clearly as we can, an "understanding of the issues," presumably our society will decide what it should do based on the values that it cherishes. Should our role then be, as advocated by Rose, the dispassionate analysis of the options available to us? Or should we try to influence society's decision-making? Although I have spent much of my professional career as an epidemiologist, striving to analyze issues and present the options for intervention as clearly and objectively as possible, I have come to feel that this dispassion ill serves us, allowing us in some ways to shirk our collective responsibilities. This is not to say that we should not present options; doing so is a core part of our remit as an academic public health enterprise. However, our actions on this front must also involve an effort to align society's values with the goals of improving the health of populations. Three realizations have brought me to this conclusion.

First, values are neither absolute nor unchanging; they evolve. Circumstances that are acceptable at one point in time may well be unacceptable at another. Because values, while influential and important, are far from set in stone, action based on these values can at times waver as a consequence of shifting foundations.

Second, if we do not seek to engage with values, others will. Society's codes of conduct are determined by laws and policies that shape how we behave and also by incentives that determine our actions. There is an array of forces that aspire to inform and influence the values that drive the production of these codes and to shape how we choose from among the options available to us. For example, within a market economy, it benefits food companies to promote calorie-dense, nutrient-poor products if doing so will maximize profits. It is also in the industry's interest to argue against laws restricting its capacity to promote its products to children, and so it does. It therefore falls to an activist public health to provide a counterargument—to actively engage in shaping the values that, in turn, inform the parameters set by legislation on whether marketing to children is, or is not, acceptable. For an illuminating read about how the medical industry shaped the values that have elevated physician-based curative care above all other health approaches in the United States, see Paul Starr's *The Social Transformation of American Medicine* [7].

Finally, my thoughts in this area are informed by a concern I have long had. I have worried that by attempting to shape societal values, I would draw inference from data that were explicitly intended to influence or bias the reader in a particular way, undermining my empiric work. This concern is not unique to me—several authors have written eloquently about the ineluctable role of personal biases and values in our scholarship [8]. However, I have come to appreciate the fact that while we, collectively as an academic public health, may have a responsibility to shape societal values, it does not fall to each individual scientist to do so. This speaks to the need for a certain degree of compartmentalizing. It also suggests that we may indeed best serve the cause by articulating the options clearly, even as we are part of an enterprise—population health scholarship—that aims to inform the values society employs to underpin its decisions. It strikes me as not implausible that some scholars among us are comfortable (and adept at) doing both—creating empiric evidence that presents options and engaging in work that aspires to influence societies—while others may be more comfortable doing one or the other.

Ultimately, values emerge from an ongoing societal conversation. As this conversation evolves, values, predictably, shift. In the midst of this change, societies must determine what they should do based on a set of priorities that are constantly in flux and subject—for better or for worse—to outside influence. It thus falls to us in academic public health to contribute to those conversations and to shape values, elevating health.

REFERENCES

1. Rose G. *The Strategy of Preventive Medicine.* Oxford, UK: Oxford University Press; 1992.
2. Keyes K, Galea S. What matters most: Quantifying an epidemiology of consequence. *Annals of Epidemiology.* 2015; 25(5): 305–11. doi:10.1016/j.annepidem.2015.01.016
3. Brill S. *America's Bitter Pill: Money, Politics, Backroom Deals, and the Fight to Fix Our Broken Healthcare System.* New York, NY: Random House; 2015.
4. The Universal Declaration of Human Rights. The United Nations Web site. http://www.un.org/en/universal-declaration-human-rights. Accessed August 31, 2016.
5. Woolf SH, Aron L, eds. Panel on Understanding Cross-National Health Differences Among High-Income Countries; Committee on Population; Division of Behavioral and Social

Sciences and Education; Board on Population Health and Public Health Practice; Institute of Medicine; National Research Council. *US Health in International Perspective: Shorter Lives, Poorer Health*. Washington, DC: The National Academies Press; 2013.

6. Health Expenditure, Total (% of GDP). The World Bank Web site. http://data.worldbank.org/indicator/SH.XPD.TOTL.ZS. Accessed September 23, 2016.

7. Starr P. *The Social Transformation of American Medicine: The Rise of a Sovereign Profession and the Making of a Vast Industry*. New York, NY: Basic Books; 1982.

8. Krieger N. *Epidemiology and the People's Health*. New York, NY: Oxford University Press; 2011.

8

Toward a Culture of Health

IN 2015, THE Robert Wood Johnson Foundation unveiled a forward-looking agenda that detailed the foundation's efforts to foster a culture of health [1]. This agenda included a comprehensive action portfolio designed to support this goal, as well as outcomes to assess culture and health in the United States. There is much that is interesting and praiseworthy about the foundation's efforts and much about their approach that echoes the priorities of public health. Inspired, in part, by the foundation's focus on culture and health, I reflect here on the meaning and importance of culture, both in the broader sense and in terms of its implications for our work.

First, what do we mean by "culture"? That question has many answers, and it has fueled countless academic discussions. In 1952, anthropologists Alfred Kroeber and Clyde Kluckhohn compiled a list of 164 definitions of culture; this list was later expanded to include more than 300 definitions in *Redefining Culture: Perspectives Across the Disciplines* [2, 3]. In 1976, the Welsh Marxist academic Raymond Williams opined that culture is "one of the two or three most complicated words in the English language" [4]. Williams, however, broadly suggested that three predominant meanings of culture are (1) the symbols that inform our intellectual and spiritual development, (2) our specific ways of life, and (3) artistic activity [4]. The latter is likely the term's most common present-day connotation, although maybe not the one most relevant for public health. Despite, or perhaps because of, more than 60 years of lexical analysis, the word retains much currency. In 2014, Merriam–Webster announced "culture" as the word of the year, noting that "culture is a word that we seem to be relying on more and more" [5]. This attention was followed, perhaps inevitably, by more social comment [6].

The definition of culture that is most directly relevant to public health is likely the one provided by the United Nations Educational, Scientific, and Cultural Organizations (UNESCO), which characterized culture as "that complex whole which includes knowledge, beliefs, arts, morals, laws, customs, and any other capabilities and habits acquired by [a human] as a member of society" [7].

These definitions suggest the ubiquity of culture. Given this ubiquity, it is not surprising that culture is an important driver of health. Indeed, a body of empiric work in population health science has long grappled with the role that cultural changes can play in shaping well-being. For example, a UK study found a significant increase in adolescent conduct problems, among both males and females, in the last 25 years of the 20th century [8]. These problems were observed in adolescents from all social groups and family types [8]. Another study found a strong positive correlation between male youth suicide rates and indices of individualism such as personal freedom and control, and it argued that the increase in suicide rates can be explained by a shift toward individualism in Western nations [9].

These are not the only potent examples of culture's capacity to influence health. Consider smoking. The national, and increasingly global, decline in smoking has been clearly linked to the growing public appreciation of the dangers of cigarettes, as well as to policy changes and a slow but inexorable shift in cultural perceptions of tobacco use, with the glamor and ubiquity associated with smoking in an earlier era giving way to the current stigma that is attached to it in many sectors of American society [10, 11, 12, 13, 14]. There is little question that culture—once so tolerant of smoking—has changed, to the benefit of public health [15]. This provides much hope.

A recognition of the power of culture to shape well-being then begs the question: Can we change culture in other ways to improve population health, creating, to quote the Robert Wood Johnson Foundation, "a culture of health"? If so, what would this culture of health look like? Definitionally, it must promote population health as an overriding value, one that is central to societal decisions about the conditions that shape how we live. In some respects, ours is a culture that takes the opposite view, far undervaluing population health. This is most readily evidenced, perhaps, by our absence of a national health insurance that extends coverage to all Americans. As articulated by Richard Wilkinson, elements of our society suggest that we have created a "culture of inequality," informing many of the inequities that continue to undermine our health and inuring us to the existence of wide health gaps between groups [16, 17]. Wilkinson and colleagues have shown that societies with more inequality have, in addition to poorer health indicators, less trust, with the United States at the top of this list [17]. Income inequality can stem from cultural ideas of wealth, social mobility, the "American Dream," and "pulling oneself up by the bootstraps," all of which reflect a particularly American way of thinking but that may be unavoidably linked to poorer population health. Working toward a culture of health, then, would help recalibrate our values and priorities, creating the conditions for the promotion of population health and the narrowing of health gaps.

Beneficial as such a shift would be in the United States, promoting a culture of health is also urgently needed in the global arena. We see an example of this need in worldwide efforts to stop female genital mutilation (FGM). This practice, which entails partially or fully removing external female genitalia, is often carried out on young girls in the Middle East and in African countries for a range of cultural reasons, including encouraging femininity, modesty, decreased libido to maintain virginity and fidelity, social conventions, and power structures [18]. More than 125 million women are alive today who have experienced FGM, and approximately 3 million girls are at risk each year. There are no health benefits to the practice, and the risks of the procedure can be devastating, including urinary tract infections, hemorrhage, anemia, HIV, birth complications, infertility, and a need for later surgery [19, 20]. Despite all of this, the practice remains deeply embedded in certain cultural practices. The global community, including the WHO, UNICEF, and UNFPA, has therefore sought to end FGM by changing the culture surrounding it. Many of these initiatives, such as the UNICEF and UNFPA joint program to accelerate the abandonment of the practice, focus on community empowerment and involvement to eventually eliminate the cultural impetus behind FGM [21]. This movement has seen growing political support, including laws against FGM in 25 African countries [22]. These results are encouraging and speak to the potential of engaging with culture to better the lives of millions worldwide.

With this potential in mind, why has culture not played a greater and more systematic role in our population health thinking until relatively recently? To this point, a few years ago, Richard Eckersley contributed a chapter on culture to my book, *Macrosocial Determinants of Population Health*, arguing that different disciplines have contrasting positions on culture, limiting our consideration of culture as a determinant of health [23]. He suggests that epidemiology, the quantitative core of public health, is mainly concerned with "subcultures and differences" and focuses on individuals at the expense of a higher level of complexity. Thomas Glass agrees, noting, somewhat dyspeptically,

> Like the pre-20th century idea of the luminiferous ether in physics, culture has no place in a Newtonian vision of cause and effect. With few exceptions (think of herd immunity) epidemiology has great difficulty incorporating aggregate-level phenomena that exist in larger dimensional space beyond what touches or invades the individual. [24]

Eckersley, for his part, offers a useful explanation of why we sometimes underestimate or ignore the effects of culture on health. He argues that culture is often invisible to those living within it, that we tend to recognize cultural influences only when they are viewed in unfamiliar societies, and that specific factors such as personal circumstances affect the influence of culture on people. In other words, culture is ubiquitous and yet experienced quite subjectively. This poses challenges to the social determinant of health framework that has broadly found acceptance as a guide to our public health thinking [25].

In summary, culture shapes our values, expectations, norms, priorities, and behaviors, all of which in turn influence the health of populations and the health gaps that can exist within these populations. The ubiquity of culture represents an enormous opportunity to improve health; indeed, an engagement with culture strikes me as an unavoidable part of the business of creating population health. As such, culture should be a central concern for those of us responsible for generating knowledge about the production of health in populations, for conveying that knowledge to our students, and for translating it to stakeholders whose actions can make change happen on a global scale.

REFERENCES

1. In It Together—Building a Culture of Health. The Robert Wood Johnson Foundation Web site. http://www.rwjf.org/en/library/annual-reports/presidents-message-2015.html. Accessed September 23, 2016.

2. Kroeber A, Kluckhohn C. *Culture: A Critical Review of Concepts and Definitions.* Cambridge, MA: The Peabody Museum of American Archeology and Ethnology, Harvard University; 1952.

3. Baldwin JR, Faulkner SL, Hecht ML, Lindsley SL, eds. *Redefining Culture: Perspectives Across the Disciplines.* Mahwah, NJ: Taylor & Francis e-Library; 2008.

4. Excerpts from Raymond Williams, *Keywords.* University of New Hampshire Web site. https://pubpages.unh.edu/~dml3/880williams.htm. Accessed September 23, 2016.

5. Steinmetz K. Merriam–Webster Announces Its Word of the Year. *TIME.* December 15, 2014. http://time.com/3632231/merriam-webster-word-of-the-year-2014. Accessed September 23, 2016.

6. Rothman J. The meaning of "culture." *The New Yorker.* December 26, 2014. http://www.newyorker.com/books/joshua-rothman/meaning-culture. Accessed September 23, 2016.

7. Cultural Diversity. United Nations Educational, Scientific and Cultural Organization Web site. http://www.unesco.org/new/en/social-and-human-sciences/themes/international-migration/glossary/cultural-diversity. Accessed September 23, 2016.

8. Collishaw S, Maughan B, Goodman R, Pickles A. Time trends in adolescent mental health. *Journal of Child Psychology and Psychiatry.* 2004; 45(8): 1350–62.

9. Eckersley R, Dear K. Cultural correlates of youth suicide. *Social Science & Medicine.* 2002; 55(11): 1891–904.

10. Hennessey M. The culture of smoking is just about extinct. *Chicago Tribune.* November 6, 2014. http://www.chicagotribune.com/news/opinion/commentary/ct-cigarette-lighter-bic-chidlren-charcoal-perspec-1107-20141106-story.html. Accessed September 23, 2016.

11. Allen J. New York City marks 10th anniversary of smoking ban. *Reuters.* March 28, 2013. http://www.reuters.com/article/us-usa-smoking-newyork-idUSBRE92R0UU20130328. Accessed September 23, 2016.

12. Rodrigues J. When smoking was cool, cheap, legal and socially acceptable. *The Guardian.* March 31, 2009. https://www.theguardian.com/lifeandstyle/2009/apr/01/tobacco-industry-marketing. Accessed September 23, 2016.

13. Briggs B. Coming of age in the years of living dangerously. *NBC News.* July 6, 2009. http://www.nbcnews.com/id/31670059/ns/health-childrens_health/t/coming-age-years-living-dangerously/#.V-WNAso5h-J. Accessed September 23, 2016.

14. Stuber J, Galea S, Link BG. Smoking and the emergence of a stigmatized social status. *Social Science & Medicine.* 2008; 67(3): 420–30. doi:10.1016/j.socscimed.2008.03.010

15. Stuber J, Galea S. Who conceals their smoking status from their health care provider? *Nicotine & Tobacco Research.* 2009; 11(3): 303–7. doi:10.1093/ntr/ntn024

16. Bales SN. The culture of inequality. *Nonprofit Quarterly.* March 12, 2015. https://nonprofit-quarterly.org/2015/03/12/the-culture-of-inequality. Accessed September 23, 2016.

17. How Economic Inequality Harms Societies. TED Web site. http://www.ted.com/talks/richard_wilkinson?language=en#t-991955. Accessed September 23, 2016.

18. Female Genital Mutilation. World Health Organization Web site. http://www.who.int/mediacentre/factsheets/fs241/en. Updated February 2016. Accessed September 23, 2016.

19. Kaplan A, Hechavarría S, Martín M, Bonhoure I. Health consequences of female genital mutilation/cutting in the Gambia, evidence into action. *Reproductive Health.* 2011; 8: 26. doi:10.1186/1742-4755-8-26

20. Health Risks of Female Genital Mutilation (FGM). World Health Organization Web site. http://www.who.int/reproductivehealth/topics/fgm/health_consequences_fgm/en. Accessed September 23, 2016.

21. Female Genital Mutilation. United Nations Population Fund Web site. http://www.unfpa. org/female-genital-mutilation. Accessed September 23, 2016.

22. Status of African Legislations of FGM. No Peace Without Justice Web site. http://www. npwj.org/FGM/Status-african-legislations-FGM.html. Accessed September 23, 2016.

23. Galea S, ed. *Macrosocial Determinants of Population Health*. New York, NY: Springer; 2007.

24. Glass TA. Commentary: Culture in epidemiology—The 800 pound gorilla? *International Journal of Epidemiology*. 2006; 35(2): 259–61; discussion 263–65.

25. Marmot M, Allen JJ. Social determinants of health equity. *American Journal of Public Health*. 2014; 104(Suppl 4): S517–519. doi:10.2105/AJPH.2014.302200

9

Paternalism

UNAVOIDABLE, PERHAPS DESIRABLE

DURING THE PAST decade, public health has often been accused of being "paternalistic," or engaging in actions that suggest the intrusion of a "nanny state." This charge was particularly difficult to avoid in New York City during the mayoral tenure of Michael Bloomberg; no more so than during his 2012 effort to amend the NYC Health Code so that "food service establishments" would be required to limit the size of containers used to sell sugary drinks [1]. The intent of the Sugary Drinks Portion Cap Rule, as the measure was called, was to elevate public awareness of the role that these beverages play in driving the obesity epidemic. At the time, I had the privilege of sitting on the NYC Health Board and voted for this rule [2]. The effort came on the heels of other public health initiatives enacted by Bloomberg, including an indoor smoking ban and a ban on trans-fat [3]. The soda rule, however, proved something of a bridge too far. Its opponents made the case that it was wrong-headed and paternalistic, and the measure was ultimately struck down by the New York Court of Appeals [4, 5].

Why has the charge of "nanny state" been such a potent rallying cry for opponents of public health? How might we best respond to accusations of paternalism? Is public health, in fact, inherently paternalistic [6]? If so, is this necessarily a bad thing?

Both the word "paternalism" and the phrase "nanny state" suggest the actions of a parent looking after a child. Whereas for some this may be comforting, and perhaps consistent with the role of government in general, for many it is precisely the problem [7]. Critics are liable to suggest that there is an infantilization at work here, a finger-wagging in the face of the individual. The citizen is deemed unfit to make her own decisions and must therefore be told what to do by a small group of "elites." It is not difficult to grasp why this conception of paternalism might upset people. Indeed, in some cases, public health has been its own worst enemy in furthering this view. In recent years, for example, advice by the Centers for Disease Control and Prevention (CDC) that all women of childbearing age should avoid drinking alcohol has been widely, and perhaps justifiably, criticized as being unnecessarily paternalistic [8, 9].

What was missing in the controversy surrounding the CDC's recommendation, however, was the *form* of the CDC's recommendation. The CDC's advice was just that—advice. The report did not advocate banning alcohol, nor was it in any way coercive. It was designed to inform, not to interfere. This is an important distinction to make. It is the difference between a paternalism that guides people's choices through suggestion, or "nudges," and a mode that relies on penalties and outright prohibitions. Because our critics sometimes fail to acknowledge this distinction, it is all the more important that we continue to point it out.

To illustrate the difference, I use a metaphor borrowed liberally from John Stuart Mill's *On Liberty*, a work that attempts, among other things, to determine to what extent the state may be permitted to interfere in the lives of citizens "for their own good" [10].

A man is backpacking in a foreign country where he does not speak the language. As he hikes a mountain trail, he approaches a steep gorge with a bridge running across it. There is a sign next to the bridge, but because the words on the sign are written in the country's native tongue, the man cannot understand what they mean. If he could, he would recognize them as a warning: "Stay off this bridge! It is unsafe."

Now imagine that you are a native of this country, watching this scene unfold. You speak the language and can understand the sign, and the peril the traveler faces. Will you intervene and explain the danger to the man? Or will you let him take his chances? Say you were to intervene and inform him of the risk he would run in proceeding. You then ask him if, knowing what he now knows, he would still like to cross the bridge. He answers "yes." Having heard his response, you decide, for his own safety, not to let him cross. This is what is known as "hard paternalism." Its political equivalent is when a government places laws between the citizen and his poor choices [11]. In his treatise *The Moral Limits of the Criminal Law*, political philosopher Joel Feinberg writes, "Hard paternalism will accept as a reason for criminal legislation that it is necessary to protect competent adults, against their will, from the harmful consequences even of their fully voluntary choices and undertakings" [12].

But say you did not choose to restrain the traveler. Say you just stepped forward and helpfully translated the sign for him, and he—now fully cognizant of his situation—decided to turn back. You would have saved his life without having had to resort to anything more drastic than simply providing a bit of information. You would have interfered with his choice only to make sure that it was truly voluntary—after all, if a man does not know that a bridge is unsound, he does not know that his decision to cross or not is actually a choice between life and possible death. His ignorance therefore becomes a kind of coercion, forcing him to make a call he never intended to make. From this perspective, your interference actually increases his autonomy. When he knows what he is getting into and can plan accordingly, he is able to exercise more direct control over his own life. This is the function of "soft paternalism"—to make sure that an individual's choices are fully informed so that they can indeed be fully voluntary [13].

Cigarette warning labels are a clear example of how soft paternalism stands to improve population health. Recalling my previous thoughts on culture, consider the status of smoking as it existed 50 years ago. With all the marketing savvy of the tobacco industry working to make smoking seem like a glamorous lark, a consumer might have been forgiven for not knowing that the activity can lead to some truly grisly health outcomes. Back then, it was possible to consider buying a pack of cigarettes without knowing that the question "to smoke, or not to smoke?" is, more realistically, the question "to lose a lung and possibly harm my family with toxic fumes, or to avoid all that?" The introduction of warning labels allowed the consumer to make a decision that was truly informed. Additional regulation has stopped short of hard paternalism (the sale of cigarettes is still legal in the United States), but labels ensure that the consumer is now aware of the risk. Perhaps this knowledge might even nudge her behavior in a healthier direction.

Such nudges are all around us. We are, in fact, regulated at all times and on all fronts—we just do not always think about it [14]. From seat belt laws to food safety initiatives, our society is full of measures designed to promote well-being through benign, commonsense regulations [15, 16]. With this in mind, the uproar occasionally provoked by a given public health effort can start to seem a bit arbitrary, not to mention inaccurate. The much-decried Portion Cap Rule, for example, was widely known as a "soda ban." Actually, it was not a ban at all—merely a limit on how much soda could be sold in a single container. Nothing about the rule would have prevented the consumer from buying a second beverage, if she so desired. The intent was that by changing the default soda size, most people—inertia being what it is—would not have made the extra effort to order more [17]. Thus, health might have been improved without infringing on anyone's freedom of choice. It is worth noting, too, that food companies regularly cut back on the amount of product they provide, although for perhaps less public-spirited reasons than those enumerated by Mayor Bloomberg [18, 19].

As Cass Sunstein, former Administrator of the White House Office of Information and Regulatory Affairs, has written, "Paternalism comes in a lot of shapes and sizes" [20]. It can be hard or soft, obtrusive or subtle. The concept of the "nudge," as explored by Sunstein and his colleague Richard Thaler, represents an opportunity to safeguard and improve the health of populations while at the same time respecting individual autonomy [21]. The nudge can take many forms, from a food label that tells you how long it will take to burn off the calories contained therein to a tax hike on a harmful substance [22, 23]. These measures, for all their modesty, stand to do much good. It is worth noting, too, that far from being an assault on liberty, nudges like these actually promote individual freedom in the short and long term, for the simple reason that healthy people, generally, have more options than sick people.

Finally, it is important to remember that the so-called nanny state is not the only actor at play here. From corporate interests to other public sectors' agenda, there are a broad range of efforts that aim to influence consumers' decisions. As Janet Hoek has argued in the pages of *Public Health*, "Rather than depriving individuals of freedoms, state intervention maintains and defends those freedoms against commercial interests, which potentially pose a much greater threat to free and informed choice" [24]. If we, fearing the accusation of "paternalism" or "nanny state," choose not to nudge the public toward a higher standard of living, there are others who will be all too happy to steer us down a more hazardous road. Facing this choice, I favor efforts to nudge us in the direction of healthier populations. If mild, conscientious regulation stands to help people sidestep the emotional, financial, and physical burdens of disease, then it is an option we ought to embrace.

REFERENCES

1. Mayor Bloomberg soda ban. *The Huffington Post.* http://www.huffingtonpost.com/news/michael-bloomberg-soda-ban. Accessed September 23, 2016.

2. Grynbaum MM. Health panel approves restriction on sale of large sugary drinks. *The New York Times.* September 13, 2012. http://www.nytimes.com/2012/09/14/nyregion/health-board-approves-bloombergs-soda-ban.html?mtrref=undefined&gwh=4B45051B586E1B8D7B5031E4E734145D&gwt=pay. Accessed September 23, 2016.

3. Kliff S. Mayor Mike Bloomberg, public health autocrat: A brief history. *The Washington Post.* June 4, 2012. https://www.washingtonpost.com/blogs/ezra-klein/post/mayor-mike-bloomberg-public-health-autocrat-a-brief-history/2012/06/04/gJQArSJbDV_blog.html. Accessed September 23, 2016.

4. Roff P. Michael Bloomberg's soda ban won't solve the obesity problem. *US News & World Report.* June 5, 2012. http://www.usnews.com/opinion/blogs/peter-roff/2012/06/05/michael-bloombergs-soda-ban-wont-solve-the-obesity-problem. Accessed September 23, 2016.

5. Galoozis C. A new kind of paternalism. *Harvard Political Review.* October 27, 2012. http://harvardpolitics.com/united-states/a-new-kind-of-paternalism. Accessed September 23, 2016.

6. Kass NE. An ethics framework for public health. *American Journal of Public Health.* 2001; 91(11): 1776–82.

7. Conn S. Central government: 13 reasons why big government matters. *The Huffington Post.* August 16, 2012. http://www.huffingtonpost.com/steven-conn/central-government-book_b_1777321.html. Updated October 16, 2012. Accessed September 23, 2016.

8. Alcohol and Pregnancy. Centers for Disease Control and Prevention Web site. http://www.cdc.gov/vitalsigns/fasd. Accessed September 23, 2016.

9. Brice A. Is CDC's alcohol warning paternalistic? Why some women think so. *Berkeley News.* February 18, 2016. http://news.berkeley.edu/2016/02/18/is-cdc-alcohol-warning-paternalistic. Accessed September 23, 2016.

10. Mill JS. *On Liberty.* London: Longman, Roberts, & Green Co; 1859 (first pub date) 1869.

11. Pope TM. Counting the dragon's teeth and claws: The definition of hard paternalism. *Georgia State University Law Review.* Spring 2004. https://litigation-essentials.lexisnexis.com/webcd/app?action=DocumentDisplay&crawlid=1&doctype=cite&docid=20+Ga.+St.+U.L.+Rev.+659&srctype=smi&srcid=3B15&key=a09113538e85ef1eb17c7c73409eec18. Accessed September 23, 2016.

12. Feinberg J. *Harm to Self (The Moral Limits of the Criminal Law).* New York, NY. Oxford University Press; 1986.

13. Soft paternalism: The state is looking after you. *The Economist.* April 6, 2006. http://www.economist.com/node/6772346. Accessed September 23, 2016.

14. Quigley M. Nudging for health: On public policy and designing choice architecture. *Medical Law Review.* 2013; 21(4): 588–621. doi:10.1093/medlaw/fwt022

15. Achievements in public health, 1900–1999 motor-vehicle safety: A 20th century public health achievement. *Morbidity and Mortality Weekly Report (MMWR).* 1999; 48(18): 369–74.

16. Achievements in public health, 1900–1999: Safer and healthier foods. *Morbidity and Mortality Weekly Report (MMWR).* 1999; 48(40): 905–13.

17. Surowiecki J. Downsizing supersize. *The New Yorker.* August 13, 2012. http://www.newyorker.com/magazine/2012/08/13/downsizing-supersize. Accessed September 23, 2016.

18. Dickler J. The incredible shrinking cereal box. *CNN Money.* September 10, 2008. http://money.cnn.com/2008/09/09/pf/food_downsizing. Accessed September 23, 2016.

19. Grynbaum MM. New York plans to ban sale of big sizes of sugary drinks. *The New York Times.* May 30, 2012. http://www.nytimes.com/2012/05/31/nyregion/bloomberg-plans-a-ban-on-large-sugared-drinks.html?_r=0&mtrref=undefined&gwh=D5B9778828EB64CF EAA0F8CFCE621EE5&gwt=pay. Accessed September 23, 2016.

20. Sunstein CR. Why paternalism is your friend. *New Republic.* April 8, 2013. https://newrepublic.com/article/112817/cass-sunstein-simpler-book-excerpt-why-paternalism-your-friend. Accessed September 23, 2016.

21. Wallace-Wells B. Cass Sunstein wants to nudge us. *The New York Times Magazine.* May 13, 2010. http://www.nytimes.com/2010/05/16/magazine/16Sunstein-t.html?mtrref=undefined& gwh=9A826C1CCB524CE25584A62140C83208&gwt=pay. Accessed September 23, 2016.

22. Dwyer L. Will people lose weight if labels show how long it takes to burn off calories? Alternet Web site. http://www.alternet.org/food/will-people-lose-weight-if-labels-show-how-long-it-takes-burn-calories. Published January 18, 2016. Accessed September 23, 2016.

23. Cauchon D. Tax hike cuts tobacco consumption. *USA Today.* September 13, 2012. http://usatoday30.usatoday.com/news/nation/story/2012-09-10/cigarette-tax-smoking/57737774/1. Accessed September 23, 2016.

24. Hoek J. Informed choice and the nanny state: Learning from the tobacco industry. *Public Health.* 2015; 129(8): 1038–45.

10

At the Heart of It All, Empathy

ON MARCH 25, 1911, a fire began to blaze at the Triangle Shirtwaist Factory in Manhattan. The factory workers, mostly young immigrant girls, rushed for the exits, only to find that the doors had been locked. This was done to prevent unauthorized breaks, discourage theft, and keep out union organizers [1]. As a consequence, 146 women died that day, from fire, smoke inhalation, and, perhaps most horribly, falling to their deaths as the flames forced them to jump out of the windows [2]. What turned this tragedy into an outrage, however, was the fact that it could easily have been prevented. For years, workers had complained about the unsafe conditions that would eventually lead to the catastrophe—the locked doors, the close quarters, and the lack of proper safety systems—but to no avail. Despite their efforts, it took the fire on March 25 to galvanize public opinion and lead to a host of reforms. Too late for the girls of the Triangle Shirtwaist Factory, these reforms would nevertheless greatly improve the lives of workers throughout the country [1].

Why did these reforms not happen sooner? Terrible factory conditions were an open secret at the time [3]. Yet for years nothing changed. What made the difference? By way of answering that question, let us consider another example—one that is more topical but, in a way, no less tragic.

Since the conflict in Syria began, more than 4 million refugees have fled the country [4]. During the course of this flight, these refugees often trade one desperate situation for another. In urban Jordan, for example, 86 percent of Syrian refugees are living below the local poverty line [4]. Despite these stark statistics, the international community has not rallied to the aid of these desperate people. By the end of 2015, just 61 percent of the United Nation's humanitarian appeal for Syrian refugees had been funded [4]. There was, however, one notable uptick in donations in recent years. It occurred after the dead body of a 3-year-old Syrian boy named Alan Kurdi was photographed lying on a beach. He had drifted there after the boat carrying him and his family away from the conflict apparently capsized [5]. So shocking was the image of the boy that donations to help migrants surged in. One charitable organization, the Migrant Offshore Aid Station, reported a 15-fold donation increase within a day of the photograph's release [6].

In the case of both the Triangle Shirtwaist Factory fire and the death of Alan Kurdi, we are confronted with the same question: Why did these individual deaths rouse public sympathy in a way that statistics, and broader advocacy attempts, did not? I suggest that it is because both stories resonate with our human instinct to imagine ourselves in the place of the person, or people, affected by terrible events. Our capacity for this kind of imagining is called empathy.

Empathy is "the action of understanding, being aware of, being sensitive to, and vicariously experiencing the feelings, thoughts, and experience of another . . . without having the feelings, thoughts, and experience fully communicated in an objectively explicit manner" [7]. It is a quality that has been observed throughout history as a key trait of many celebrated artists and leaders. We see it in Shakespeare, for example, when his characters plead fiercely for a more empathetic society [8]. More recently, Nelson Mandela has shown us the power of empathy when it is allowed to play out on a global, political scale [9]. But perhaps the example of empathy that is most resonant in our cultural consciousness are the words of Atticus Finch, from the novel *To Kill a Mockingbird:* "You never really understand a person until you consider things from his point of view . . . until you climb into his skin and walk around in it" [10].

We are literally hardwired for empathy—it has its structural basis in neuroscience [11]. When we see someone suffering, the victim's facial expression, pupil size, and body language can directly stimulate the "mirror neuron" system to trigger an empathetic response, especially if that person's situation is similar to one we have faced in the past [12, 13, 14]. For a complete understanding of empathy, we must take into account these underlying neurological mechanisms. But brain chemistry alone does not fully explain moments of fellow-feeling. There are also psychological reasons why people experience (or do not experience) empathy. Psychological and neurological theories suggest that there are two fundamental systems in human cognition: the experiential system and the analytic system [15]. The experiential system is triggered when we see the individual victim of some misfortune. When we witness suffering, our experiential system triggers the empathic part of the brain, perhaps even moving us to help the person in need.

Just as it is easy for us to connect with individuals, it is, by contrast, often difficult for us to empathize with large numbers of people. This difficulty has much to do with the other fundamental system in human cognition: the analytic mode [15, 16]. The analytic mode is triggered when we contemplate populations in the abstract, often in the form of statistics. This perspective can blunt our empathetic impulse and lead to "compassion fatigue" [17].

This suggests that, in many ways, our efforts to understand and safeguard the health of populations are hindered by our own neurobiology. It falls to us, then, to ensure that people do not become "just numbers"—to ourselves or to anyone else. To stop this from happening, we must engage with empathy on the individual level, even as we work to improve the health of whole populations.

What can we in public health take from an understanding of empathy? First, we must never lose sight of how compelling individual stories can be. We cannot assume that data alone will sway opinions in our favor. Recognizing the powerful role that empathy plays in mobilizing action, and, conversely, how difficult it is to act absent a clear focus for our empathy, is a reminder of the hard work we must do to engage others in our project—the creation of the social, economic, and cultural conditions that are needed to safeguard health.

Second, we must work even harder to communicate the ongoing narrative of population health. At core, this means telling our story, with energy and creativity, always taking care to foreground the humanity at the heart of a particular problem or initiative. For example, perhaps the broader tale of Syrian mass migration is indeed too big for any one person to process all at once. On the other hand, the story of little Alan Kurdi, dying scared and alone in the middle of the sea, is almost impossible not to connect with on an emotional level. We need to make sure that people hear these stories—taking great care, of course, not to be exploitative—in order to convey to the world the events and circumstances that are putting populations at risk. We must make storytelling and empathy a key part of our armamentarium.

REFERENCES

1. Dreier P, Cohen D. Have we forgotten the lessons of the triangle fire? *The Huffington Post.* March 24, 2014. Updated May 24, 2014. http://www.huffingtonpost.com/peter-dreier/triangle-shirtwaist-fire-lessons-anniversary_b_5019431.html. Accessed September 23, 2016.

2. Leap for Life, Leap of Death. California State University, Northridge Web site. https://www.csun.edu/~ghy7463/mw2.html. Accessed September 23, 2016.

3. Triangle Shirtwaist Factory Fire. The History Channel Web site. http://www.history.com/topics/triangle-shirtwaist-fire. Accessed September 23, 2016.

4. Syria's Refugee Crisis in Numbers. Amnesty International Web site. https://www.amnesty.org/en/latest/news/2016/02/syrias-refugee-crisis-in-numbers. Published February 3, 2016. Accessed September 23, 2016.

5. Walsh B. Alan Kurdi's story: Behind the most heartbreaking photo of 2015. *TIME.* December 29, 2015. http://time.com/4162306/alan-kurdi-syria-drowned-boy-refugee-crisis. Accessed September 23, 2016.

6. Henley J, Grant H, Elgot J, McVeigh K, O'Carroll L. Britons rally to help people fleeing war and terror in Middle East. *The Guardian.* September 3, 2015. https://www.theguardian.com/uk-news/2015/sep/03/britons-rally-to-help-people-fleeing-war-and-terror-in-middle-east. Accessed September 23, 2016.

7. Empathy (definition). Merriam–Webster Web site. http://www.merriam-webster.com/dictionary/empathy. Accessed September 23, 2016.

8. The Book of Sir Thomas More: Shakespeare's Only Surviving Literary Manuscript. The British Library Web site. https://www.bl.uk/collection-items/shakespeares-handwriting-in-the-book-of-sir-thomas-more. Accessed September 23, 2016.

9. Eze C. *Nelson Mandela and the Politics of Empathy:* Reflections on the moral conditions for conflict resolutions in Africa. *African Conflict and Peacebuilding Review.* 2012; 2(1): 122–35. doi:10.2979/africonfpeacerevi.2.1.122

10. Lee H. *To Kill a Mockingbird.* New York, NY: Grand Central Publishing; 1960.

11. Carr L, Iacoboni M, Dubeau MC, Mazziotta JC, Lenzi GL. Neural mechanisms of empathy in humans: A relay from neural systems for imitation to limbic areas. *Proceedings of the National Academy of Sciences of the United States of America.* 2003; 100(9): 5497–502.

12. Harrison NA, Singer T, Rotshtein P, Dolan RJ, Critchley HD. Pupillary contagion: Central mechanisms engaged in sadness processing. *Social Cognitive and Affective Neuroscience*. 2006; 1(1): 5–17.

13. Preston SD, de Waal FB. Empathy: Its ultimate and proximate bases. *Brain and Behavioral Sciences*. 2002; 25(1): 1–20; discussion 20–71.

14. Marsh J. Do mirror neurons give us empathy? Greater Good: The Science of a Meaningful Life Web site. http://greatergood.berkeley.edu/article/item/do_mirror_neurons_give_empathy. Published March 29, 2012. Accessed September 23, 2016.

15. Slovic P, Finucane ML, Peters E, MacGregor DG. Risk as analysis and risk as feelings: Some thoughts about affect, reason, risk, and rationality. *Risk Analysis*. 2004; 24(2): 311–22.

16. Empathy Represses Analytic Thought, and Vice Versa: Brain Physiology Limits Simultaneous Use of Both Networks. Science Daily Web site. https://www.sciencedaily.com/releases/2012/10/121030161416.htm. Published October 30, 2012. Accessed September 23, 2016.

17. Carey B. Becoming compassionately numb. *The New York Times*. October 1, 2011. http://www.nytimes.com/2011/10/02/sunday-review/compassion-fatigue.html?_r=0&mtrref=undefined&gwh=ADDC438F7FDDB5DA90C235D79BB271DD&gwt=pay&assetType=opinion. Accessed September 23, 2016.

11

On Courage

IT CAN TAKE considerable courage to face the world as it is. It can take even more to imagine how society could be made better and to undertake the often difficult task of trying to implement positive change. When facing this difficulty in my own work, I have often found myself looking back to the examples of history for both inspiration and perspective. For this chapter, I spotlight two stories from the past that I think embody the kind of moral and physical courage that is absolutely essential to the work of public health. One story demonstrates this courage in the context of the individual, the other in the context of a social movement. Both involve work that improved the health of the public tremendously; in each case, this achievement took many years and required immense courage in the face of many obstacles. I present these two cases—the story of Ignaz Semmelweis and a brief history of the movement to fight HIV/AIDS in the United States—as examples of the kind of fortitude that we would do well to emulate in our own work.

In the 19th century, puerperal fever—caused by a bacterial uterine infection—was a common postpartum killer in both Europe and the United States, claiming many lives [1]. The disease was also called "childbed fever," and it would strike women in the days immediately following childbirth [2]. A horrifying condition, both to witness and to experience, puerperal fever has been described as "raging fevers, putrid pus emanating from the birth canal, painful abscesses in the abdomen and chest, and an irreversible descent into an absolute hell of sepsis and death—all within 24 hours of the baby's birth" [3].

Ignaz Semmelweis, a Hungarian obstetrician, was determined to find the cause of these childbed fever epidemics. He began collecting data in the 1840s, while he was the director of the maternity clinic at the Vienna General Hospital in Austria [4]. Between two maternity wards in the hospital, one staffed by midwives and the other by doctors and medical students, he noted that the death rate was nearly five times higher in the ward staffed by doctors and students [5]. This led him to hypothesize that the difference in mortality was due to the fact that the doctors often performed autopsies elsewhere in the hospital prior to their work in the maternity clinic. Although Semmelweis developed his hypothesis years before the confirmation of germ theory, he nevertheless speculated that childbed fever was caused by some type of "morbid poison" on the hands of the doctors, which they transferred from cadavers to the bodies of the women giving birth [6, 7]. With this in mind, Semmelweis began requiring his staff to wash their hands in a chlorine solution, causing mortality rates in the most afflicted wards to drop from 18.27 percent to 1.27 percent [8].

Despite these dramatic results, the medical community did not rush to embrace the practice of handwashing. Many derided Semmelweis's work and resented the implication that they themselves might be responsible for transmitting disease [9]. The American obstetrician Charles Meigs summed up prevailing attitudes when he said, "Doctors are gentlemen, and gentlemen's hands are clean" [9]. The pushback was so strong that it led to the coining of a new phrase, the "Semmelweis reflex," which refers to the human tendency to reject innovation out of hand whenever it contradicts widely held beliefs or established paradigms. To make matters worse, Semmelweis had a difficult personality, refusing to publish his findings for more than a decade because he considered them to be "self-evident" [10]. His increasingly volatile behavior led to him being committed to a mental institution, where, in 1865, at the age of 47 years, he died apparently of sepsis, a condition similar to the very infection he had spent his life fighting to prevent [5]. In a final irony, the death of Semmelweis came shortly before the publication of Louis Pasteur's work on bacteria, which ushered in a wider acceptance of the germ theory of disease. Joseph Lister would later use Pasteur's research as a starting point for his own experiments in applying new standards of cleanliness to surgical practice [11]. Semmelweis, troubled though he was, is now regarded as a medical pioneer and a courageous figure in the ongoing struggle to safeguard population health.

Now, we move from puerperal fever to another deadly disease of the more recent past: HIV/AIDS. In the United States, more than 1.2 million people are living with HIV [12], a diagnosis that is now, fortunately, far less dire than it once was. Advances in treatment have changed the face of the illness, although some groups still face disproportionate rates of infection [13, 14, 15]. Although HIV is now viewed as a chronic condition that can be managed and lived with, it is important that we do not forget just how bad the AIDS crisis was at its peak in the last decades of the 20th century [16]. Remembrance is particularly vital when we consider how hard communities of people with HIV/AIDS had to fight to make their voices heard at all. Horrific as the physical reality of HIV/AIDS was and is, the stigma associated with the condition during the 1980s made a terrible situation even worse [17]. Because the disease disproportionally affected men who have sex with men, intravenous drug users, and Haitian immigrants, some saw it as "God's punishment" for "immorality" and found affected populations easy to marginalize [18, 19, 20, 21]. Because of this stigma, people were able to create psychological barriers between themselves and individuals with HIV/AIDS [22]. Government, too, was widely ineffective in coming to grips with the plague. The Reagan administration was slow to even acknowledge it, much less confront the entrenched homophobia and misinformation that allowed it to flourish [23, 24, 25, 26].

In the face of government inaction, the gay community mobilized to do for itself what the political establishment would not. This led to the rise of activist groups such as the Gay

Men's Health Crisis, the AIDS Coalition to Unleash Power (ACT UP), and the AIDS Action Committee, which formed to advocate for individuals living with HIV/AIDS [27, 28, 29]. These groups pursued their goals with energy and creativity. In 1988, ACT UP protested the US Food and Drug Administration's (FDA) slow drug-approval procedure, prompting the FDA to accelerate the process [30]. In addition to widespread organization, countless individuals committed themselves to the cause, including ACT UP founder Larry Kramer and Craig Harris, co-founder of the National Minority AIDS Council [31, 32, 33]. Randy Shilts was the first journalist to cover the US AIDS crisis full-time, and he went on to publish *And the Band Played On*, a seminal look at the first 5 years of the epidemic [34, 35]. Meanwhile, media coverage of several high-profile HIV-positive activists, including Alison Gertz, Elisabeth Glaser, and Ryan White, also did much to dispel the stigma of the disease [36, 37, 38]. Magic Johnson, too, has been an effective advocate, and he is an example of how it is possible to live a full, active life after being diagnosed with HIV [39]. And the illness of public figures such as Rock Hudson and Arthur Ashe helped millions of people put a familiar face to the plight of the gay community, making the crisis of that community unignorable [40, 41].

The courage and ingenuity of the AIDS movement also found ample expression in the arts world, with many iconic works emerging from that era of fear. Plays such as Kramer's *The Normal Heart* and Tony Kushner's *Angels in America* and visual art such as Keith Haring's 1988 *Silence = Death* and the NAMES Project AIDS Memorial Quilt (conceived by activist Cleve Jones) have conveyed the experience of HIV/AIDS to the wider world [42, 43, 44, 45, 46]. Coupled with ongoing political activism, these artistic efforts helped to build social momentum, lessen stigma, and create the conditions for ever-better HIV prevention measures and treatments, bringing us to where we can now realistically hope to eliminate this disease within the coming decades [47].

As both Semmelweis and the HIV/AIDS movement exemplify, having courage often means taking action even when we know that change might not come within a single lifetime. It means trying to engage with a social/political/medical establishment that can be, at times, indifferent or even actively hostile to the voices of advocates and innovators.

In the face of this reality, courage is no minor factor. It is central to the work of public health. To advance our ideas and create healthier populations, we must be willing to occasionally take stands that are perhaps at the moment unpopular and to shine a light on uncomfortable truths. As an idea, this may sound noble, romantic even, but the day-to-day enactment of it can be a brutal grind. It cost Semmelweis his reputation, maybe his health; it cost the energy, reputations, and lives of countless HIV/AIDS activists in this country.

The centrality of courage to public health action means that we need to teach it as a core competency of a public health education, using the context of our scholarship and study as an opportunity to ask ourselves some difficult questions. Just what, for example, are the moral and intellectual risks entailed by our aspirations? How far are we willing to go—as individuals and as a field—to achieve our goal of improved population health? How much progress can we reasonably expect to see over the course of a lifetime or a career, and can we live with the likelihood that this progress will be incremental? These are not easy questions to consider—to ask them takes a kind of courage, to answer them honestly takes even more.

REFERENCES

1. Busowski MT, Lee M, Busowski JD, Akhter K, Wallace MR. Puerperal group A streptococcal infections: A case series and discussion. *Case Reports in Medicine*. 2013; 2013: Article ID: 751329. doi:10.1155/2013/751329

2. Hallett C. The attempt to understand puerperal fever in the eighteenth and early nineteenth centuries: The influence of inflammation theory. *Medical History*. 2005; 49(1): 1–28.

3. Markel H. In 1850, Ignaz Semmelweis saved lives with three words: Wash your hands. *PBS NewsHour*. May 15, 2015. http://www.pbs.org/newshour/updates/ignaz-semmelweis-doctor-prescribed-hand-washing. Accessed September 24, 2016.

4. Ignaz Semmelweis (1818–65). Science Museum, London Web site. http://www.sciencemuseum.org.uk/broughttolife/people/ignazsemmelweis. Accessed September 24, 2016.

5. Davis R. The doctor who championed hand-washing and briefly saved lives. *NPR*. January 12, 2015. http://www.npr.org/sections/health-shots/2015/01/12/375663920/the-doctor-who-championed-hand-washing-and-saved-women-s-lives. Accessed September 24, 2016.

6. Dr. Semmelweis' Biography. Semmelweis Society International Web site. http://semmelweis.org/about/dr-semmelweis-biography. Accessed September 24, 2016.

7. Germ Theory. Science Museum, London Web site. http://www.sciencemuseum.org.uk/broughttolife/techniques/germtheory Accessed September 24, 2016.

8. Zoltán I. Ignaz Philipp Semmelweis. Encyclopaedia Britannica Web site. https://www.britannica.com/biography/Ignaz-Semmelweis. Accessed September 24, 2016.

9. Hendrick C. The Semmelweis reflex: Why does education ignore important research? *chronotope*. June 6, 2015. https://chronotopeblog.com/2015/06/06/the-semmelweis-reflex-why-does-education-ignore-important-research. Accessed September 24, 2016.

10. Markel H. The doctor who made his students wash up. *The New York Times*. October 7, 2003. http://www.nytimes.com/2003/10/07/health/the-doctor-who-made-his-students-wash-up.html. Accessed September 24, 2016.

11. Joseph Lister (1827–1912). Science Museum, London Web site. http://www.sciencemuseum.org.uk/broughttolife/people/josephlister. Accessed September 24, 2016.

12. HIV in the United States: At a glance. Centers for Disease Control and Prevention Web site. http://www.cdc.gov/hiv/statistics/overview/ataglance.html. Accessed September 24, 2016.

13. Griffin RM. Advances in HIV treatment: Understanding ART. WebMD Web site. http://www.webmd.com/hiv-aids/features/hiv-aids-treatment-advances-art. Accessed September 24, 2016.

14. Young S. HIV no longer considered death sentence. *CNN*. December 1, 2013. http://www.cnn.com/2013/12/01/health/hiv-today. Accessed September 24, 2016.

15. McCollum R. The perfect storm facing black men on HIV. *The Advocate*. May 2, 2016. http://www.advocate.com/current-issue/2016/5/02/perfect-storm-facing-black-men-hiv. Accessed September 24, 2016.

16. Deeks SG, Lewin SR, Havlir DV. The end of AIDS: HIV infection as a chronic disease. *The Lancet*. 2013; 382 (9903): 1525–33.

17. Stigma, discrimination and HIV. Avert Web site. http://www.avert.org/professionals/hiv-social-issues/stigma-discrimination. Accessed September 24, 2016.

18. HIV among gay and bisexual men. Centers for Disease Control and Prevention Web site. http://www.cdc.gov/hiv/group/msm. Accessed September 24, 2016.

19. DrugFacts: HIV/AIDS and drug abuse: Intertwined epidemics. National Institute on Drug Abuse Web site. https://www.drugabuse.gov/publications/drugfacts/hivaids-drug-abuse-intertwined-epidemics. Updated May 2012. Accessed September 24, 2016.

20. Avasthi A. AIDS virus traveled to Haiti, then US, study says. *National Geographic*. October 29, 2007. http://news.nationalgeographic.com/news/2007/10/071029-aids-haiti.html. Accessed September 24, 2016.

21. 23 Percent see AIDS as God's punishment for immorality. Pew Research Center Web site. http://www.pewresearch.org/daily-number/see-aids-as-gods-punishment-for-immorality. Published May 7, 2007. Accessed September 24, 2016.

22. Barnhart G. The stigma of HIV/AIDS. American Psychological Association Web site. http://www.apa.org/pi/about/newsletter/2014/12/hiv-aids.aspx. Published December 2014. Accessed September 24, 2016.

23. Lawson R. The Reagan Administration's unearthed response to the AIDS crisis is chilling. *Vanity Fair*. December 1, 2015. http://www.vanityfair.com/news/2015/11/reagan-administration-response-to-aids-crisis. Accessed September 24, 2016.

24. White A. Reagan's AIDS legacy/silence equals death. *San Francisco Chronicle*. June 8, 2004. http://www.sfgate.com/opinion/openforum/article/Reagan-s-AIDS-Legacy-Silence-equals-death-2751030.php. Accessed September 24, 2016.

25. Halkitis PN. Discrimination and homophobia fuel the HIV epidemic in gay and bisexual men. American Psychological Association Web site. http://www.apa.org/pi/aids/resources/exchange/2012/04/discrimination-homophobia.aspx. Published April 2012. Accessed September 24, 2016.

26. Geiling N. The confusing and at-times counterproductive 1980s response to the AIDS epidemic. The Smithsonian Web site. http://www.smithsonianmag.com/history/the-confusing-and-at-times-counterproductive-1980s-response-to-the-aids-epidemic-180948611/?no-ist. Published December 4, 2013. Accessed September 24, 2016.

27. GMHC Web site. http://www.gmhc.org. Accessed September 24, 2016.

28. ACT UP accomplishments and partial chronology. ACT UP New York Web site. http://actupny.com/actions/index.php/the-community. Accessed September 24, 2016.

29. AIDS Action Committee Web site. http://www.aac.org. Accessed September 24, 2016.

30. Crimp D. Before occupy: How AIDS activists seized control of the FDA in 1988. *The Atlantic*. December 6, 2011. http://www.theatlantic.com/health/archive/2011/12/before-occupy-how-aids-activists-seized-control-of-the-fda-in-1988/249302. Accessed September 24, 2016.

31. Green J. 4,000 Pages and counting. *New York Magazine*. December 27, 2009. http://nymag.com/news/features/62887. Accessed September 24, 2016.

32. Stephens C. On the greatest generation: The black gay '80s. *The Huffington Post*. December 2, 2013. Updated February 2, 2016. http://www.huffingtonpost.com/charles-stephens/on-the-greatest-generatio_b_4333993.html. Accessed September 24, 2016.

33. National Minority AIDS Council Web site. http://www.nmac.org. Accessed September 24, 2016.

34. Grimes W. Randy Shilts, author, dies at 42; One of first to write about AIDS. *The New York Times*. February 18, 1994. http://www.nytimes.com/1994/02/18/obituaries/randy-shilts-author-dies-at-42-one-of-first-to-write-about-aids.html. Accessed September 24, 2016.

35. Shilts R. *And the Band Played On: Politics, People, and the AIDS Epidemic*. New York, NY: St. Martin's Press; 1987.

36. Lambert B. Alison L. Gertz, whose infection alerted many to AIDS, dies at 26. *The New York Times*. August 9, 1992. http://www.nytimes.com/1992/08/09/nyregion/alison-l-gertz-whose-infection-alerted-many-to-aids-dies-at-26.html. Accessed September 24, 2016.

37. Elizabeth's story. Elizabeth Glaser Pediatric AIDS Foundation Web site. http://www.ped-aids.org/pages/elizabeths-story. Accessed September 24, 2016.

38. Markel H. Remembering Ryan White, the teen who fought against the stigma of AIDS. *PBS NewsHour*. April 8, 2016. http://www.pbs.org/newshour/updates/remembering-ryan-white-the-teen-who-fought-against-the-stigma-of-aids. Accessed September 24, 2016.

39. Jaslow R. Magic Johnson's HIV activism hasn't slowed 22 years since historic announcement. *CBS News*. November 29, 2013. http://www.cbsnews.com/news/magic-johnsons-hiv-activism-hasnt-slowed-22-years-since-historic-announcement. Accessed September 24, 2016.

40. Smith L. How America woke up to AIDS: Rock Hudson's death, 30 years later. *CNN*. October 1, 2015. http://www.cnn.com/2015/10/01/entertainment/rock-hudson-anniversary-death. Accessed September 24, 2016.

41. Rhoden WC. An emotional Ashe says that he has AIDS. *The New York Times*. April 9, 1992. http://www.nytimes.com/1992/04/09/sports/an-emotional-ashe-says-that-he-has-aids.html?pagewanted=all. Accessed September 24, 2016.

42. Kramer L. *The Normal Heart*. New York, NY: Samuel French, Inc.; 1985.

43. "Angels in America," 20 years later. *NPR*. September 13, 2011. http://www.npr.org/2011/09/13/140438370/angels-in-america-twenty-years-later. Accessed September 24, 2016.

44. Leitsinger M. Keith Haring, activist: Artist's politics on display in exhibit. *NBC News*. November 8, 2014. http://www.nbcnews.com/news/us-news/keith-haring-activist-artists-politics-display-exhibit-n243866. Accessed September 24, 2016.

45. The Names Project—AIDS Memorial Quilt Web site. http://www.aidsquilt.org. Accessed September 24, 2016.

46. LGBT activist Cleve Jones: 'I am old, but I am not cynical.' *WBUR*. October 27, 2015. http://www.wbur.org/hereandnow/2015/10/27/cleve-jones-gay-lgbt-rights. Accessed September 24, 2016.

47. Justman J. We can eliminate HIV by 2030: Regular testing is a crucial part of the solution. *The Guardian*. August 10, 2015. https://www.theguardian.com/commentisfree/2015/aug/08/eliminate-hiv-by-2030-regular-testing. Accessed September 24, 2016.

SECTION 2

The World as It Is

12

More Hate, More Harm

⌒ ──

IN JANUARY 2015, three men killed 12 people and injured 11 others in Paris at the offices of the satirical news magazine *Charlie Hebdo* [1]. The attackers were purportedly motivated by a desire to avenge satirical cartoons demeaning the Prophet Muhammad [1]. In total, 20 people were killed between January 7 and January 9, as the initial shootings were followed by police involvement and subsequent shoot-outs on the outskirts of Paris [1]. These events galvanized France, and large-scale demonstrations were held in Paris, protesting extremism and violence [1]. The subsequent terrorist attacks in the city in November of that same year, which killed a staggering 130 people, only compounded this grief and galvanization [2].

During the past two decades, population health scholarship has illustrated how prejudice, discrimination, and segregation—linked along multiple axes to interpersonal hatred and antagonism—have a harmful and wide-ranging effect on population health. Duncan and Hatzenbuehler, for example, linked Boston-area lesbian, gay, bisexual, and transgender (LGBT) youth suicide with neighborhood-level LGBT hate crimes involving assaults [3]. They found that reports of suicide ideation or attempts were significantly likelier among sexual minority high school students living in neighborhoods with higher rates of assault [3]. They also found evidence for an increased prevalence of marijuana use among these same LGBT students living in higher hate crime neighborhoods compared to their counterparts living in neighborhoods with a lower rate of hate crimes [4]. Another study found that "structural stigma," defined using the General Social Survey as anti-gay prejudice at the community level, was associated with higher all-cause mortality among sexual minorities [5]. Ilan Meyer put forward a conceptual framework linking stigma and prejudice to mental health disorders among LGBT people through hostile social environments [6].

Looking at respondents to the MIDUS national survey, Kessler and colleagues found that individuals who personally perceived any kind of major lifetime discrimination were likelier to have major depression [7, 8]. Moving beyond a focus on individuals, discrimination against groups following a specific collective event has also been studied. For example, Arab

Americans living in the United States who perceived abuse after the September 11, 2001, terrorist attacks were likelier to report high levels of psychological distress as well as lower levels of happiness [9].

The literature on the consequences of discrimination and hate extends well beyond the negative health effects suffered by minorities who are targeted by specific discrimination. One study found that racial resentment, also referred to as "symbolic racism," was associated with smoking among non-Hispanic whites [10]. This association suggests that the harmful effects of hate reach out-groups, with negative health consequences for those in the majority groups. In the case of cigarette use, these effects are clear, with a well-established link between smoking and a host of physical health problems [11]. There is also a robust literature about the relationship between segregation—often a proxy for racial tension in a community—and health outcomes, with one systematic review finding isolation segregation to be associated with poor pregnancy outcomes and mortality [12]. Additional research has further explored the link between racial segregation and mortality. In 2011, I was involved with a study that estimated that approximately 176,000 deaths annually may be attributed to racial segregation [13].

The terrorism in Paris captured the world's attention, demonstrating how acts of hatred can tear at the fabric of a society. But hatred and intolerance are not confined to isolated incidents such as terror attacks. They pervade our daily lives, shaping the health of populations. Their influence speaks to the fundamental causes of population health—the social processes and structures that form the conditions that produce health. This suggests that a concern with the health of the public is inextricable from a concern with the conditions that make people healthy. There are, of course, many reasons, beyond the promotion of health, why hatred and intolerance should have no place in a pluralistic, enlightened society. But because health is a shared and universal aspiration, our common goal of maximizing the health of populations should push us to engage with the social fractures, such as hate, that threaten the collective well-being. This argues strongly for an activist public health agenda—one that is motivated by a concern for social justice and committed to mitigating the effects of hatred and intolerance in our society.

REFERENCES

1. 2015 Charlie Hebdo attacks fast facts. *CNN*. November 23, 2015. http://www.cnn.com/2015/01/21/europe/2015-paris-terror-attacks-fast-facts. Accessed October 8, 2016.

2. 2015 Paris terror attacks fast facts. *CNN*. April 13, 2016. http://www.cnn.com/2015/12/08/europe/2015-paris-terror-attacks-fast-facts. Accessed October 8, 2016.

3. Duncan DT, Hatzenbuehler ML. Lesbian, gay, bisexual, and transgender hate crimes and suicidality among a population-based sample of sexual-minority adolescents in Boston. *American Journal of Public Health*. 2014; 104(2): 272–8. doi:10.2105/AJPH.2013.301424

4. Duncan DT, Hatzenbuehler ML. Johnson RM. Neighborhood-level LGBT hate crimes and current illicit drug use among sexual minority youth. *Drug and Alcohol Dependence*. 2014; 135: 65–70. doi:10.1016/j.drugalcdep.2013.11.001

5. Hatzenbuehler ML, et al. Structural stigma and all-cause mortality in sexual minority populations. *Social Science & Medicine*. 2014; 103: 33–41.

6. Meyer IH. Prejudice, social stress, and mental health in lesbian, gay, and bisexual populations: Conceptual issues and research evidence. *Psychological Bulletin*. 2003; 129(5): 674–97.

7. Kessler RC, Mickelson KD, Williams DR. The prevalence, distribution, and mental health correlates of perceived discrimination in the United States. *Journal of Health and Social Behavior*. 1999; 40(3): 208–30.

8. History & Overview of MIDUS. MIDUS—Midlife in the United States: A National Longitudinal Study of Health & Well-being Web site. http://www.midus.wisc.edu/scopeof-study.php. Accessed April 5, 2016.

9. Padela AI, Heisler M. The association of perceived abuse and discrimination after September 11, 2001, with psychological distress, level of happiness, and health status among Arab Americans. *American Journal of Public Health*. 2010; 100(2): 284–91.

10. Samson FL. Racial resentment and smoking. *Social Science & Medicine*. 2015; 126: 164–8. doi:10.1016/j.socscimed.2014.12.033

11. Forey BA, Thornton AJ, Lee PN. Systematic review with meta-analysis of the epidemiological evidence relating smoking to COPD, chronic bronchitis and emphysema. *BMC Pulmonary Medicine*. 2011; 11: 36. doi:10.1186/1471-2466-11-36

12. Kramer MR, Hogue CR. Is segregation bad for your health? *Epidemiologic Reviews*. 2009; 31: 178–94. doi:10.1093/epirev/mxp001

13. Galea S, Tracy M, Hoggatt KJ, Dimaggio C, Karpati A. Estimated deaths attributable to social factors in the United States. *American Journal of Public Health*. 2011; 101(8): 1456–65. doi:10.2105/AJPH.2010.300086

13

The Burden of Incarceration

PUBLIC HEALTH AS an organized enterprise emerged from a concern with unsanitary living conditions in the mid-19th century [1]. This early concern foreshadowed the field's long engagement with the social forces that shape the health of populations. However, despite our historical engagement with these forces, there is still a range of social issues that public health has not tackled as forcefully as it perhaps might, especially given the degree to which many of them influence well-being. In this chapter, I discuss such an issue—one that has been, in my estimation, overlooked relative to the impact it has on the health of the public: incarceration in the United States.

In 2012, there were nearly 1.6 million prisoners in US state and federal prisons [2]. At 716 per 100,000 people, the incarceration rate in the United States is higher than that of any other country [3]. What is the reason for this astronomical incarceration rate? A key driver appears to be the Rockefeller drug laws. Implemented in 1973 in New York State, these laws targeted drug offenders and became a model for national policy [4]. In the three decades after the laws were introduced, the incarceration rate of drug offenders rose explosively, as did the proportion of drug-related prison commitments [5]. At a perhaps more fundamental level, we seem as a society to regard incarceration as a form of retribution, deeming it an acceptable, maybe even desirable, way to cope with our fears about violence. This acceptance comes at the expense of choosing alternative forms of punishment or conflict resolution that minimize the recourse to incarceration.

Why should public health engage with the issue of incarceration? There is ample evidence that incarceration is associated with the health of populations, both directly and indirectly, shaping the health of not only the incarcerated but also their families and communities.

Viewed as a disease, the disability-adjusted life year (DALY) rate for mass incarceration is more than double the DALY rate attributed to other conditions commonly experienced by the general population [4]. Much of this burden of disability is due to the bars to social resources and civic participation imposed by incarceration, including access to employment and social welfare benefits such as housing and public assistance [4]. Prison also increases the risk of specific exposures, with the cramped spaces, injection drug use, and unprotected sex endemic among incarcerated populations enhancing the transmission of infectious diseases such as tuberculosis and viral hepatitis [4]. Making matters worse, approximately one in seven Americans with HIV/AIDS pass through the prison system, representing a convergence of uptick in drug-related incarceration coupled with the emergence of this blood-borne virus [6]. Incarceration and mental illness represent another convergence leading to substantial morbidity and—in the case of suicides—mortality among the incarcerated. A review of the evidence suggests that the prevalence of mental illness among incarcerated populations is substantially higher than estimates from community samples. Although there is little question that adverse social experiences such as incarceration contribute to the onset of mental illness, the relationship between incarceration and mental illness is more complex than a straight line from cause to effect, reflecting, rather, a rising incarceration rate that is paralleled by a decline in institutionalization for mental disorders [7, 8].

This suggests that many individuals who require mental health care are instead being diverted to the prison system, which cannot effectively cope with their health needs. Despite the fact that prisoners are the only US citizens who have a constitutional right to health care, they often face delays accessing this care, as well as restrictive medication formularies, a lack of acute care options, and understaffing of specialty care medical providers. Female prisoners, especially, encounter challenges in getting appropriate and timely care [4, 9, 10]. Substance use disorders are another threat to the health of the incarcerated; of the estimated 70 to 85 percent of prisoners in need of treatment, only 10 percent receive such services [11].

But the burden of physical and mental illness associated with incarceration, and the limited attention we pay to these issues, is unfortunately only the tip of the iceberg when it comes to the health consequences of incarceration. Growing evidence indicates that the effects of incarceration extend well beyond imprisoned populations. Fragmented families of the incarcerated face intergenerational consequences, with children experiencing years of separation from their parents. Recent parental incarceration is also associated with a 30 percent increase in the infant mortality rate, with a stronger effect among black children than whites [12]. The mental health consequences of incarceration are likewise widespread, touching whole communities. Non-incarcerated residents of neighborhoods with high incarceration rates have a two- to threefold odds of current or lifetime major depression and generalized anxiety disorder compared to residents of neighborhoods with low incarceration rates [13]. This likely reflects a combination of the social strain incarceration places on families and the social circumstances that drive high community incarceration rates in the first place.

It is important to note that any discussion of the effects of incarceration must recognize that the health consequences of incarceration are borne unevenly across US society, disproportionately affecting minority populations—particularly blacks and Hispanics [14]. The following is an illustration of this inequality: Among children born in 1990, 1 in 25 whites and 1 in 4 blacks had a parent imprisoned by age 14 years—an increase in magnitude and racial disparity compared with children born in 1978 [15]. This extreme disproportion in incarceration rates is a product of the systematic marginalization faced by minority communities, representing what is, to my mind, one of the most significant threats to health in the United States.

How, then, do we most effectively frame incarceration as a public health issue so that we can mitigate its consequences? There is a growing literature on the epidemiology of incarceration, as well as some journalism examining the link between incarceration and public health and reports from organizations such as the Vera Institute discussing how we can improve health in an era of mass incarceration [4, 16, 17]. This encouragingly suggests that incarceration is increasingly more often being viewed as a public health matter—a change of focus that has inflected the broader conversation around this issue. I worry, however, that this conversation risks tacitly reinforcing the status quo, implying that if we could minimize the public health consequences of mass incarceration, our goal would be achieved. It would be far better for us to recognize that incarceration is a symptom of the foundational social conditions that influence health and that to solve the problem of mass incarceration, we need to come to grips with the underlying structural forces that shape the health of populations.

REFERENCES

1. Duffy J. *The Sanitarians: A History of American Public Health*. Champaign, IL: University of Illinois Press; 1990.
2. Fact Sheet: Trends in US Corrections. The Sentencing Project Web site. http://sentencingproject.org/wp-content/uploads/2016/01/Trends-in-US-Corrections.pdf. Accessed September 28, 2016.
3. States of Incarceration: The Global Context. Prison Policy Initiative Web site. https://www.prisonpolicy.org/global. Accessed September 28, 2016.
4. Drucker E. *A Plague of Prisons: The Epidemiology of Mass Incarceration in America*. New York, NY: The New Press; 2011.
5. Drucker E. Commentary: Population impact of mass incarceration under New York's Rockefeller drug laws: An analysis of years of life lost. *Journal of Urban Health: Bulletin of the New York Academy of Medicine*. 2002; 79(3).
6. HIV Among Incarcerated Populations. Centers for Disease Control and Prevention Web site. http://www.cdc.gov/hiv/group/correctional.html. Updated July 22, 2015. Accessed September 28, 2016.
7. Prins SJ. Prevalence of mental illnesses in US state prisons: A systematic review. *Psychiatric Services*. 2014; 65(7): 862–72.
8. Harcourt B. From the asylum to the prison: Rethinking the incarceration revolution. *Texas Law Review*. 2006; 84: 1751–86.
9. Know Your Rights: Medical, Dental and Mental Health Care, ACLU National Prison Project. American Civil Liberties Union Web site. https://www.aclu.org/files/assets/know_your_rights_--_medical_mental_health_and_dental_july_2012.pdf. Accessed September 28, 2016.
10. Daniel AE. Care of the mentally ill in prisons: Challenges and solutions. *Journal of the American Academy of Psychiatry and the Law Online*. 2007; 35(4): 406–10.
11. Executive Office of the President, Office of National Drug Control Policy: ONDCP Drug Policy Information Clearinghouse Fact Sheet. National Criminal Justice Reference Service Web site. https://www.ncjrs.gov/ondcppubs/publications/pdf/94406.pdf. Published March 2001. Accessed September 28, 2016.

12. Wildeman C. Imprisonment and (inequality in) population health. *Social Science Research*. 2012; 41(1): 74–91.

13. Hatzenbuehler ML, Keyes K, Hamilton A, Uddin M, Galea S. The collateral damage of mass incarceration: Risk of psychiatric morbidity among nonincarcerated residents of high-incarceration neighborhoods. *American Journal of Public Health*. 2015; 105(1): 138–43.

14. Alexander M. *The New Jim Crow: Mass Incarceration in the Age of Colorblindness*. New York, NY: The New Press; 2012.

15. Wildeman C. Parental imprisonment, the prison boom, and the concentration of childhood disadvantage. *Demography*. 2009; 46(2): 265–80.

16. The New York Times Editorial Board. Mass imprisonment and public health. *The New York Times*. November 26, 2014. http://www.nytimes.com/2014/11/27/opinion/mass-imprisonment-and-public-health.html. Accessed September 28, 2016.

17. On Life Support: Public Health in the Age of Mass Incarceration. Vera Institute of Justice Web site. https://www.vera.org/publications/on-life-support-public-health-in-the-age-of-mass-incarceration. Published November 2014. Accessed September 28, 2016.

14

Finding a Way Out

SUICIDE AND THE HEALTH OF POPULATIONS

IN A 2015 study published in *Proceedings of the National Academy of Sciences*, Anne Case and Angus Deaton reported that the death rate among white, non-Hispanic middle-aged Americans has recently risen [1]. This rise represents a phenomenon that is unique to this racial group and that is distinct from mortality trends in all other high-income countries [1].

What are the reasons for this sharp rise in mortality? Case and Deaton suggest that there are two major factors: increases in drug use and suicide [1]. Deadly as both these hazards are, the latter has been far less talked about than the former. Whereas there has been much recent media attention given to the problem of drug-related deaths—as drug overdoses have soared, particularly from the nonmedical use of prescription opioids—there has been substantially less focus on suicides [2, 3]. Some thoughts, then, on suicide and the challenge it poses to the health of populations are presented in this chapter.

More than 40,000 Americans take their own lives each year, and it is estimated that approximately 500,000 attempt to do so [4, 5]. In 2012, suicide was the second leading cause of death globally among people aged 15 to 29 years [6]. Three-fourths of these deaths occurred in low- and middle-income countries.

The challenge presented by suicide is twofold: It is intractable, and it is unpredictable. Starting with the former, suicide mortality has been quite constant throughout the decades [7]. As noted previously, suicides have come into greater focus recently due to a concern for rising suicide rates among less educated middle-aged adults. However, suicide among this age group is only part of the problem. In the United States, there are more than 40,000 suicide deaths annually, represented by a 13 per 100,000 rate [8]. During the past 10 years, the highest rates have been among 40- to 64-year-olds, whereas youth suicide has remained relatively stable [9]. However, in recent years, rates among the 20- to 39-year-old age group have increased [9]. The majority of suicides occur among whites, with a rate of 14.75 per 100,000 [9].

Research has also focused on particular subgroups of suicide victims. A case in point is the recently observed clustering of suicides among students at Palo Alto, California, area high schools, in one of the wealthiest areas of the country [10]. Attention has also been paid to rising rates of suicide among military populations. In the past, suicide rates in the Army were lower than demographically matched civilian rates [11]. This changed, however, by 2008, when the Army saw close to 20 suicide deaths per 100,000 people compared to approximately 19 among civilians [11]. In 2012, the number of deaths from suicide in the Army surpassed the number of deaths from combat [12]. This rise is driven by several factors. As a consequence of their work, military personnel can face exposure to potentially traumatic events during deployment that can lead to conditions such as post-traumatic stress disorder, substance use disorder, and depression. Worsening the problem, military personnel are often reluctant to seek help due to pressure and fear of losing their position. Many soldiers also enter the military having already experienced suicidal thoughts, risk factors, and mental disorders prior to enlistment [13]. Separation from the military may also be associated with increased suicide risk, especially in the absence of an honorable discharge [14].

The second feature of suicides, their unpredictability, is borne out by the vast majority of predictive models that show quite poor predictive validity at the individual level [15]. This begs the question: What do we know about those in the general population who commit or attempt suicide? Importantly, a dose–response relationship has been suggested among a number of psychiatric disorders and long-term suicide risk [16]. The majority of people who attempt suicide also seek some kind of medical care in the months preceding their attempt, and approximately 80 percent of people contemplating suicide give some sign of their intentions, including talking to loved ones about suicide [5, 17]. In addition to these indicators, 20 to 40 percent of people who actually complete suicide have attempted it in the past. Other proposed population-level risk factors for suicide include a history of sexual abuse, financial strain or unemployment, as well as LGBT status and low family support [18, 19, 20]. It is important, however, to note that these factors are useful predictors at the level of populations rather than at the level of individuals. Further challenging the field is the large number of studies that aim to understand the drivers of suicide by using suicidal ideation as a proxy for the act of suicide. The limitation here is that suicidal ideation does not necessarily inform completion, and studies have suggested that the link between suicidal ideation and subsequent completion is weak [21].

In the growing field of suicide prevention, there have been some potentially successful interventions aimed at decreasing the rate of people who take their own life. One randomized controlled trial of suicide attempters in low- and middle-income countries compared individual education sessions focused on alternatives to suicide, repetition, and referrals to usual care, observing in follow-up among the treatment group significantly fewer deaths from suicide [22]. Although such results are encouraging, less work has been done among groups that have not already attempted suicide.

Despite research in the area of prevention, suicide remains a substantial threat to the health of populations—one to which we have paid little attention relative to the scale of the challenge. Let us hope that a growing focus on population mental and behavioral health will lead to commensurately greater interest in suicide, prompting new insights and preventive approaches that can help to solve this perplexing and stubborn problem.

REFERENCES

1. Case A, Deaton A. Rising morbidity and mortality in midlife among white non-Hispanic Americans in the 21st century. *Proceedings of the National Academy of Sciences of the United States of America.* 2015; 112(49): 15078–83. doi:10.1073/pnas.1518393112

2. Kounang N. Drug overdose deaths reach all-time high. December 18, 2015. *CNN.* http://www.cnn.com/2015/12/18/health/drug-overdose-deaths-2014. Accessed October 2, 2016.

3. Prescription Opioid Overdose Data. Centers for Disease Control and Prevention Web site. http://www.cdc.gov/drugoverdose/data/overdose.html. Updated June 21, 2016. Accessed October 2, 2016.

4. Suicide Statistics. American Foundation for Suicide Prevention Web site. https://afsp.org/about-suicide/suicide-statistics. Accessed October 2, 2016.

5. Suicide. Mental Health America Web site. http://www.mentalhealthamerica.net/suicide. Accessed October 2, 2016.

6. Suicide Data. World Health Organization Web site. http://www.who.int/mental_health/prevention/suicide/suicideprevent/en. Accessed October 2, 2016.

7. National Suicide Prevention Month: Update 2015. National Institute of Mental Health Web site. https://www.nimh.nih.gov/news/science-news/2015/national-suicide-prevention-month-update-2015.shtml. Published September 28, 2015. Accessed October 2, 2016.

8. Suicide and Self-Inflicted Injury. Centers for Disease Control and Prevention Web site. http://www.cdc.gov/nchs/fastats/suicide.htm. Updated June 13, 2016. Accessed October 2, 2016.

9. Suicide in the USA Fact Sheet Based on 2012 Data. 2014. American Association of Suicidology Web site. http://www.suicidology.org/Portals/14/docs/Resources/FactSheets/USA2012.pdf. Accessed October 2, 2016.

10. Rosin H. The Silicon Valley suicides. *The Atlantic.* December 2015. http://www.theatlantic.com/magazine/archive/2015/12/the-silicon-valley-suicides/413140. Accessed October 2, 2016.

11. Suicide in the Military: Army-NIH Funded Study Points to Risk and Protective Factors. National Institute of Mental Health Web site. https://www.nimh.nih.gov/news/science-news/2014/suicide-in-the-military-army-nih-funded-study-points-to-risk-and-protective-factors.shtml. Published March 3, 2014. Accessed October 2, 2016.

12. Chappell B. US Military's suicide rate surpassed combat deaths in 2012. *NPR.* January 14, 2013. http://www.npr.org/sections/thetwo-way/2013/01/14/169364733/u-s-militarys-suicide-rate-surpassed-combat-deaths-in-2012. Accessed October 2, 2016.

13. Nock MK, et al. Prevalence and correlates of suicidal behavior among soldiers: Results from the Army Study to Assess Risk and Resilience in Servicemembers (Army STARRS). *JAMA Psychiatry.* 2014; 71(5): 514–22. doi:10.1001/jamapsychiatry.2014.30

14. Reger MA, et al. Risk of suicide among US military service members following Operation Enduring Freedom or Operation Iraqi Freedom deployment and separation from the US military. *JAMA Psychiatry.* 2015; 72(6): 561–9. doi:10.1001/jamapsychiatry.2014.3195

15. Sher L. Is it possible to predict suicide? *Australian & New Zealand Journal of Psychiatry.* 2011; 45(4): 341. doi:10.3109/00048674.2011.560136

16. Holmstrand C, Bogren M, Mattisson C, Brådvik L. Long-term suicide risk in no, one or more mental disorders: The Lundby Study 1947–1997. *Acta Psychiatrica Scandinavica*. 2015; 132(6): 459–69. doi:10.1111/acps.12506

17. Ahmedani BK. Racial/ethnic differences in health care visits made before suicide attempt across the United States. *Medical Care*. 2015; 53(5): 430–35. doi:10.1097/MLR.0000000000000335

18. Bae S, Ye R, Chen S, Rivers PA, Singh KP. Risky behaviors and factors associated with suicide attempt in adolescents. *Archives of Suicide Research*. 2005; 9(2): 193–202.

19. Unemployment among post-9/11 veterans still running heavy. *NBC News*. March 8, 2013. http://usnews.nbcnews.com/_news/2013/03/08/17237011-unemployment-among-post-911-veterans-still-running-heavy?lite. Accessed October 2, 2016.

20. Mustanski B, Liu RT. A longitudinal study of predictors of suicide attempts among lesbian, gay, bisexual, and transgender youth. *Archives of Sexual Behavior*. 2013; 42(3): 437–48. doi:10.1007/s10508-012-0013-9

21. Silverman MM, Berman AL. Suicide risk assessment and risk formulation Part I: A focus on suicide ideation in assessing suicide risk. *Suicide and Life-Threatening Behavior*. 2014; 44(4): 420–31. doi:10.1111/sltb.12065

22. Fleischmann A, et al. Effectiveness of brief intervention and contact for suicide attempters: A randomized controlled trial in five countries. *Bulletin of the World Health Organization*. 2008; 86(9): 703–9.

15

The Heavy Toll of Substance Use

THE ABUSE OF alcohol and drugs has become a worldwide public health crisis. Nearly 5 percent of total years of life lost globally has been attributed to alcohol and illicit drug use [1]. Estimates suggest that there are 185 million illicit drug users among the world's population, with opioid dependence the primary driver of this epidemic [2]. The harm caused by substance use disorders is extensive, and substance use disorders have been associated with substantial morbidity and mortality, loss of economic productivity, unemployment, and intimate partner violence; substance use disorders also go hand in hand with psychiatric disorders and other comorbidities, including obesity [3, 4, 5, 6, 7, 8].

Substance use disorders represent only one of the many population health consequences of substance use. Even in the absence of such disorders, alcohol and drugs can still pose challenges to health. Binge drinking, for example, is a very common problem in the United States that can lead to liver disease, injury, neurological damage, sexually transmitted diseases, and unintended pregnancy [9]. The problem of binge drinking is especially common among particular populations. One such group is military personnel, for whom binge drinking has been associated with psychiatric comorbidity and risky behavior [10, 11, 12].

There is also the challenge of drug-related incidents, principally overdoses and deaths, which have informed much of the recent concern regarding opioid use. In a 2015 study, colleagues and I reviewed the available literature on unintentional drug overdose globally, concluding that global overdose is unequivocally on the rise [13]. This trend is especially pronounced in rural areas and is driven by prescription opioids. To date, the rise in overdoses has had an appreciable cost, and not just in lives. From 1999 to 2008, hospitalization rates for overdoses in the United States increased by 55 percent, costing approximately $737 million in 2008—a figure that is undoubtedly dwarfed today [14].

As prescription opioids become more available throughout the United States, illicit drug use has decreased in many areas. One unexpected consequence of this shift is that many individuals who may not have been likely to use heroin are introduced to opioids through prescription medication [15]. As their tolerance for the substance increases or they no longer have access to the medication, these individuals are liable to turn to heroin [15]. As a consequence, heroin use is actually beginning to increase again [16]. This is especially the case among affluent people living in the suburbs, a demographic that has not historically been associated with widespread heroin use [16].

How does this epidemic relate to law enforcement? Stricter policing practices, not atypically linked to the rise in drug-related overdoses, can themselves contribute to a rise in drug-related deaths [17]. This happens when drug users move their activities underground and overdose witnesses become reluctant to call for help [17]. However, there is cause for optimism. The growing burden of drug-related overdose has made it clear that this hazard is no longer simply a legal matter but, rather, a public health issue [18]. Overdose is usually preventable, and individuals rarely overdose alone, providing a unique opportunity for intervention. Provision of the opioid antagonist naloxone to drug users, a practice that is being implemented in many areas, is one example of how public health efforts could potentially stop an overdose from leading to death [19, 20]. Hearteningly, community intervention programs are taking the initiative in the United States to move beyond thinking of substance use as a legal issue, recontextualizing it within the realm of public health [21].

The 2015 Case and Deaton study referenced in Chapter 14 reinforced the tremendous population health consequences of drug use by demonstrating how, if the substance use-driven death rate among those aged 45 to 54 years had continued to decline the way it had between 1979 and 1998, half a million deaths between 1999 and 2013 would have been avoided, comparable to the number of lives lost to AIDS in the United States [22].

Again, however, these figures represent merely the "tip of the iceberg." Mortality is far from the only consequence of drug use. Other associated outcomes include the cost of hospitalization and lost work productivity [23]. Also, the problem of overdose presents its own unique set of hazards. The consequences of nonfatal overdose can include cardiac and muscular problems, cognitive impairment, renal failure, and other injuries [24]. Moreover, following the life course paradigm, the effects of substance use can be intergenerational: Maternal smoking during pregnancy is associated with low birth weight in offspring, and the use of alcohol and other substances during pregnancy is associated with a myriad of undesirable outcomes, including preterm birth, placental abruption, neonatal withdrawal, and cognitive deficits [25, 26].

The burden of substance use has long been underappreciated, existing on the fringes of mainstream public health. Going forward, it is important that we view this problem for what it is—a chronic challenge to population health. Unfortunately, the historical marginalization of this issue has been accompanied by substantial shortage in treatment opportunities for substance-dependent populations. This has led to an unmet need and a lack of engagement with the prevention of substance use and misuse. The recent attention to the issue is an important, if halting, step in the right direction [27, 28].

REFERENCES

1. The Global Burden. World Health Organization Web site. http://www.who.int/substance_abuse/facts/global_burden/en. Accessed October 2, 2016.

2. Degenhardt L, et al. Global burden of disease attributable to illicit drug use and dependence: Findings from the Global Burden of Disease Study 2010. *The Lancet*. 2013; (382)9904: 1564–74. doi:http://dx.doi.org/10.1016/S0140-6736(13)61530-5

3. Whiteford HA, Ferrari AJ, Degenhardt L, Feigin V, Vos T. The global burden of mental, neurological and substance use disorders: An analysis from the Global Burden of Disease Study 2010. *PLoS One*. 2015; 10(2): e0116820. doi:10.1371/journal.pone.0116820

4. Montgomery SM, Cook DG, Bartley MJ, Wadsworth MEJ. Unemployment, cigarette smoking, alcohol consumption and body weight in young British men. *European Journal of Public Health*. 1998; 8(1): 21–7. doi:http://dx.doi.org/10.1093/eurpub/8.1.21

5. Choenni V, Hammink A, van de Mheen D. Association between substance use and the perpetration of family violence in industrialized countries: A systematic review. *Trauma, Violence, & Abuse*. 2015: 1–14. doi:10.1177/1524838015589253

6. DrugFacts: Comorbidity—Addiction and Other Mental Disorders. National Institute on Drug Abuse Web site. https://www.drugabuse.gov/publications/drugfacts/comorbidity-addiction-other-mental-disorders. Updated March 2011. Accessed October 2, 2016.

7. Kalichman SC, et al. Continued substance use among people living with HIV-hepatitis-C co-infection and receiving antiretroviral therapy. *Substance Use & Misuse*. 2015; 50(12): 1536–43. doi:10.3109/10826084.2015.1023451

8. Huang DY, Lanza HI, Anglin MD. Association between adolescent substance use and obesity in young adulthood: A group-based dual trajectory analysis. *Addictive Behaviors*. 2013; 38(11): 2653–60. doi:10.1016/j.addbeh.2013.06.024

9. Binge Drinking. Centers for Disease Control and Prevention Web site. http://www.cdc.gov/alcohol/fact-sheets/binge-drinking.htm. Updated October 16, 2015. Accessed October 2, 2016.

10. Calhoun PS, et al. The prevalence of binge drinking and receipt of provider drinking advice among US veterans with military service in Iraq or Afghanistan. *American Journal of Drug and Alcohol Abuse*. 2016; 42(3): 269–78. doi:10.3109/00952990.2015.1051185

11. LeardMann CA, et al. Risk factors associated with suicide in current and former US military personnel. *JAMA: The Journal of the American Medical Association*. 310(5): 496–506. doi:10.1001/jama.2013.65164

12. Vander Weg MW, DeBon M, Sherrill-Mittleman D, Klesges RC, Relyea GE. Binge drinking, drinking and driving, and riding with a driver who had been drinking heavily among Air National Guard and Air Force Reserve personnel. *Military Medicine*. 2006; 171(2): 177–83.

13. Martins SS, Sampson L, Cerdá M, Galea S. Worldwide prevalence and trends in unintentional drug overdose: A systematic review of the literature. *American Journal of Public Health*. 2015; 105(11): e29–49. doi:10.2105/AJPH.2015.302843

14. White AM, Hingson RW, Pan IJ, Yi HY. Hospitalizations for alcohol and drug overdoses in young adults ages 18–24 in the United States, 1999–2008: Results from the Nationwide Inpatient Sample. *Journal of Studies on Alcohol and Drugs*. 2011; 72(5): 774–86.

15. Gupta S. Unintended consequences: Why painkiller addicts turn to heroin. *CNN*. June 2, 2016. http://www.cnn.com/2014/08/29/health/gupta-unintended-consequences. Accessed October 2, 2016.

16. Cicero TJ, Kuehn BM. Driven by prescription drug abuse, heroin use increases among suburban and rural whites. *JAMA: The Journal of the American Medical Association*. 2014; 312(2): 118–9. doi:10.1001/jama.2014.7404

17. Bohnert AS, et al. Policing and risk of overdose mortality in urban neighborhoods. *Drug and Alcohol Dependence.* 2011; 113(1): 62–8. doi:10.1016/j.drugalcdep.2010.07.008

18. Paulozzi LJ. Overdoses are injuries too. *Injury Prevention.* 2007; 13(5): 293–4. doi:10.1136/ip.2007.016113

19. Wheeler E, Davidson PJ, Jones TS, Irwin KS. Community-based opioid overdose prevention programs providing naloxone—United States, 2010. *Morbidity and Mortality Weekly Report (MMWR).* 2012; 61(6): 101–5.

20. Cosgrove J. Naloxone available in Oklahoma without a prescription. *NewsOK.* June 18, 2015. http://newsok.com/article/5428372. Accessed October 2, 2016.

21. Gloucester police department offers heroin addicts amnesty, treatment. *WCVB.* August 14, 2015. http://www.wcvb.com/health/gloucester-police-department-offers-heroin-addicts-amnesty-treatment/34715948. Accessed October 2, 2016.

22. Case A, Deaton A. Rising morbidity and mortality in midlife among white non-Hispanic Americans in the 21st century. *Proceedings of the National Academy of Sciences of the United States of America.* 2015; 112(49): 15078–83. doi:10.1073/pnas.1518393112

23. Trends & Statistics. National Institute on Drug Abuse Web site. https://www.drugabuse.gov/related-topics/trends-statistics. Updated August 2015. Accessed October 2, 2016.

24. Warner-Smith M, Darke S, Lynskey M, Hall W. Heroin overdose: Causes and consequences. *Addiction.* 2001; 96(8): 1113–25. doi:10.1080/09652140120060716

25. Wang X, et al. Maternal cigarette smoking, metabolic gene polymorphism, and infant birth weight. *JAMA: The Journal of the American Medical Association.* 2002; 287(2): 195–202. doi:10.1001/jama.287.2.195

26. Forray A, Foster D. Substance use in the perinatal period. *Current Psychiatry Reports.* 2015; 17(11): 91. doi:10.1007/s11920-015-0626-5

27. Choi NG, DiNitto DM, Marti CN. Alcohol and other substance use, mental health treatment use, and perceived unmet treatment need: Comparison between baby boomers and older adults. *American Journal on Addictions.* 2015; 24(4): 299–307. doi:10.1111/ajad.12225

28. Benningfield MM, Riggs P, Stephan SH. The role of schools in substance use prevention and intervention. *Child and Adolescent Psychiatric Clinics of North America.* 2015; 24(2): 291–303. doi:10.1016/j.chc.2014.12.004

16

The Health Effects of War

FROM PRE-ROMAN DAYS until now, it seems as though humanity has always been engaged in war [1]. In Syria alone, more than 200,000 people were killed in the first 5 years of the recent conflict in that country. In 2014, nearly 21,000 lives were lost in the Iraqi government's battle against Islamic State terrorists [2]. Similar conflicts can be observed all over the globe [2].

When we consider the consequences of war from a public health perspective, we often focus on the substantial negative health outcomes that soldiers and veterans face, from post-traumatic stress disorder (PTSD) to traumatic brain injury and depression. Less frequently discussed are the more indirect effects of war and how these effects shape the health of civilians and societies as a whole, across time.

In recent years, a survey commissioned by the International Committee of the Red Cross of more than 4,000 civilians in Afghanistan, Colombia, Liberia, Lebanon, Haiti, the Democratic Republic of Congo, Georgia, and the Philippines found that approximately 66 percent of respondents in these countries reported feeling the effects of violence even if they were not directly involved in the hostilities [3]. This speaks to how the experience of simply being a civilian in a country at war can be devastating, leading to psychological trauma. Additional research bears this out. A review of studies examining Lebanese adolescents during times of heavy war found among the young people a high prevalence of PTSD from various traumas such as the destruction of homes, bereavement, and economic hardships [4]. Another review summarized literature across several different countries, examining the impact of war on mental health [5]. It found that women, children, and elderly civilians are particularly vulnerable to poor health outcomes in times of war. In my work,

I have studied the mental health outcomes of civilians after the September 11, 2001, terrorist attack in New York City, and others have done similar research in the wake of civilian-targeted mass killings [6, 7].

Another key consideration is how media exposure complicates the consequences of war. During the American Civil War, the first widely-photographed conflict in history, images of the battlefield dead shocked the nation, swaying public opinion [8]. More than 150 years later, all it takes is a quick Google search for a detailed look at the horrors of such conflict. Technology has made it easier for civilians to gain access to pictures and film of violence, spreading the impact of war across geographic boundaries, often far from where the fighting is actually taking place [9]. These technologies make it difficult for people to keep the reality of war "at arm's length," and studies are beginning to examine whether exposure to war through the media can lead to mental illness [10, 11].

There are also known environmental health exposures related to war, including pollution, pesticides, radiation, and susceptibility to infectious disease agents among both soldiers and civilians [12]. Speaking to these hazards, Roberta White has identified toxic exposures from the 1991 Gulf War that likely contributed to the Gulf War illness seen in soldiers that for many years was poorly understood [13, 14]. Armed conflict can also have a harmful effect on the physical environment, damaging entire ecosystems [15].

Often, another more immediate effect of war is the outpouring of refugees who escape a war zone to enter another area. It is a sad truth that these populations often find themselves living in camps with conditions almost as bad as those they escaped. I address the health of refugees, including their high risk of mental health disorders, infectious disease, malnutrition, poor birth outcomes, and abuse, in a later chapter.

More broadly, war is tremendously consequential for national economies, both in terms of actual dollars spent on combat and preparedness and in terms of related expenditures. The Watson Institute of International and Public Affairs at Brown University found that between 2001 and 2011, the US ratio of federal debt held by the public to gross domestic product increased by almost 37 percentage points, due in part to financing the wars in Iraq and Afghanistan [16]. The Institute also projected that if the US government had invested the amount of money it spent on the military between 2001 and 2014 on health care coverage, the clean energy industry, and education, between 1 and 3 million more jobs could have been created in nonmilitary sectors.

The economic cost of war always represents a diversion of resources away from the necessary projects of a peacetime society. The price of conflict will inevitably be borne by the population, at the expense of its neglected needs. This was well expressed by President Dwight Eisenhower when he said, "Every gun that is made, every warship launched, every rocket fired signifies, in the final sense, a theft from those who hunger and are not fed, those who are cold and are not clothed" [17]. This "theft" is not limited to the duration of the conflict itself. The aftermath of war can also include food shortages and lack of medical care or other social services [18, 19].

The destruction of war is comprehensive. It wears away at a country's economy, its environment, its infrastructure, and the physical and mental health of its citizens. It should therefore be a key responsibility of public health to clearly communicate the challenges to health imposed by war, wherever and whenever conflicts arise.

REFERENCES

1. Barash DP. Are we hard-wired for war? *The New York Times*. September 28, 2013. http://www.nytimes.com/2013/09/29/opinion/sunday/are-we-hard-wired-for-war.html?_r=1. Accessed October 4, 2016.

2. Sim D. The world's 15 deadliest conflicts including Syria, Iraq and Afghanistan [Photo report]. *International Business Times*. March 20, 2015. http://www.ibtimes.co.uk/worlds-15-deadliest-conflicts-photo-report-1492815. Accessed October 4, 2016.

3. ICRC stresses burden on civilians in war. *SWI swissinfo.ch*. June 23, 2009. http://www.swissinfo.ch/eng/icrc-stresses-burden-on-civilians-in-war/225368. Accessed October 4, 2016.

4. Shaar KH. Post-traumatic stress disorder in adolescents in Lebanon as wars gained in ferocity: A systematic review. *Journal of Public Health Research*. 2013; 2(2): e17. doi:10.4081/jphr.2013.e17

5. Murthy RS, Lakshminarayana R. Mental health consequences of war: A brief review of research findings. *World Psychiatry*. 2006; 5(1): 25–30.

6. Boscarino JA, Adams RE, Galea S. Alcohol use in New York after the terrorist attacks: A study of the effects of psychological trauma on drinking behavior. *Addictive Behaviors*. 2006; 31(4): 606–21.

7. Whalley MG, Brewin CR. Mental health following terrorist attacks. *The British Journal of Psychiatry*. 2007; 190(2): 94–6. doi:10.1192/bjp.bp.106.026427

8. The Impact of Civil War Photos on the Public. The Civil War Trust Web site. http://www.civilwar.org/resources/the-impact-of-civil-war.html. Accessed October 4, 2016.

9. Wing N, McGonigal C. Look at these photos before you say we can't take in Syrian refugees. *The Huffington Post*. November 16, 2015. http://www.huffingtonpost.com/entry/syrian-refugee-photos_us_564a319ee4b045bf3df04d49. Updated November 18, 2015. Accessed October 4, 2016.

10. Feinstein A, Audet B, Waknine E. Witnessing images of extreme violence: A psychological study of journalists in the newsroom. *Journal of the Royal Society of Medicine*. 2014; 5(8). doi:10.1177/2054270414533323

11. Viewing Violent News on Social Media Can Cause Trauma. The British Psychological Society Web site. http://www.bps.org.uk/news/viewing-violent-news-social-media-can-cause-trauma. Published July 5, 2015. Accessed October 4, 2016.

12. Brown VJ. Battle scars: Global conflicts and environmental health. *Environmental Health Perspectives*. 2004; 112(17): A994–1003.

13. White RF, et al. Recent research on Gulf War illness and other health problems in veterans of the 1991 Gulf War: Effects of toxicant exposures during deployment. *Cortex*. 2016; 74: 449–75. doi:10.1016/j.cortex.2015.08.022

14. Gulf War Veterans' Medically Unexplained Illnesses. US Department of Veterans Affairs Web site. http://www.publichealth.va.gov/exposures/gulfwar/medically-unexplained-illness.asp. Accessed October 4, 2016.

15. DeWeerdt S. War and the environment. *World Watch*. http://www.worldwatch.org/node/5520. Accessed October 4, 2016.

16. Costs of War: Macroeconomic Impact. The Watson Institute for International and Public Affairs Web site. http://watson.brown.edu/costsofwar/costs/economic/economy/macroeconomic. Updated June 2011. Accessed October 4, 2016.

17. Schlesinger R. The origins of that Eisenhower "Every gun that is made . . ." quote. *US News & World Report*. September 30, 2011. http://www.usnews.com/opinion/blogs/robert-schlesinger/2011/09/30/the-origins-of-that-eisenhower-every-gun-that-is-made-quote. Accessed October 4, 2016.

18. Armed Conflict and Hunger—How Conflict Causes Hunger. Hunger Notes Web site. http://www.worldhunger.org/armed-conflict-and-hunger-how-conflict-causes-hunger. Accessed October 4, 2016.

19. Fieldstadt E. War leaves Syrian children without adequate health care. *NBC News*. March 9, 2014. http://www.nbcnews.com/storyline/syrias-children/war-leaves-syrian-children-without-adequate-health-care-n48456. Accessed October 4, 2016.

17

Out in the Cold

THE US DEPARTMENT of Housing and Urban Development, which conducts an annual count of homeless people in the United States, found an average of 564,708 people per night were living on the streets in January 2015 [1]. Although this number represents an overall decline in homelessness during the past few years (651,142 people were homeless in 2007), it is important to note that the number of homeless has actually increased in certain areas—importantly in New York City, where approximately 14 percent of the national homeless population resides [2, 3].

Although most homeless people are only considered homeless for a short time, a subpopulation of the homeless are chronically homeless for 30 to 40 years. According to the 2015 nationwide count, 83,170 individuals and 13,105 people in families with children had either been continuously homeless for a year or experienced a minimum of four episodes of homelessness in the past 3 years [1].

There is no shortage of evidence demonstrating the health consequences of homelessness. The homeless have higher premature mortality than those who are appropriately housed; key drivers of this mortality are injuries, unintentional overdose, and extreme weather events [4]. The homeless also have poor quality of life, characterized by chronic pain associated with poor sleeping conditions and limited access to medications and other salutary resources [5]. Skin and foot issues, dental problems, and chronic infectious diseases are also well-described among homeless populations [6].

The intractability of this problem challenges us to examine how we think of homelessness and its consequences, and how we might envision solutions. One useful perspective is to consider homelessness across the life course by way of highlighting the factors that are coincident with, and contribute to, this condition.

Twenty-three percent of the homeless population in the United States is younger than the age of 18 years. These homeless youth are especially vulnerable to drug use. An *American*

Journal of Public Health study found that 55 percent of street youth and 34 percent of shelter youth have used illicit drugs since leaving home, compared to 13 percent of youth who have never been homeless [7].

Mental illness is also intertwined with the problem of homelessness. A sample of homeless adolescents in Los Angeles showed that 32 percent reported a need for help with mental health problems and 15 percent met criteria for emotional distress [8]. The proportion of those with emotional distress was higher among gay, lesbian, or bisexual youth, as well as black youth. It has been estimated that roughly three times as many homeless adolescents suffer from depression compared to other adolescents. Homeless adolescents are also likely to experience violence: 21 to 42 percent report sexual abuse compared to 1 to 3 percent of the general population, and approximately 40 percent have reported being assaulted with a weapon [9, 10]. Roughly 40 percent of these homeless adolescents identify as LGBT [10].

Homeless adults, like homeless youth, are at greater risk of substance use disorders and overdose compared to the general population [11, 12]. Homeless adults are also disproportionately affected by psychiatric disorders. However, it is difficult to estimate the true burden of mental illness among this population because they are usually excluded from national surveys [13]. In addition, homeless individuals suffering from mental illnesses tend to have less contact with family or friends and are more likely to remain homeless for a longer time period [14].

One key driver of homelessness among individuals is lack of income [14]. Individuals younger than age 65 years who do not yet receive Medicare or social security benefits, and are unemployed, may be especially vulnerable. Older veterans also make up a large portion of the homeless population, although the proportion of veterans who are homeless has decreased since 2009 [1]. In January 2015, 47,725 veterans were considered homeless on a given night [1].

It is clear that homelessness is overwhelmingly coincident with socioeconomic vulnerability and with poor behavioral health—that is, mental illness and substance use. It is therefore unsurprising that much of the literature in this area suggests that interventions that provide case management for substance use and mental illness, and critical time intervention approaches that mitigate the consequences of acute stressors, can be effective in the reduction of homelessness [15]. Yet these approaches rest on health care and interventions embedded in health care systems. They do not obviate, nor supplant, the centrality of approaches that tackle the social policies and structural factors—including absence of affordable housing and of social safety nets that target vulnerable and low-income individuals—that ultimately drive homelessness and unstable housing among marginalized populations. To mitigate, and ultimately solve, the problem of homelessness, we must embrace solutions that engage with these upstream causes.

REFERENCES

1. Henry M, et al. *The 2015 Annual Homeless Assessment Report (AHAR) to Congress: Part 1—Point-in-Time Estimates of Homelessness*. Washington, DC: US Department of Housing & Urban Development; 2015.

2. National Alliance to End Homelessness, Homelessness Research Institute. *The State of Homelessness in America 2015*. Washington, DC: Author; 2015.

3. Stewart N. New York's rise in homelessness went against national trend, US report finds. *New York Times*. November 19, 2015. http://www.nytimes.com/2015/11/20/nyregion/new-yorks-rise-in-homelessness-went-against-national-trend-us-report-finds.html. Accessed July 26, 2016.

4. Baggett TP, et al. Mortality among homeless adults in Boston: Shifts in causes of death over a 15-year period. *JAMA Internal Medicine*. 2013; 173(3): 189–95. doi:10.1001/jamainternmed.2013.1604

5. Hwang SW, et al. Chronic pain among homeless persons: Characteristics, treatment, and barriers to management. *BMC Family Practice*. 2011; 12(73). doi:10.1186/1471-2296-12-73

6. Hwang SW. Homelessness and health. *Canadian Medical Association Journal*. 2001; 164(2): 229–33.

7. Greene JM, Ennett ST, Ringwalt CL. Substance use among runaway and homeless youth in three national samples. *American Journal of Public Health*. 1997; 87(2): 229–35.

8. Solorio MR, Milburn NG, Andersen RM, Trifskin S, Rodríguez MA. Emotional distress and mental health service use among urban homeless adolescents. *Journal of Behavioral Health Services & Research*. 2006; (4): 381–93.

9. Homeless Youth & Sexual Violence: Infographic. National Sexual Violence Resource Center Web site. http://www.nsvrc.org/publications/nsvrc-publications-infographic/homeless-youth-sexual-violence-infographic. Published September 2014. Accessed July 26, 2016.

10. Homeless Youth Statistics & Facts. Safe Horizon Web site. http://www.safehorizon.org/page/homeless-youth-statistics--facts-69.html. Accessed July 26, 2016.

11. Bassuk EL, Buckner JC, Perloff JN, Bassuk SS. Prevalence of mental health and substance use disorders among homeless and low-income housed mothers. *American Journal of Psychiatry*. 1998; 155(11): 1561–4.

12. Bohnert ASB, Tracy M, Galea S. Characteristics of drug users who witness many overdoses: Implications for overdose prevention. *Drug and Alcohol Dependence*. 2012; 120(1–3): 168–73.

13. Health & Homelessness. American Psychological Association Web site. http://www.apa.org/pi/ses/resources/publications/homelessness-health.aspx. Accessed July 26, 2016.

14. Homelessness Assessment: What Is the Current Situation? Community Advancement Network Web site. http://canatx.org/homeless/documents/2001Assessment/WhatIs.htm. Updated October 18, 2010. Accessed July 26, 2016.

15. Hwang SW, Burns T. Health interventions for people who are homeless. *The Lancet*. 2014; 384(9953): 1541–7.

18

Priced out of Health

A SMALL MIRACLE took place during the early months of the 2016 US presidential race. In that season of insults, feuds, and partisan rancor, candidates Hillary Clinton, Marco Rubio, and Donald Trump all found something to agree on. The issue was the high, and seemingly ever-increasing, cost of prescription medications. Trump expressed the opinion that Medicare should negotiate price discounts, Rubio accused drug companies of profiteering, and Clinton unveiled an "aggressive plan" designed to save more than $100 billion on pharmaceutical costs over the course of a decade [1, 2, 3]. The reason why the issue of drug pricing is so politically potent is well captured by a report from Express Scripts, the US pharmacy benefit management organization. The report found that the average price for common, brand-name prescription drugs has increased 164 percent since 2008, even as the price of generic drugs has declined [4].

These kinds of data, along with tales of industry "price hiking"—as exemplified by the widely reported actions of former Turing Pharmaceuticals CEO Martin Shkreli, who has been criticized for his company's decision to boost the price of the antiparasitic drug Daraprim by more than 5,000 percent—have kept the issue of drug costs at the forefront of the public debate [5].

This debate has played out on both the national and the state level. In Massachusetts, the state Attorney General Maura Healey wrote a letter to then Gilead Sciences CEO John Martin, asking that the company consider lowering the price of Sovaldi, a drug capable of curing hepatitis C [6]. Healey warned that Solvaldi's $1,000 price tag may constitute an unfair trade practice under state law. Staying in Massachusetts, Boston-based Vertex Pharmaceuticals has also attracted criticism for the $259,000 annual cost of its cystic fibrosis drug, Orkambi. The company has pushed back against this criticism, stating that the price of Orkambi reflects the high overhead costs of developing such a drug over a period of many years. Continuing this work, the company states, will require "a very significant investment" [7].

This is not an unreasonable claim. It can take many years—often more than a decade—for a medication to be developed to the point at which it can be licensed for human consumption, and the expense of this process can be considerable [8]. A 2014 study conducted by the Tufts Center for the Study of Drug Development suggested that the average cost to bring a drug to market had increased to nearly $2.6 billion; the study, however, has been challenged, having been funded, in large part, by the pharmaceutical industry [9, 10, 11].

But the full story is not so straightforward—there is the matter of federal funding for drug research and development. Often, the costs for pharmaceutical innovation are subsidized by the taxpayer [12]. The National Institutes of Health, for example, makes an annual investment of nearly $32.3 billion on medical research [13]. This spending allows drug companies to offload much of the risk involved in pharmaceutical development, freeing them to invest more of their budgets in marketing [14].

Despite this federal assistance, it is nevertheless a fact that the cost of drug development—in both money and time—remains high [15].

An additional reason for rising drug costs could well be the high number of mergers in the pharmaceutical industry [16]. Mergers can lessen competition, driving innovation down and prices up [17, 18, 19]. These mergers have come under fire for leading to "bad science" (due to cuts in research and development spending), and they have been decried by some voices in the press as nothing more than cynical attempts to get a better corporate tax rate [18, 20].

Finally, a key driver of high drug costs in the United States is the fact that, quite simply, there are no regulatory efforts to lower prices. This lack of regulation is, in many ways, unique to the United States. In Europe, price controls for drugs are commonplace [21]. In Switzerland, drugs are only approved if they are proven to be both medically successful and cost-effective [22]. Australia's Pharmaceutical Benefits Scheme provides government-subsidized drugs and lists the medications, and their fixed prices, online [23]. Canada has a drug review board that examines the effectiveness of a given drug and makes recommendations to public drug plans about reimbursement [24]. Not only does the United States lack anything like these measures but also, in 2003, the US Congress refused to even permit Medicare to negotiate prices with drug companies [25].

The current political climate makes it unlikely that we will see the problem of pricing solved legislatively any time soon [26]. Given the unlikelihood of sweeping policy solutions, the question facing us here is perhaps narrower: What is the role of public health in the debate over drug costs?

I suggest that the role of public health here is clear. Rising drug prices, and the high cost of treatment in the United States, has created a real market demand for just the kind of prevention agenda that should be at the heart of our field. Circling back to Sovaldi, we see a case in point. Sovaldi stands to make a tremendous difference in the lives of those affected by hepatitis C, and it would be a shame if the drug's cost prevented these people from receiving care. But how much better off would they be if they did not have hepatitis C to begin with? What if the disease, in fact, no longer existed, rendering the debate over Sovaldi's pricing moot?

We in public health know that this is possible through prevention. Needle exchanges and education campaigns can go far toward reducing the incidence of hepatitis C in populations, without the use of expensive drugs that cost $1,000 per pill [27, 28].

Hidden in the political rancor around drug pricing is an implicit acceptance of our fundamental reliance on drugs and medical curative strategies as the cornerstone of our national approach to health. A well-articulated prevention agenda, therefore, is positioned to make real gains. Prevention represents a "third way" between the extremes of paying high costs or going without needed care. This is a case we must continue to make. It falls to public health to articulate the importance of prevention so that populations can reap the benefits of this approach. We need to convey the message that prevention is not simply cancer screening, or environmental regulation, or even working to improve health by reducing poverty. It is all of these measures and more—the sum of its parts. For this approach to reach its full potential, it must be carefully calibrated to target the specific social, political, economic, and environmental causes of disease. This means that we must communicate, through our scholarship and through our broader translation of our public health agenda, that when we talk about prevention, we are talking about a comprehensive engagement with the fundamental drivers of population health.

I recognize that this discussion may touch a nerve and that in some respects a call for lower drug prices is an easy reflection of a contemporary hot button issue. However, it is also true that the pharmaceutical industry presents extraordinary opportunities for investment in curative care, particularly as novel developments create ever more dynamic opportunities to target disease. This spotlights the fundamental difference between medicine and public health, with the former focused on treating diseases that have already taken root and the latter committed to preventing diseases altogether. The challenges posed by high drug prices suggest the importance of a public health preventive approach, both toward improving health in general and, specifically, toward minimizing our reliance on medications, obviating the demand for expensive treatments.

REFERENCES

1. Politico Pro Staff. Trump backs Medicare negotiating drug prices. *Politico*. January 25, 2016. http://www.politico.com/story/2016/01/trump-backs-medicare-negotiating-drug-prices-218215. Accessed October 4, 2016.

2. Karlin S, Norman B. Rubio attacks drug costs. *Politico*. October 19, 2015. http://www.politico.com/tipsheets/prescription-pulse/2015/10/rubio-attacks-drug-costs-210798. Accessed October 4, 2016.

3. Norman B. Hillary Clinton taking on drug industry. *Politico*. September 22, 2015. http://www.politico.com/story/2015/09/hillary-clinton-prescription-drugs-health-care-213910. Accessed October 4, 2016.

4. Express Scripts Lab. Express Scripts 2015 drug trend report. https://lab.express-scripts.com/lab/drug-trend-report. March 2016. Accessed October 4, 2016.

5. Seidman B. Drug price increases 5,000 percent overnight. *CBS News*. September 21, 2015. http://www.cbsnews.com/news/generic-drug-price-increases-5000-percent-overnight. Accessed October 4, 2016.

6. Dumcius G. Massachusetts Attorney General Maura Healey urges Gilead to reconsider charging $1,000 per pill for hepatitis C drug in US. *MassLive*. January 27, 2016. http://www.masslive.com/news/index.ssf/2016/01/massachusetts_attorney_general_26.html. Accessed October 4, 2016.

7. Weisman R. Doctors challenge Vertex over high price of cystic fibrosis drug. *The Boston Globe*. July 20, 2015. https://www.bostonglobe.com/business/2015/07/20/researcher-and-group-doctors-challenge-vertex-price-new-cystic-fibrosis-drug/d5PZMlj6T6uzqousm2x-LEL/story.html. Accessed October 4, 2016.

8. Clinical Trials 101. Crohn's & Colitis Foundation of America Web site. http://www.ccfa.org/resources/clinical-trials-101.html. Accessed October 4, 2016.

9. Weisman R. Group hits Tufts Center's drug development figure. *The Boston Globe*. December 2, 2014. https://www.bostonglobe.com/business/2014/12/02/critics-question-tufts-research-team-estimate-that-costs-billion-develop-drug/Y34czSIKnmfcfiNpV5EQlI/story.html. Accessed October 4, 2016.

10. Cost to Develop and Win Marketing Approval for a New Drug Is $2.6 Billion. Tufts Center for the Study of Drug Development Web site. http://csdd.tufts.edu/news/complete_story/pr_tufts_csdd_2014_cost_study. Published November 18, 2014. Accessed October 4, 2016.

11. Financial Disclosure. Tufts Center for the Study of Drug Development Web site. http://csdd.tufts.edu/about/financial_disclosure. Accessed October 4, 2016.

12. Five More Pharmaceutical Companies Join NIH Initiative to Speed Therapeutic Discovery. National Institutes of Health Web site. https://www.nih.gov/news-events/news-releases/five-more-pharmaceutical-companies-join-nih-initiative-speed-therapeutic-discovery. Published June 12, 2012. Accessed October 4, 2016.

13. Budget. National Institutes of Health Web site. https://www.nih.gov/about-nih/what-we-do/budget. Accessed October 4, 2016.

14. Swanson A. Big pharmaceutical companies are spending far more on marketing than research. *The Washington Post*. February 11, 2015. https://www.washingtonpost.com/news/wonk/wp/2015/02/11/big-pharmaceutical-companies-are-spending-far-more-on-marketing-than-research. Accessed October 4, 2016.

15. Adams CP, Brantner VV. Estimating the cost of new drug development: Is it really 802 million dollars? *Health Affairs*. 2006; 25(2): 420–8.

16. Wieczner J. The real reasons for the pharma merger boom. *Fortune*. July 28, 2015. http://fortune.com/2015/07/28/why-pharma-mergers-are-booming. Accessed October 4, 2016.

17. Competitive Effects. Fair Trade Commission Web site. https://www.ftc.gov/tips-advice/competition-guidance/guide-antitrust-laws/mergers/competitive-effects. Accessed October 4, 2016.

18. Lo C. Pharma mergers: Big business, bad science? *Pharmaceutical-Technology.com*. January 7, 2015. http://www.pharmaceutical-technology.com/features/featurepharma-mergers-big-business-bad-science-4467897. Accessed October 4, 2016.

19. Lazarus D. Firms should stop pretending that high-profile mergers will benefit consumers. *Los Angeles Times*. July 28, 2015. http://www.latimes.com/business/la-fi-lazarus-20150728-column.html. Accessed October 4, 2016.

20. Cassidy J. The Pfizer–Allergen merger is a disgrace. *The New Yorker*. November 23, 2015. http://www.newyorker.com/news/john-cassidy/the-pfizer-allergan-merger-is-a-disgrace. Accessed October 4, 2016.

21. Why do drugs cost less in Canada? *Slate*. 2000. http://www.slate.com/articles/news_and_politics/explainer/2000/05/why_do_drugs_cost_less_in_canada.html. Accessed October 4, 2016.

22. Emanuel EJ. The solution to drug prices. *The New York Times*. September 9, 2015. http://www.nytimes.com/2015/09/09/opinion/the-solution-to-drug-prices.html?_r=1. Accessed October 4, 2016.

23. Pharmaceutical Benefits Scheme (PBS). The Pharmaceutical Benefits Scheme Web site. http://www.pbs.gov.au/pbs/home. Accessed October 4, 2016.

24. CADTH Common Drug Review (CDR). CADTH Common Drug Review (CDR) Web site. https://www.cadth.ca/about-cadth/what-we-do/products-services/cdr. Accessed October 4, 2016.

25. Morgan D. Obama administration seeks to negotiate Medicare drug prices. *Reuters*. February 2, 2015. http://www.reuters.com/article/us-usa-budget-medicare-idUSKBN0L61OW20150202. Accessed October 4, 2016.

26. Glantz LH. US drug companies failing to offer affordable drugs. *BU Today*. October 26, 2015. http://www.bu.edu/today/2015/pov-us-drug-companies-failing-to-produce-affordable-drugs. Accessed October 4, 2016.

27. Syringe Exchange Programs and Hepatitis C Fact Sheet. Harm Reduction Coalition Web site. http://harmreduction.org/syringe-access/syringe-access-tools/seps-and-hepatitis-c. Accessed October 4, 2016.

28. Weinbaum C, Lyerla R, Margolis HS. Prevention and control of infections with hepatitis viruses in correctional settings. *Morbidity and Mortality Weekly Report (MMWR)*. 2003; 52(RR01): 1–33.

19

When Disaster Strikes

DISASTERS ARE SUDDEN, large-scale events that disrupt communities and cause death, destruction, and trauma [1]. Globally, the number of disasters—both natural and human-made—is increasing, primarily as a consequence of climate change and urbanization [2]. In 2012, there were nearly 360 natural disasters registered worldwide [3]. Disasters can strike anywhere, without warning; no geographic area is immune. China is the country most frequently affected by disasters, followed by the United States, the Philippines, India, and Indonesia. In the United States, an estimated 13 to 19 percent of adults have reported having experienced a disaster in their lifetime [4].

Between 2003 and 2012, natural disasters killed an average of 106,654 people per year [5]. This loss of life was driven, in part, by several major, destructive storms. These include the 2011 Japanese tsunami, which killed more than 15,000 and left more than 2,500 people missing; the 2010 Haitian earthquake, which led to a death toll of more than 230,000; the 2008 earthquake in China's Sichuan province, which killed approximately 70,000 and left more than 18,000 missing; and the 2004 Indian Ocean tsunami, which killed approximately 230,000, displaced 1.7 million people, and injured more than half a million [6, 7, 8, 9, 10]. The United States has also seen its share of disasters. In the past 15 years alone, the country has endured Hurricanes Katrina, Ike, and Sandy. These combined events resulted in tragic loss of life, as well as billions of dollars in damage.

The burden of disasters is extensive. It includes death, property loss, infrastructural damage, monetary loss, years lost to disability, interruption of services, and damage to individual and population health [11, 12, 13]. The health effects of disasters are twofold: There are the immediate effects of the event itself, and then there are the long-term consequences. Physical injury and death after a disaster tend to be immediate, happening within minutes of the event onset. They also tend to be just the beginning of the harm a disaster can cause. Indeed, much of the health burden following disasters relates to the psychological damage inflicted by these events, which can unfold over time and be debilitating. In reviewing the post-traumatic stress disorder (PTSD) literature, for example, colleagues and I previously found that 30 to 60 percent of direct victims of disasters experience PTSD [4]. This prevalence was smaller among rescue workers (10 to 15 percent) and the general public (approximately 5 to 10 percent). PTSD prevalence varies greatly between studies due to different scales of disasters, degree of exposure, timing, and methods.

There are several factors that determine mental health risk among populations in the wake of disasters. Many studies have found PTSD symptoms to be associated with younger age, female gender, and a history of mental illness [14, 15, 16]. Following disasters, there is also an increase in the risk of depression and substance use disorders. These substances, which tend to be used more by men, often function as coping mechanisms [17]. After the September 11, 2001, terrorist attacks in New York City, for example, many studies found an uptick in the use of alcohol, cigarettes, and drugs [18]. Finally, a study of Hurricane Sandy survivors in New Jersey found that high hurricane exposure, physical health limitations, and environmental health concerns were all associated with worse mental health outcomes [19]. Other risk factors found to be associated with post-hurricane mental health include ongoing stressors, lower social support, and financial loss [20].

It is important to note that most individuals who are faced with disaster tend to be resilient, or to regain functioning relatively soon after experiencing a traumatic event, even after initially experiencing symptoms of mental health trouble [21]. Longitudinal work allows us to observe this phenomenon over time. Pietrzak and colleagues followed Hurricane Ike survivors at three time points after the storm and found that the prevalence of past-month mental disorder, specifically hurricane-related PTSD, decreased over time [22]. However, this capacity for resilience can vary. Most studies suggest that the course of mental health after disasters is different for different groups of people. A majority may exhibit few symptoms of mental disorder at any time point, whereas others may demonstrate rapid resolution of symptoms, ongoing moderate symptoms, ongoing substantial burden of psychopathology, or, occasionally, increases in psychopathology over time [23, 24]. For example, a study of children affected by the 2008 Sichuan earthquake found that the proportion of participants who used mental health services dropped substantially between follow-up periods, although PTSD and depression prevalence remained stable [25].

It is also becoming clear that social context plays a role in shaping the health of populations after disasters. In post-tsunami Indonesia, community-wide destruction has been shown to have worsened PTSD, even when taking into account a range of individual exposures and loss [26]. On the other hand, community social capital can promote resilience in individuals in the wake of sudden, catastrophic events [27]. Also, although the initial disaster can be devastating, many post-disaster events can also affect psychopathology. For example, displacement and lack of order in a community can increase the likelihood of violence, especially violence toward women and children [28]. At a more macro level, disasters affecting less economically advantaged communities, and places that have experienced more overall destruction, are associated with worse health outcomes. This was particularly the case after Hurricane Katrina, when the economically vulnerable were among those most affected by storm [29]. There has also been some evidence that human-made disasters and mass violence may have a more profound psychological impact on survivors compared to natural or technological disasters, although this finding is debatable, and it is complicated by a paucity of longitudinal data in disaster studies [14, 30].

Looking at population health in the aftermath of disasters raises an intriguing, broader question: How can we expect populations to behave in the wake of these events? After Hurricane Katrina, the media paid significant attention to the sometimes extreme behavior prompted by unprecedented circumstances. But is post-disaster population behavior really so unpredictable? Recent work has articulated a model of population behavior following large-scale disasters [31]. This model is grounded in theory and based on a data set of 339 disasters from 1950 to 2005 [31]. The results of this work suggest replicable and consistent patterns of behavior after large-scale, traumatic events [31]. The model posits five overlapping behavioral stages. Stage 1, group preservation, involves directly affected people acting to preserve life and secure safety. This means both information-seeking (from friends, employers, the media, government, etc.) and action (targeting the source of the hazard, evacuating, etc.). Stage 2, population preservation, is similar to Stage 1 but occurs among the larger population, not just those directly affected by the hazard. Stage 2 can include disseminating information to people who may be at risk and the activity of leaders who take charge to determine what actions are necessary after a disaster has struck. Also included in this stage are volunteers and formal response agencies that lend assistance to the directly affected group.

Stage 3 begins after the initial danger has passed. Its components include mourning the loss of people and property, memorialization, recognizing a new set of norms, and creating a narrative. Stage 4, externalizing, involves seeking redress and addressing vulnerabilities. These actions can take a variety of shapes. Formal investigations or criminal charges are examples of how a society might seek redress after a terrorist attack. We have also seen externalization manifest as anger at the government for a perceived lack of preparedness leading up to a disaster [32]. Addressing vulnerabilities can include plans for preventive measures to mitigate the effects of future disasters. The final stage, renormalization, includes cultural adaption to post-disaster circumstances, normalization of vulnerability, and new modes of behavior. This phase lasts until new post-disaster modes of behavior become dominant. This could be when new technology is adopted or new security policies become regular, such as heightened airline security in the wake of the September 11, 2001, attacks [33].

Each of these stages has implications for health. For example, volunteerism as part of Stage 2 may improve the mental health of those who choose to volunteer after a disaster, even if these volunteers were not themselves directly affected by the event [34]. There are also other suggested models of behavior following disasters, including models that focus on community response, as well as evidence-based post-disaster policy recommendations [35, 36].

Disasters do happen and, unfortunately, will continue to happen. We cannot stop them, but we can work to minimize the damage they can cause. The difference between disasters with devastating consequences (e.g., Hurricane Katrina) and those with much milder outcomes (e.g., Hurricane Sandy) frequently comes down to the fundamental salutary conditions that promote or undermine population health before and after disasters strike. This suggests that, ultimately, the most effective step we can take to mitigate the consequences of disasters is to engage with the factors that drive health every day.

REFERENCES

1. What Is a Disaster? International Federation of Red Cross and Red Crescent Societies Web site. http://www.ifrc.org/en/what-we-do/disaster-management/about-disasters/what-is-a-disaster. Accessed October 4, 2016.

2. Intergovernmental Panel on Climate Change. *Climate Change 2014—Impacts, Adaptation and Vulnerability: Part A: Global and Sectoral Aspects, Working Group II Contribution to the IPCC Fifth Assessment Report.* New York, NY: Cambridge University Press; 2014.

3. Guha-Sapir D, Hoyois P, Below R. *Annual Disaster Statistical Review 2012: The Numbers and Trends.* Brussels: Centre for Research on the Epidemiology of Disasters; 2013.

4. Galea S, Nandi A, Vlahov D. The epidemiology of post-traumatic stress disorder after disasters. *Epidemiologic Reviews.* 2005; 27: 78–91.

5. Centre for Research on the Epidemiology of Disasters (CRED) Web site. http://www.cred.be/publications. Accessed October 4, 2016.

6. Oskin B. Japan earthquake & tsunami of 2011: Facts and information. *Live Science.* May 7, 2015. http://www.livescience.com/39110-japan-2011-earthquake-tsunami-facts.html. Accessed October 4, 2016.

7. CNN Library. Haiti earthquake fast facts. *CNN.* http://www.cnn.com/2013/12/12/world/haiti-earthquake-fast-facts. Updated December 13, 2015. Accessed October 4, 2016.

8. Sichuan Earthquake. *The New York Times.* http://www.nytimes.com/topic/subject/sichuan-earthquake. Accessed October 4, 2016.

9. CNN Library. Tsunami of 2004 fast facts. *CNN.* http://www.cnn.com/2013/08/23/world/tsunami-of-2004-fast-facts. Updated December 16, 2015. Accessed October 4, 2016.

10. Osborne H. 2004 Indian Ocean earthquake and tsunami: Facts about the Boxing Day disaster. *International Business Times.* December 22, 2014. http://www.ibtimes.co.uk/2004-indian-ocean-earthquake-tsunami-facts-1480629. Accessed October 4, 2016.

11. Kliesen KL. The economics of natural disasters. *The Regional Economist.* April 1994. https://www.stlouisfed.org/Publications/Regional-Economist/April-1994/The-Economics-of-Natural-Disasters. Accessed October 4, 2016.

12. Fewtrell L, Kay D. An attempt to quantify the health impacts of flooding in the UK using an urban case study. *Public Health.* 2008; 122(5): 446–51. doi:10.1016/j.puhe.2007.09.010

13. Wang PS, et al. Disruption of existing mental health treatments and failure to initiate new treatment after Hurricane Katrina. *American Journal of Psychiatry.* 2008; 165(1): 34–41.

14. Norris FH, et al. 60,000 disaster victims speak: Part I. An empirical review of the empirical literature, 1981–2001. *Psychiatry.* 2002; 65(3): 207–39.

15. North CS, et al. Psychiatric disorders among survivors of the Oklahoma City bombing. *JAMA: The Journal of the American Medical Association.* 1999; 282(8): 755–62. doi:10.1001/jama.282.8.755

16. Berenz EC, et al. Pretyphoon panic attack history moderates the relationship between degree of typhoon exposure and posttyphoon PTSD and depression in a Vietnamese sample. *Depression and Anxiety.* 2013; 30(5): 461–8. doi:10.1002/da.22096

17. Galea S, Goldmann E. Mental health consequences of disasters. *Annual Review of Public Health.* 2014; 35: 169–83. doi:10.1146/annurev-publhealth-032013-182435

18. Vlahov D, et al. Increased use of cigarettes, alcohol, and marijuana among Manhattan, New York, residents after the September 11th terrorist attacks. *American Journal of Epidemiology*. 2002; 155(11): 988–96.

19. Boscarino JA, et al. Mental health outcomes at the Jersey Shore after Hurricane Sandy. *International Journal of Emergency Mental Health and Human Resilience*. 2013; 15(3): 147–58.

20. Nillni YI, et al. Unique and related predictors of major depressive disorder, posttraumatic stress disorder, and their comorbidity after Hurricane Katrina. *Journal of Nervous and Mental Disease*. 2013; 201(10): 841–7. doi:10.1097/NMD.0b013e3182a430a0

21. Bonanno GA. Loss, trauma, and human resilience: Have we underestimated the human capacity to thrive after extremely aversive events? *American Psychologist*. 2004; 59(1): 20–8.

22. Pietrzak RH, et al. Resilience in the face of disaster: Prevalence and longitudinal course of mental disorders following Hurricane Ike. *PLoS One*. 2012; 7(6): e38964. doi:10.1371/journal.pone.0038964

23. Norris FH, Tracy M, Galea S. Looking for resilience: Understanding the longitudinal trajectories of responses to stress. *Social Science & Medicine*. 2009; 68(12): 2190–8. doi:10.1016/j.socscimed.2009.03.043

24. Kessler RC, et al. Trends in mental illness and suicidality after Hurricane Katrina. *Molecular Psychiatry*. 2008; 13(4): 374–84. doi:10.1038/sj.mp.4002119

25. Jia Z, et al. Traumatic experiences and mental health consequences among child survivors of the 2008 Sichuan earthquake: A community-based follow-up study. *BMC Public Health*. 2013; 13: 104. doi:10.1186/1471-2458-13-104

26. Frankenberg E, Nobles J, Sumantri C. Community destruction and traumatic stress in post-tsunami Indonesia. *Journal of Health and Social Behavior*. 2012; 53(4): 498–514. doi:10.1177/0022146512456207

27. Wind TR, Komproe IH. The mechanisms that associate community social capital with post-disaster mental health: A multilevel model. *Social Science & Medicine*. 2012; 75(9): 1715–20. doi:10.1016/j.socscimed.2012.06.032

28. Gupta J, Agrawal A. Chronic aftershocks of an earthquake on the well-being of children in Haiti: Violence, psychosocial health and slavery. *Canadian Medical Association Journal*. 2010; 182(18): 1997–9. doi:10.1503/cmaj.100526

29. Zoraster RM. Vulnerable populations: Hurricane Katrina as a case study. *Prehospital and Disaster Medicine*. 2010; 25(1): 74–8.

30. Neria Y, DiGrande L, Adams BG. Posttraumatic stress disorder following the September 11, 2001, terrorist attacks: A review of the literature among highly exposed populations. *American Psychologist*. 2011; 66(6): 429–46. doi:10.1037/a0024791

31. Rudenstine S, Galea S. Behavioral consequences of disasters: A five-stage model of population behavior. *Disaster Medicine and Public Health Preparedness*. 2014; 8(6): 497–504. doi:10.1017/dmp.2014.114

32. Egan M, Farragher T. Angry America asks why more isn't done. *The Sydney Morning Herald*. September 4, 2005. http://www.smh.com.au/news/world/angry-america-asks-why-more-isnt-done/2005/09/03/1125302783624.html. Accessed October 6, 2016.

33. Airlines security policies post 9/11. *Boston.com*. http://archive.boston.com/news/nation/specials/sept_11_anniversary/gallery/changed_airline_security_policies. Accessed October 6, 2016.

34. Adams RE, Boscarino JA. Volunteerism and well-being in the context of the World Trade Center terrorist attacks. *International Journal of Emergency Mental Health and Human Resilience.* 2015; 17(1): 274–82.

35. Patterson O, Weil F, Patel K. The role of community in disaster response: Conceptual models. *Population Research and Policy Review.* 2010; 29(2): 127–41. doi:10.1007/s11113-009-9133-x

36. Beaton RD, et al. The role of public health in mental and behavioral health in children and families following disasters. *Journal of Public Health Management and Practice.* 2009; 15(6): E1–11. doi:10.1097/PHH.0b013e3181a8c307

20

Climate Change and Our Health

DURING THE PAST century, the temperature on the surface of the earth increased by approximately 0.85°C, while the global sea level rose by approximately 0.19 m [1]. The key features of climate change, in addition to rising global temperatures and sea levels, include increases in temperature variability, extreme precipitation, and heat waves; acidification of the oceans; and the reduction of glacier mass and sea ice [1]. Climate change has also been projected to amplify the effects of existing climatologic risks to human, plant, and animal ecosystems [1].

Given the wide-ranging influence of environmental climate change on all global systems, it is not surprising that this phenomenon stands to shape human health on a large scale. To illustrate this influence, I focus here on two key mechanisms through which climate change will likely affect population health: disasters and forced migration. Both disasters and forced migration will increase over time as a consequence of climate change, and both represent significant threats to population health worldwide. Indeed, they are already on the rise. In the past two decades, the number of natural disasters doubled from approximately 200 to 400 per year [2]. Related, migration patterns have shifted populations toward coastal regions, which are most vulnerable to extreme weather events [3].

In Chapter 19, I touched on the consequences of the type of natural disasters caused by climate change. These consequences include mortality, physical morbidity, and psychiatric problems. There may also be exacerbations of pre-existing health problems among those who survive disasters, as well as the onset of new problems [4]. These new concerns, such as injuries and acute renal failure, can manifest in the immediate aftermath of disaster, whereas other issues, such as gastrointestinal symptoms, musculoskeletal pain, and psychiatric disorders, can arise in the weeks following the initial event [4]. Still other problems, such as increased risk of cardiovascular disease and diabetes, may be elevated in the longer term (≥1 year) post-disaster [4].

The consequences of disasters can also extend beyond the physical, affecting mental health. These psychological effects can include post-traumatic stress disorder (PTSD), depression, substance use disorders, and suicidality [5]. In the aftermath of Hurricane Katrina, for example, approximately 49.1 percent of individuals living in the New Orleans Metropolitan Area—the population most directly exposed to hurricane-related trauma— were estimated to have experienced a *Diagnostic and Statistical Manual of Mental Disorders*, fourth edition, anxiety or mood disorder in the prior 30 days, compared to 26.4 percent in less directly exposed areas [6]. Similarly, 30.3 percent of individuals living in the New Orleans Metropolitan Area were estimated to have PTSD, whereas the PTSD estimate in other areas was less than half that, at 12.5 percent [6].

In addition to these concerns, forced migration, one of the sentinel consequences of climate change, is emerging at an unprecedented scale [2]. A variety of climate change-driven factors contribute to the problem of forced migration, including natural disasters, desertification of previously arable land, and rising sea levels. Bangladesh is a case in point. The country has already experienced forced migration as a consequence of climate change, and it is poised to experience a great deal more, given its coastal location and vast river delta network [7, 8].

Forced migration affects health in a number of ways. The sheer adversity of forced migration and the attendant processes of adaptation constitute a powerful set of stressors that may exacerbate pre-existing health problems and increase the risk of new-onset health issues. Relations between health and the process of migration can be conceptualized in terms of the stage of migration [9]. Lack of access to medical care is a particular feature of the migration process, placing those with pre-existing health problems at risk of disease progression [10]. Lack of care also means that minor health issues that arise during migration are at greater risk of developing into long-term problems [10]. Worse, migrants are highly vulnerable to deep exploitation, both physical (e.g., sexual trauma, violence, and forced labor) and financial [11]. These traumas are themselves associated with increased risk of health problems—including psychiatric disorders such as PTSD and depression— independent of the ordeal of migration [12]. I further discuss the issue of forced migration in a later chapter.

As the consequences of climate change unfold, we are faced with the central concern that the burden of these consequences will be disproportionately borne by the poor and the disadvantaged. This concern is particularly relevant to public health, given its special focus on the well-being of low-income populations. Poverty and relative disadvantage are fundamental causes of health disparities between groups [13]. Wealth and social position also determine risk of exposure to harm because more vulnerable low-lying coastal areas tend to be occupied by the poor, whereas the wealthy tend to occupy safer, more elevated areas [14]. Socioeconomic status can also shape vulnerability to poor mental health outcomes. This was evident in the United States as a consequence of Hurricane Katrina, when those who were black and had lower pre-disaster income suffered from an elevated risk of PTSD [6]. Within the context of climate change, we can therefore see how social and financial resources buffer both the risk of exposure to natural disasters and the deleterious effects that follow such exposure. Similarly, financial resources insulate and protect against forced migration by providing a safer base and more contingency options in the event of disaster. As concluded in the International Panel on Climate Change's *Climate Change 2014: Synthesis Report*, risks associated with climate change are "generally greater for disadvantaged people and communities at all levels of development" [1].

Climate change is unequivocally progressing [15]. As it does, it is emerging as one of the greatest threats to population health in the 21st century [15]. The danger of this phenomenon speaks, I think, to the need to engage with the foundational drivers of health in societies. Unless we pay attention to the fundamental issue at hand—in this case, climate change driven by energy consumption patterns—we cannot hope to arrive at a sustainable, long-term solution [16, 17]. Despite our best attempts to mitigate the public health risks associated with climate change, any efforts that do not tackle the root causes of this problem are bound to come up short.

REFERENCES

1. Contribution of Working Groups I, II and III to the Fifth Assessment Report of the Intergovernmental Panel on Climate Change, Core Writing Team Pachauri RK, Meyer LA, eds. *Climate Change 2014: Synthesis Report.* Geneva, Switzerland: Intergovernmental Panel on Climate Change; 2014.

2. Guterres A. *Climate Change, Natural Disasters and Human Displacement: A UNHCR Perspective.* Geneva, Switzerland: UNHCR; 2009.

3. McGranahan G, Balk D, Anderson B. The rising tide: Assessing the risks of climate change and human settlements in low elevation coastal zones. *Environment & Urbanization.* 2007; 19(1): 17–37.

4. Neria Y, Galea S, Norris FH, eds. *Mental Health and Disasters.* New York, NY: Cambridge University Press; 2009.

5. Galea S, Goldmann E. Mental health consequences of disasters. *Annual Review of Public Health.* 2014; 35: 169–83. doi:10.1146/annurev-publhealth-032013-182435

6. Galea S, et al. Exposure to hurricane-related stressors and mental illness after Hurricane Katrina. *Archives of General Psychiatry.* 2007; 64(12): 1427–34.

7. Lobell DB, et al. Prioritizing climate change adaptation needs for food security in 2030. *Science.* 2008; 319(5863): 607–10. doi:10.1126/science.1152339

8. Poncelet A, Gemenne F, Martiniello M, Bousetta H. A country made for disasters: Environmental vulnerability and forced migration in Bangladesh. In Afifi T, Jäger J, eds.: *Environment, Forced Migration and Social Vulnerability.* Heidelberg, Germany: Springer-Verlag; 2010: 211–22.

9. World Health Organization, Office of the High Commissioner for Human Rights and the International Organization for Migration. *International migration, health and human rights.* 2013.

10. Gushulak B, Weekers J, Macpherson D. Migrants and emerging public health issues in a globalized world: Threats, risks and challenges, an evidence-based framework. *Emerging Health Threats Journal.* 2009; 2: e10. doi:10.3134/ehtj.09.010

11. Belser P, Andrees B, eds. *Forced Labor: Coercion and Exploitation in the Private Economy.* Boulder, CO: Lynne Rienner; 2009.

12. Fink DS, Galea S. Life course epidemiology of trauma and related psychopathology in civilian populations. *Current Psychiatry Reports.* 2015; 17(5): 31. doi:10.1007/s11920-015-0566-0

13. Link BG, Phelan J. Social conditions as fundamental causes of disease. *Journal of Health and Social Behavior*. 1995; Spec No: 80–94.

14. Cutter SL, Emrich CT. Moral hazard, social catastrophe: The changing face of vulnerability along the hurricane coasts. *The Annals of the American Academy of Political and Social Science*. 2006; 604(1): 102–112. doi:10.1177/0002716205285515

15. McMichael AJ, Woodruff RE, Hales S. Climate change and human health: Present and future risks. *The Lancet*. 2006; 367(9513): 859–69.

16. Patz JA, Frumkin H, Holloway T, Vimont DJ, Haines A. Climate change: Challenges and opportunities for global health. *JAMA: The Journal of the American Medical Association*. 2014; 312(15): 1565–80. doi:10.1001/jama.2014.13186

17. Costello A, et al. Managing the health effects of climate change: Lancet and University College London Institute for Global Health Commission. *The Lancet*. 2009; 373(9676): 1693–733. doi:10.1016/S0140-6736(09)60935-1

21

Reproductive Health, Reproductive Justice

THE UNITED NATIONS Population Fund defines sexual and reproductive health in the following terms:

> A state of complete physical, mental, and social well-being in all matters relating to the reproductive system. It implies that people are able to have a satisfying and safe sex life, the capability to reproduce, and the freedom to decide if, when, and how often to do so. [1]

This definition is, I think, comprehensive, expressing the clear link between reproductive health and the broader well-being of individuals, families, and populations across generations [2]. At core, reproductive rights are human rights; the struggle for reproductive justice is inextricable from the fight for gender equality and the empowerment of women and girls all over the world [3].

Globally, there have been many encouraging developments in reproductive health during the past few decades. For example, the worldwide number of women who died during pregnancy or childbirth fell by almost half during the past 25 years [4]. In the United States, the teenage pregnancy rate reached a record low in 2013, registering a 10 percent drop from the previous year [5]. This decline was largely attributable to birth control use among sexually active teens [5].

This progress in the United States, however, does not obviate the unmet sexual and reproductive health needs that exist in many other areas of the world. Complications related to pregnancy and childbirth, a large proportion of which are preventable, remain the most common killer of reproductive-age women, causing almost 300,000 deaths worldwide, with most of this mortality concentrated in low-income countries [6].

The provision of safe, effective abortions is a core reproductive right. Unfortunately, this right remains elusive for women in many countries—a list which includes the United States.

And although abortion is often opposed in the name of preserving life, lack of access to safe abortion can, tragically, have the opposite effect. It has been estimated that 13 percent of maternal mortality worldwide is due to unsafe abortions, resulting in the deaths of approximately 47,000 women [7]. With this in mind, I present a few thoughts on the past, present, and future of abortion as a core reproductive right in the United States.

On January 22, 1973, the Supreme Court decision *Roe v. Wade* transformed reproductive health in the United States. The ruling declared unconstitutional a state law that banned all abortions except for those that would save the life of the mother [8]. The decision made clear that states were permitted to regulate abortions only after the first trimester of pregnancy, and only in cases explicitly linked to maternal health or to laws protecting the lives of fetuses during the third trimester. The lawsuit was brought on by a pregnant woman in Dallas, "Jane Roe," whose lawyers argued that the Texas ban on abortions violated Roe's constitutional rights [9]. Written by Justice Harry Blackmun, the Court's 7 to 2 decision argued that contraception and childbirth are covered in constitutional "zones of privacy" and are therefore protected by the First, Fourth, Ninth, and Fourteenth Amendments. The decision of a companion case, *Doe v. Bolton*, was released on the same day and overturned a Georgia abortion law that placed many barriers between women and the procedure, including requiring a licensed physician to perform an abortion only under his "best clinical judgment" [10].

Despite the watershed of *Roe v. Wade*, the provision of abortion care in the United States remains under threat. The Hyde Amendment, originally passed in 1976, bans the use of federal funds for abortion services in all circumstances except for those of rape, incest, or life endangerment [11]. Worse, many states have defied the decision of *Roe v. Wade* outright by passing new laws prohibiting abortions or enacting measures that make abortions difficult to obtain. For example, in 1982, Pennsylvania passed the Abortion Control Act, which required women seeking abortions to provide informed consent and minors to get informed consent from their parents (except in cases of "hardship") [12]. It also placed a 24-hour waiting period on abortions, during which time women were to be given information about the procedure [12]. Finally, the act required that a wife must inform her husband of her plans to abort, except in medical emergencies, and that all Pennsylvania abortion clinics report themselves to the state. In 1992, *Planned Parenthood v. Casey* addressed such obstructive logistical hurdles, affirming *Roe v. Wade*'s basic ruling and keeping states from placing unnecessary burdens or obstacles on women seeking abortions. However, it also stated that states may outlaw the abortions of "viable" fetuses, and it ruled that most of Pennsylvania's laws were in fact constitutional [13].

The challenge of states placing barriers between women and safe medical abortions is perhaps most vividly illustrated by the battles that have been fought over this issue in Texas. The average county in Texas is currently 111 miles from the nearest clinic that will perform abortions, and there were, in 2016, only 17 abortion clinics in the entire state, a marked decline from the 41 clinics in existence in 2012 [14]. Almost all of these clinics are located in major urban areas, making it very difficult for rural, low-income women to receive the service [14]. As a consequence of this lack of access, the Texas Policy Evaluation Project estimates that 1.7 percent of Texas women aged 18 to 49 years reported having attempted to end a pregnancy on their own without medical assistance [15].

Encouragingly, abortion is declining overall in the United States [16]. Abortion rates decreased from 2002 to 2011 for women in all age groups except for those younger than age 15 years, for whom they increased. Despite this limited success, approximately half of all pregnancies in the United States each year are unplanned, and almost one-third of women will have an abortion in their lifetime. The rates of abortion vary by economic and age demographic. Adolescents aged 15 to 19 years accounted for 13.5 percent of all abortions in 2011, 58 percent of women who have abortions are in their 20s, and 69 percent are economically disadvantaged. In 2011, there were 1,720 abortion providers in the United States, a slight decrease from 1,787 in 2008 [16, 17].

Roe v. Wade occurred at a time when most states had strict abortion policies, rendering abortions, for many, difficult or impossible to obtain. The freedoms codified by *Roe v. Wade* are therefore a critical part of a population reproductive health armamentarium. The Title X Family Planning program represents a similar bulwark against threats to reproductive health [18]. Title X was enacted in 1970 as part of the Public Health Service Act (Public Law 91-572, Population Research and Voluntary Family Planning Programs) [18]. It is a grant program aimed at providing comprehensive family planning, prioritizing low-income individuals and those not eligible for Medicaid or who are otherwise uninsured [18]. Although Title X funds, by statute, cannot be used to pay for abortions, it continues to this day to finance a range of counseling, contraceptive methods, cancer screening, pregnancy testing, HIV testing, as well as screening and treatment for sexually transmitted infections [18]. These services are overseen by the US Department of Health and Human Services' Office of Population Affairs and serve approximately 4.5 million clients per year. Public expenditures for family planning services in the United States overall totaled $2.37 billion in 2010, with Medicaid accounting for 75 percent of total expenditures, state appropriations for 12 percent, and Title X for 10 percent [19].

Title X's contribution to population health is well illustrated by two key pieces of evidence. First, women using Title X reproductive services are generally young, members of a minority, and poor. Significantly, these are the populations that most need access to safe, effective reproductive health services; they are also the populations that are least likely to get it, absent government services. Among the 20 million women in need of publicly funded contraceptive care, 77 percent are considered low-income [19]. Among women in need of publicly funded services from 2000 to 2010, the proportion of Hispanic women increased by 47 percent, the proportion of black women increased by 17 percent, and the proportion of white women increased by 4 percent. Title X's second contribution is economic. It is estimated that every public dollar spent on contraceptive services in 2008 resulted in approximately $3.74 in savings that would have been spent on Medicaid costs related to pregnancy care and delivery or to infants in their first year of life [18].

Reproductive rights remain challenged throughout the country. The debate over abortion, in particular, has been characterized by great contention, even though a clear majority of Americans favor abortion rights [20, 21]. In 2015, tensions around the issue reached a new level following a shooting at a Planned Parenthood in Colorado [22]. This incident occurred after an anti-abortion organization released a series of edited videos claiming that Planned Parenthood was illegally selling body parts of aborted fetuses [22]. Other worrying developments include the Trump administration's decision to reinstate the Mexico City policy, or "global gag rule," denying federal funds to non-governmental organizations that provide abortions.

Notwithstanding this turn of events, there are still reasons to hope that we can perhaps enter a new era of reproductive rights and reproductive health in this country. This hope arises in part from shifts in the political and legal landscapes, including the Supreme Court's landmark *Whole Woman's Health v. Hellerstedt* ruling—the Supreme Court's first major abortion case since 2007—which struck down a Texas law that would have shuttered many of the state's remaining abortion clinics through the use of "medically unnecessary restrictions" [23]. Heartening as this ruling was, however, the fact that it was needed at all demonstrates both the persistence of the opposition to reproductive rights in the United States and the need for public health to be a forceful voice for the continued defense of these vital services and the freedom of all women to access them.

REFERENCES

1. Sexual & Reproductive Health. United Nations Population Fund Web site. http://www.unfpa.org/sexual-reproductive-health. Accessed October 11, 2016.

2. Quinn K, Ejlak J. *Women's Sexual and Reproductive Health: A Literature Review*. Melbourne, Australia: Women's Health Victoria; 2008.

3. Gender Equality. United Nations Population Fund Web site. http://www.unfpa.org/gender-equality. Accessed October 11, 2016.

4. MDG 5: Improve Maternal Health. World Health Organization Web site. http://www.who.int/topics/millennium_development_goals/maternal_health/en. Reviewed May 2015. Accessed October 11, 2016.

5. Reproductive Health: Teen Pregnancy. Centers for Disease Control and Prevention Web site. http://www.cdc.gov/teenpregnancy. Updated August 31 2016. Accessed October 11, 2016.

6. Women's Health. World Health Organization Web site. http://www.who.int/mediacentre/factsheets/fs334/en. Updated September 2013. Accessed October 11, 2016.

7. Preventing Unsafe Abortion. World Health Organization Web site. http://www.who.int/reproductivehealth/topics/unsafe_abortion/magnitude/en. Accessed October 11, 2016.

8. *Roe v. Wade*, 410 US. 113 (1973).

9. McBride A. Landmark cases: Roe v. Wade (1973). PBS Web site. http://www.pbs.org/wnet/supremecourt/rights/landmark_roe.html. Published December 2006. Accessed October 11, 2016.

10. *Doe v. Bolton*, 410 US. 179 (1973).

11. Hyde Amendment. Planned Parenthood Action Fund Web site. https://www.plannedparenthoodaction.org/issues/abortion/hyde-amendment. Accessed October 11, 2016.

12. McBride A. Landmark cases: *Casey v. Planned Parenthood* (1992). PBS Web site. http://www.pbs.org/wnet/supremecourt/rights/landmark_casey.html. Published December 2006. Accessed October 11, 2016.

13. *Planned Parenthood of Southeastern Pennsylvania v. Casey. Oyez*. Chicago-Kent College of Law at Illinois Tech Web site. https://www.oyez.org/cases/1991/91-744. Accessed October 11, 2016.

14. Soffen K. How Texas could set national template for limiting abortion access. *The New York Times*. August 19, 2015. http://www.nytimes.com/2015/08/20/upshot/how-texas-could-set-national-template-for-limiting-abortion-access.html?_r=0. Accessed October 11, 2016.

15. Welch A. Study: 100,000 Texas women have tried to self-induce abortion. *CBS News*. November 19, 2015. http://www.cbsnews.com/news/100000-texas-women-have-tried-to-self-induce-abortion. Accessed October 11, 2016.

16. Pazol K, Creanga AA, Burley KD, Jamieson DJ. Abortion surveillance—United States, 2011. *Morbidity and Mortality Weekly Report (MMWR)*. 2014; 63(SS11); 1–41.

17. State Facts About Abortion: Texas. Guttmacher Institute Web site. https://www.guttmacher.org/fact-sheet/state-facts-about-abortion-texas. Published June 2015. Accessed October 11, 2016

18. History of Title X. US Department of Health & Human Services Web site. http://www.hhs.gov/opa/title-x-family-planning. Accessed October 11, 2016.

19. Publicly Funded Family Planning Services in the United States. Guttmacher Institute Web site. https://www.guttmacher.org/fact-sheet/publicly-funded-family-planning-services-united-states. Published September 2016. Accessed October 11, 2016.

20. Tarico V. After Roe: It's hard to believe now, but the abortion debate wasn't always so toxic. What happened? *Salon*. December 20, 2015. http://www.salon.com/2015/12/20/after_roe_its_hard_to_believe_now_but_the_abortion_debate_wasnt_always_so_toxic_what_happened. Accessed October 11, 2016.

21. Saad L. Americans Choose "Pro-Choice" for First Time in Seven Years. Gallup, Inc. Web site. http://www.gallup.com/poll/183434/americans-choose-pro-choice-first-time-seven-years.aspx. Published May 29, 2015. Accessed October 11, 2016.

22. Turkewitz J, Healy J. 3 are dead in Colorado Springs shootout at Planned Parenthood center. *The New York Times*. November 27, 2015. http://www.nytimes.com/2015/11/28/us/colorado-planned-parenthood-shooting.html?mtrref=undefined&gwh=E4B3A1EC0F8F2E366CAB8BDCF5D1C86B&gwt=pay. Accessed October 11, 2016.

23. *Whole Woman's Health v. Hellerstedt*. Center for Reproductive Rights Web site. http://www.reproductiverights.org/case/whole-womans-health-v-hellerstedt. Accessed October 11, 2016.

22

Coming to Terms with Firearms

⌒——

BETWEEN THE COLUMBINE High School shooting on April 20, 1999, and December 31, 2012, there were 66 school shootings throughout the world, 50 of which took place in the United States. During this time period, only 2 school shootings occurred in Canada and 14 in all other countries combined [1]. The data are unequivocal: The United States is in the midst of a firearm epidemic. By way of further example, in 2012, 11,622 deaths were attributable to firearm homicides, and 20,666 deaths were attributable to firearm suicides, according to the National Center for Injury Prevention and Control [2]. These rates stand in stark contrast with peer nations. In 2003, compared to 23 other populous, high-income countries, the United States had the highest rates of firearm homicide (6.9 times higher) and firearm suicide (5.8 times higher) [3]. These findings are consistent with prior data from 1994, which showed that the US rate of firearm mortality is eightfold times higher than rates of other high-income countries and 1.5 times higher than rates of upper-middle-income countries [4]. In addition, a frequently forgotten element of this problem is that there are many more firearm-related nonfatal injuries than there are fatalities, and a large proportion of these injuries result in long-term, debilitating consequences for their victims [5].

The United States has a long and complex relationship with firearms, with many organizations at work advocating for unfettered firearm availability [6]. Setting aside the constitutional rights argument, this chapter is concerned with a simpler question: What is the role of public health in this debate?

Although arguments in favor of gun ownership often center around self-protection, the evidence is overwhelmingly clear that this argument is not supported by the data [7]. Extant studies on the risks of firearm mortality in the context of firearm availability have provided evidence of an increased risk of both homicide and suicide driven by proximity to guns [8, 9]. A meta-analysis of 16 observational studies, mostly conducted in the United States, estimated that firearm accessibility was associated with an odds ratio of 3.24 for suicide and 2.0 for homicide, with women at a particularly high risk of homicide victimization (odds ratio = 2.84) compared to men (odds ratio = 1.32) [10]. Adolescents, for their part, appear to be at particularly high risk of firearm suicide, relative to adults [9].

Another study examined the link by state between firearm legislation and US firearm deaths from 2007 to 2010, creating a "legislative strength score" based on five categories of legislative intent: curbing firearm trafficking, strengthening Brady background checks, improving child safety, banning military-style assault weapons, and restricting guns in public places [11]. Higher legislative strength scores were linked with less firearm mortality; adjusted multivariable models showed that those in the highest quartile had a lower firearm suicide rate and a lower firearm homicide rate compared to those in the lowest quartile of legislative strength scores.

These studies are roundly supportive of causal relationships between firearm availability and firearm mortality, and, conversely, of firearm legislation as protective against firearm deaths. It is true that some concern about "reverse causation" has been raised, centered around the view that gun availability increases as a response to rising homicide rates or personal threat. However, this is probably not the case. Although some studies indicate that higher homicide rates may indeed precede higher gun ownership, this bias is unlikely to explain away a majority of the observed effect [8]. In particular, it is not liable to account for the hazard posed to women and children—the two groups most often affected by firearm homicide [8]. By contrast, the literature on firearms and firearm-related suicide is not subject to the same potential of reverse causation, although it does suffer from a dearth of longitudinal studies [9].

Despite the clear evidence that guns undermine the health of populations, the public health community has been unable to be an effective voice on this issue. This has been due, to a large extent, to the coordinated opposition of pro-gun groups such as the National Rifle Association (NRA). As a consequence of this opposition, we have seen throughout the years the silencing of gun researchers, health practitioners, and policymakers intent on addressing the problem of gun violence [12]. In 1996, actions by Congress, prompted by the NRA, effectively defunded federal gun research, a still extant legacy [13]. And although translatable lessons from successful public health campaigns on smoking, unintentional poisonings, and car safety abound, the political will necessary to implement similar approaches in the area of gun violence has been either absent, or, where it exists, under unremitting attack [14].

In 2011, physicians and other health practitioners in Florida became subject to legislation (HB 155) that essentially restricts their ability to discuss with patients the subject of guns or gun safety; although this legislation has been challenged, it was upheld in court [15, 16]. The difficulty of mitigating gun violence is also complicated by the lack of industrial regulation for firearms. Whereas manufacturers of a wide range of products—including cars, medications, and medical devices—are subject to regulation that holds them accountable for product safety risks, gun manufacturers appear to be immune to such forces. Perhaps that lack of accountability is why we are now faced with weapons such as the Bushmaster AR-15 semiautomatic rifle, the gun used in the Sandy Hook massacre, designed to "deliver maximum carnage with extreme efficiency" [17]. Such weapons have no place in civilian settings, as the parents of several victims of Sandy Hook argued in their lawsuit against Bushmaster Firearms [17].

While acknowledging sensitivity to paternalism, and respecting strong feelings about the Second Amendment, it seems to me that it falls to public health to be a clear voice against the legal widespread availability of a pathogen—firearms [18]. I use the word "pathogen" quite deliberately here. It suggests an important question: Would we tolerate such lapses in our legal response to other prevalent health challenges, such as infectious disease? Imagine for a moment that because of emphatically articulated rights-based arguments, the United States remained alone among peer countries in not having automobile seat belt laws, resulting in an automobile death rate seven times greater than that of Canada. Would that be tolerable?

In many ways, I worry that the voice of academic public health has been far too quiet on this issue, simply because the typical mechanisms that support our scholarship—extramural funding chief among them—have not been conducive of this work—even, at times, actively discouraging it. This suggests, then, that we must organize ourselves in a way that will allow us to speak clearly, and compellingly, about gun violence. It means taking an active role in translating scholarship, to fully engage with policymakers, and the broader public conversation, to move toward effective, healthier solutions to this truly preventable epidemic.

REFERENCES

1. Follman M, Aronsen G, Pan D. US mass shootings, 1982–2016: Data from Mother Jones' investigation. *Mother Jones.* Updated September 24, 2016. http://www.motherjones.com/politics/2012/12/mass-shootings-mother-jones-full-data. Accessed October 11, 2016.

2. Fatal Injury Reports. Centers for Disease Control and Prevention Web site. http://www.cdc.gov/injury/wisqars/fatal_injury_reports.html. Updated October 7, 2016. Accessed October 11, 2016.

3. Richardson EG, Hemenway D. Homicide, suicide, and unintentional firearm fatality: Comparing the United States with other high-income countries, 2003. *Journal of Trauma.* 2011; 70(1): 238–43. doi:10.1097/TA.0b013e3181dbaddf

4. Krug EG, Powell KE, Dahlberg LL. Firearm-related deaths in the United States and 35 other high- and upper-middle-income countries. *International Journal of Epidemiology.* 1998; 27(2): 214–21.

5. Kalesan B, French C, Fagan JA, Fowler DL, Galea S. Firearm-related hospitalizations and in-hospital mortality in the United States, 2000–2010. *American Journal of Epidemiology.* 2014; 179(3): 303–12. doi:10.1093/aje/kwt255

6. Second Amendment Foundation Web site. https://www.saf.org. Accessed October 13, 2016.

7. Constitutional Rights PAC Web site. https://constitutionalrightspac.com. Accessed October 13, 2016.

8. Hepburn LM, Hemenway D. Firearm availability and homicide: A review of the literature. *Aggression and Violent Behavior.* 2004; 9(4): 417–40.

9. Miller M, Hemenway D. The relationship between firearms and suicide: A review of the literature. *Aggression and Violent Behavior.* 1999; 4(1): 59–75.

10. Anglemyer A, Horvath T, Rutherford G. The accessibility of firearms and risk for suicide and homicide victimization among household members: A systematic review and meta-analysis. *Annals of Internal Medicine.* 2014; 160(2): 101–110.

11. Fleegler EW, Lee LK, Monuteaux MC, Hemenway D, Mannix R. Firearm legislation and firearm-related fatalities in the United States. *JAMA Internal Medicine.* 2013; 173(9): 732–40. doi:10.1001/jamainternmed.2013.1286

12. Kellermann AL, Rivara FP. Silencing the science on gun research. *JAMA: The Journal of the American Medical Association*. 2013; 309(6): 549–50. doi:10.1001/jama.2012.208207

13. Thacker PD. How Congress blocked research on gun violence. *Slate*. December 19, 2012. http://www.slate.com/articles/health_and_science/science/2012/12/gun_violence_ research_nra_and_congress_blocked_gun_control_studies_at_cdc.html. Accessed October 13, 2016.

14. Mozaffarian D, Hemenway D, Ludwig DS. Curbing gun violence: Lessons from public health successes. *JAMA: The Journal of the American Medical Association*. 2013; 309(6): 551–2. doi:10.1001/jama.2013.38

15. CS/CS/HB 155—Privacy of Firearm Owners. Florida House of Representatives Web site. http://www.myfloridahouse.gov/Sections/Bills/billsdetail.aspx?BillId=44993. Accessed October 13, 2016.

16. SphericalXS. NRA wins over free speech—Florida doctors silenced on guns by court. *Daily Kos*. July 30, 2014. http://www.dailykos.com/story/2014/07/30/1317592/-NRA-Wins-Over-Free-Speech-Florida-Doctors-Silenced-On-Guns-By-Court. Accessed October 13, 2016.

17. Newtown families file lawsuit against gunmaker. *The News-Times*. http://www.newstimes.com/news/item/Newtown-families-file-lawsuit-against-gunmaker-35640.php. Accessed October 13, 2016.

18. Jones MM, Bayer R. Paternalism and its discontents: Motorcycle helmet laws, libertarian values, and public health. *American Journal of Public Health*. 2007; 97(2): 208–17.

23

The Corrosive Role of Racism

IN RECENT YEARS, the list of reported incidents in which police have injured or killed unarmed black men seems inexhaustible [1, 2]. These events have often been followed by an outpouring of anguished civic protest and by commentary on the pervasiveness of racism that still persists in American life. As we deepen our understanding of racism in the United States, it becomes clear that instances of police violence are just a single manifestation of this problem. Dramatic as these events are, they fail to capture the full extent of the racist social interactions and structures that shape the experiences of the millions of black and minority individuals whose plight does not make the news. In a particularly powerful 2015 piece, New York City Commissioner of Health and Mental Hygiene Mary Bassett commented on #BlackLivesMatter and the implications of very public demonstrations of anger around racial divides for the medical and public health communities [3]. Informed by this discussion, how should we, in the academic public health community, think about racism within the context of population health and about our responsibility to tackle this issue toward creating a safer, less fearful society?

It may be clarifying to think of racism's impact on two levels: interpersonal or individual racism and structural or institutional racism. There is ample evidence of the impact of racism on health in both domains. The iceberg metaphor well illustrates this, showing the distinction between the more readily observable (i.e., interpersonal) dimensions of racism and its structural dimensions, which can be more difficult to observe (Figure 23.1) [4].

There is ample evidence that self-reported racism is associated with poor health [5]. Such interpersonal racism can operate through a number of mechanisms, including physiologic response and/or unequal quality of care, which can be a product of implicit racial bias [6, 7]. The most consistently studied and observed positive associations are for markers of poor mental health (i.e., emotional distress and depression symptoms) and health-related behaviors (i.e., smoking and substance use)—findings that are robust to adjustment for potential confounding. Less studied, however, are negative physical outcomes. Findings in this area

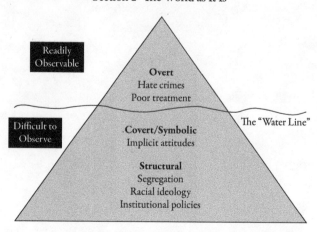

FIGURE 23.1 The discrimination iceberg. Gee GC, Ro A, Shariff-Marco S, Chae D. Racial discrimination and health among Asian Americans: Evidence, assessment, and directions for future research. *Epidemiologic Reviews.* 2009; 31: 130–151. doi: 10.1093/epirev/mxp009 [4]

have been inconsistent, although positive associations have been noted for cardiovascular risk factors and poor birth outcomes, to name two examples. Findings have been similar among youth, although greater evidence has emerged for a negative relation between self-reported racism and positive mental health outcomes (i.e., self-esteem and resilience) relative to adults [8]. Studies of racism and health have expanded in recent years and now include cancer as an outcome. This wider view has led to further evidence for links between racism and health over relatively long disease induction periods. Teletia R. Taylor, along with Yvette D. Cozier, Julie R. Palmer, and Lynn Rosenberg, found perceived racial discrimination to be related to elevated breast cancer risk among black women, particularly among women who were younger and had experienced racism in multiple forms (i.e., housing, job, and police-related) [9].

Regarding institutional and structural racism, much of the work in this area has centered around residential segregation and unequal access to health care [6, 10]. For example, a geographically weighted regression approach demonstrated that residential segregation was associated with black/white differences in congenital heart defect mortality [11]. Just as the conditions of structural racism are bad for health, the alleviation of these conditions has been shown to have a positive influence. A recent analysis demonstrated a beneficial effect of the end of Jim Crow laws (i.e., legal discrimination) toward the reduction of premature mortality for blacks, accounting for age, period, cohort, state, and county income effects; a related analysis demonstrated a similarly beneficial effect on the black infant mortality rate [12, 13]. It is important to note, however, that there is nowhere near enough research on institutional and structural racism, especially relative to the now large body of work on interpersonal racism [14].

How should we in academic public health engage with the issue of racism, at both interpersonal and structural levels? How might we best mitigate its effects? I suggest four possible approaches.

First, we must tackle racism at the community level. In this capacity, some of us may choose to express solidarity with affected groups, participating in public shows of support. Such actions ensure that the issue of racism moves to the forefront of the public debate and stays there. Indeed, peaceful public statements of concern about a pressing social issue always have a place in an open society, and our responsibility to make these statements is not in any way inconsistent with our role as members of an academic community.

Given that we are members of this community, my second suggestion relates to how our scholarship may pave the way for progress on this issue. The work of knowledge generation can help inform acute social needs, developing constructive strategies to help solve the urgent problems of our time—problems such as racism. This nudges us toward a scholarship of consequence, where we aim to shed light on the root causes of racial divides and the link between racism and the health of the public. To do this, we must prioritize our research questions accordingly. By focusing on what matters most, and orienting our scholarship toward areas of inquiry that tackle the foundational drivers of population health, we stand to make a real difference in creating a fairer, less racially fraught society [15].

Third, we are charged at our various institutions with fostering an educational environment that both teaches the foundations of our field and prepares students to engage with evolving issues of contemporary public health importance. That calls for an education that is dynamic and reflexive, but also one that is encouraging and respectful of the sharing of ideas. Such an academic climate does much to advance the goals of engendering mutual understanding and identifying solutions grounded in diversity of experience, opinion, and perspective. It is not enough to merely acknowledge disparities; we need to engage in difficult, sometimes uncomfortable discussions about these issues in order to understand one another and improve the often unacceptable conditions our scholarship makes all too apparent to us.

Finally, insofar as public health centers around shaping the conditions that make people healthy, and insofar as those conditions depend on the introduction of health in all sectors, we need to work toward a health conversation that extends well beyond the walls of academia. This agitates for an engagement with the public conversation around the issue of racism wherever the conversation may arise. Public health's unique perspective, informed by its scholarship, is well positioned to influence how we understand racism and its consequences for the well-being of populations. By clarifying the links between racism and health, by making them unignorable in the public debate, we can then begin to advance solutions.

Needless to say, racism and hate of any kind are intolerable, even when we do not take into account their health consequences. But health, as a universal aspiration, can serve as a clarifying lens for action, elevating the importance of creating a society free of racism, where health will no longer be determined by the color of a person's skin. The actions of a committed, activist public health will go far toward bringing this about.

REFERENCES

1. Wright B. Police shooting videos: 6 times unarmed black men were killed by white officers and what it means for social justice. *International Business Times*. April 9, 2015. http://www.ibtimes.com/police-shooting-videos-6-times-unarmed-black-men-were-killed-white-officers-what-it-1876156. Accessed October 13, 2016.
2. Stolberg SG. Baltimore enlists National Guard and a curfew to fight riots and looting. *The New York Times*. April 27, 2015. http://www.nytimes.com/2015/04/28/us/baltimore-freddie-gray.html?hp&action=click&pgtype=Homepage&module=second-column-region&region=top-news&WT.nav=top-news&_r=0. Accessed October 13, 2016.

3. Bassett MT. #BlackLivesMatter—A challenge to the medical and public health communities. *The New England Journal of Medicine.* 2015; 372(12): 1085–7. doi:10.1056/NEJMp1500529

4. Gee GC, Ro A, Shariff-Marco S, Chae D. Racial discrimination and health among Asian Americans: Evidence, assessment, and directions for future research. *Epidemiologic Reviews.* 2009; 31: 130–51. doi:10.1093/epirev/mxp009

5. Paradies Y. A systematic review of empirical research on self-reported racism and health. *International Journal of Epidemiology.* 2006; 35(4): 888–901.

6. Institute of Medicine. *Unequal Treatment: Confronting Racial and Ethnic Disparities in Health Care* (full printed version). Washington, DC: The National Academies Press; 2003.

7. Chapman EN, Kaatz A, Carnes M. Physicians and implicit bias: How doctors may unwittingly perpetuate health care disparities. *Journal of General Internal Medicine.* 2013; 28(11): 1504–10. doi:10.1007/s11606-013-2441-1

8. Priest N, et al. A systematic review of studies examining the relationship between reported racism and health and wellbeing for children and young people. *Social Science & Medicine.* 2013; 95: 115–27. doi:10.1016/j.socscimed.2012.11.031

9. Taylor TR, et al. Racial discrimination and breast cancer incidence in US black women: The Black Women's Health Study. *American Journal of Epidemiology.* 2007; 166(1): 46–54.

10. Williams DR, Mohammed SA. Discrimination and racial disparities in health: Evidence and needed research. *Journal of Behavioral Medicine.* 2009; 32(1): 20–47. doi:10.1007/s10865-008-9185-0

11. Gebreab SY, Diez Roux AV. Exploring racial disparities in CHD mortality between blacks and whites across the United States: A geographically weighted regression approach. *Health & Place.* 2012; 18(5): 1006–14. doi:10.1016/j.healthplace.2012.06.006

12. Krieger N, et al. Jim Crow and premature mortality among the US black and white population, 1960–2009: An age-period-cohort analysis. *Epidemiology.* 2014; 25(4): 494–504. doi:10.1097/EDE.0000000000000104

13. Krieger N, Chen JT, Coull B, Waterman PD, Beckfield J. The unique impact of abolition of Jim Crow laws on reducing inequities in infant death rates and implications for choice of comparison groups in analyzing societal determinants of health. *American Journal of Public Health.* 2013; 103(12): 2234–44. doi:10.2105/AJPH.2013.301350

14. Krieger N. Discrimination and health inequities. *International Journal of Health Services.* 2014; 44(4): 643–710.

15. Keyes K, Galea S. What matters most: Quantifying an epidemiology of consequence. *Annals of Epidemiology.* 2015; 25(5): 305–11. doi:10.1016/j.annepidem.2015.01.016

SECTION 3

On Inequities and the Health
of Marginalized Populations

24

On Health Haves and Health Have-Nots

PUBLIC HEALTH HAS long been concerned with health inequalities within and across groups. There is a substantial body of scholarship focused on health differences between populations—a body of scholarship that has been characterized as health inequalities or health disparities research. But our focus on health inequalities extends beyond the academic world and into the realm of public health practice. In this area, several efforts nationwide have been explicitly focused on narrowing health disparities, including the HHS Action Plan to Reduce Racial and Ethnic Health Disparities and the National Stakeholder Strategy for Achieving Health Equity, both through the US Department of Health and Human Services [1, 2]. We have also seen this concern at work at the level of political policy. The Minority Health and Health Disparities Research and Education Act was passed in 2000, which established the National Institute on Minority Health and Health Disparities [3]. The second goal of *Healthy People 2020* is to "achieve health equity and eliminate disparities" [4]. Some statewide efforts have also been quite visible in targeting health inequalities, including The California Campaign to Eliminate Racial and Ethnic Disparities in Health, co-chaired by the American Public Health Association and the Prevention Institute [5]. The Health Center program, which was originally funded by the Health Resources and Services Administration and recently received $11 billion from the Affordable Care Act, supports community health centers that try to overcome geographic, language, and cultural barriers to care for low-income individuals and minorities [6]. Even the Affordable Care Act itself is largely aimed at reducing health disparities by expanding insurance coverage. All of these measures reflect an interest, on the part of public health and its partners in government and other sectors, to lessen the health inequalities that exist between groups within the United States.

Given this activity, it is reasonable to ask: How are we doing on health inequalities? Are we, in fact, succeeding at narrowing health gaps between groups in this country? The answers to these questions are complex. I attempt to shed some light on them here with a number of

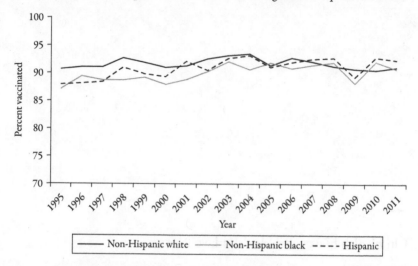

FIGURE 24.1 Estimated measles, mumps, and rubella (≥1 doses) vaccination coverage for children aged 19–35 months, National Immunization Survey, 1995–2011. Estimated measles, mumps, and rubella (≥1 doses) vaccination coverage for children aged 19–35 months, National Immunization Survey, 1995–2011. Created from table 1 of Walker AT, Smith PJ, Kolasa M. Reduction of Racial/Ethnic Disparities in Vaccination Coverage, 1995–2011. *Morbidity and Mortality Weekly Report* (*MMWR*). 2014; 63(01): 7–12 [7].

specific examples, restricting my comments to the United States to narrow the scope of the conversation, although much of this could well be extended to other countries.

On some levels, particularly process indicators, we are indeed doing well. This is particularly true in the case of access to preventive care among racial minorities, where disparities seem to be narrowing. Figure 24.1 shows data from a Centers for Disease Control and Prevention (CDC) report that compares, across racial groups, the proportion of children vaccinated for measles, mumps, and rubella [7]. Over time, there is a clear narrowing of the gap between white, black, and Hispanic children.

Another way of measuring preventive care is by examining the proportion of adults who report having no usual source of health care. This proportion has also narrowed over time across racial groups (Figure 24.2) [8].

Another encouraging development is the public's growing awareness of the existence of health disparities. According to a 1999 national survey, 55 percent of American adults said that they knew blacks and Latinos had poorer health outcomes than whites. That number increased in 2010 to 59 percent [9]. Although this represents only a modest increase, it is encouraging to observe this growing acknowledgment of the unfairness that exists in our society, even as we launch more policies and programs to try to narrow these health gaps.

But how are we doing on health indicators? In some respects, the news is less heartening here. The final *Healthy People 2010* review, which reported on health disparities for 469 population-based health objectives, showed that although there was some improvement, disparities have either increased or remained the same since baseline measures for the majority of objectives, particularly between racial and ethnic groups [10].

There is also that most basic measure of health disparities—life expectancy. Here, there is cause for both optimism and frustration. From 2003 to 2013, there was an increase in life

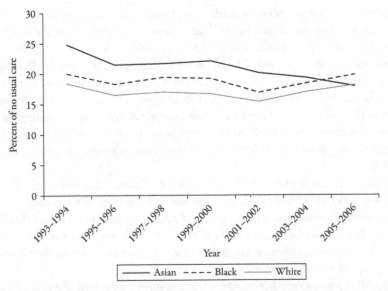

FIGURE 24.2 Percent of adults age 18–64 with no usual source of health care, 1993–2006. Created from table 78 of National Center for Health Statistics. Health, United States, 2007 With Chartbook on Trends in the Health of Americans. Hyattsville, MD; 2007 [8].

expectancy for all race/gender groups, and the gap between the white and black groups decreased slightly across years (Figure 24.3) [11, 12]. However, between blacks and non-Hispanic whites, there is still an astonishing 4.7-year difference among men and a 3.1-year difference among women [11, 12].

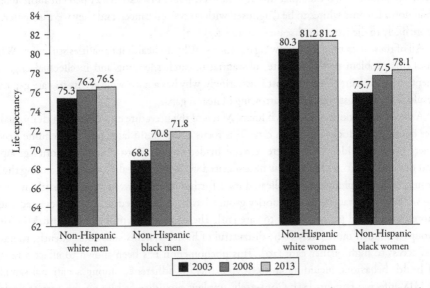

FIGURE 24.3 Life expectancy at birth in the US by race/ethnicity, 2003 and 2008. Harper S, Rushani D, Kaufman JS. Trends in the black-white life expectancy gap, 2003–2008. *JAMA: The Journal of the American Medical Association.* 2012; 307 (21): 2257–2259; and Deaths: Final data for 2013. National Vital Statistics Reports. Available at: http://www.cdc.gov/nchs/data_access/Vitalstatsonline.htm Accessed April 22, 2015 [11, 12].

Examining the top five causes of death in the United States, it can be seen that, in 2010, blacks had a higher rate of all types of death compared to whites, with the exception of chronic lower respiratory diseases and accidents [13] (Table 24.1).

Death rates, however, are only "the tip of the iceberg" when it comes to US health disparities. Examining prevalence over time, it can be seen that disparities persist across a broad range of health indicators. A clear example is obesity, one of the most common chronic conditions in the United States. Figure 24.4 shows the prevalence of obesity among black and white women from 1976 to 2004. At every time point, black women have a higher level of obesity, and the gap remains wide throughout time, even increasing for the period 2001 to 2004 [8].

Another increasingly prevalent chronic condition, diabetes, also well reflects racial and ethnic disparities in the United States. Time and again, it is racial minorities who shoulder the heaviest burden of disease. From 2010 to 2012, Hispanics, non-Hispanic blacks, and American Indians/Alaska Natives saw the highest proportions of adults with diagnosed diabetes, with the prevalence among American Indians/Alaskan Natives more than double that of non-Hispanic whites (Figure 24.5) [14].

HIV/AIDS provides another example of the disproportionate level of disease often experienced by minority populations. In this case, one minority, in particular, bears this burden more than most. The prevalence of HIV is greater among blacks than among all other racial/ethnic groups, with black men suffering a higher proportion of HIV infections at all disease stages [15]. Figure 24.6 shows estimated HIV infection rates using the CDC's national HIV surveillance system; one can see that in both 2005 and 2008, blacks had the highest rate and largest relative difference between groups [16].

The disparity between blacks and whites in terms of colorectal cancer incidence and deaths provides a final example. In 2008, non-Hispanic blacks were 23 percent more likely than non-Hispanic whites to be diagnosed with colorectal cancer, and they were 46 percent more likely to die from the disease (Figure 24.7) [17].

All of these data raise the following questions: Why do health inequalities still exist? Why does this problem persist, despite substantial research spending and intellectual engagement with this issue? Perhaps most frustratingly, why has a narrowing access-to-care gap not resulted in an across-the-board narrowing of health gaps?

A word, first, about our research focus. Much of the literature examining health inequalities continues to focus on health *care*. This focus is driven, in large part, by genuine need. There is ample evidence that there remains inadequate access to care for minority groups, and that limited access to care may be associated with poorer health indicators among these groups [18]. The picture is complicated even further by the current state of health literacy. Lower health literacy among minority groups has been observed, and it is associated with more limited, and poorer, access to care [19]. There is also the problem of trust. Minority groups are much more likely to be distrustful of health systems and, consequently, to have less access to high-quality care [20]. This phenomenon has been shown to affect a range of health behaviors, including antiretroviral therapy adherence among a national sample of HIV-infected patients [21]. Conversely, implicit prejudice or bias on the part of health care providers reinforces mistrust, placing yet another barrier between minority patients and the care they need [20]. Language can be an additional barrier. Indeed, people living in

TABLE 24.1

Percentage of Total Death, Death, Rates, and Age-Adjusted Death Rates for 2010, Percentage Change in Age-Adjusted Death Rates in 2010 from 2009, and Ratio of Age-Adjusted Death Rates by Race and Sex for the Five Leading Causes of Death for the Total Population in 2010: United States

Rank[a]	Cause of Death	No.	Percent of Total Deaths	2010 Crude Death Rate	Age-Adjusted Death Rate		Ratio	
					2010	Percent Change 2009 to 2010	Male to Female	Black[b] to White
	All causes	2,468,435	100.0	799.5	747.0	−0.3	1.4	1.2
1	Diseases of heart	597,689	24.2	193.6	179.1	−2.0	1.6	1.3
2	Malignant neoplasms	574,743	23.2	186.2	172.8	−0.4	1.4	1.2
3	Chronic lower respiratory diseases	138,080	5.6	44.7	42.2	−1.2	1.3	0.7
4	Cerebrovascular diseases	129,476	5.2	41.9	39.1	−1.3	1.0	1.4
5	Accidents (unintentional injuries)	120,859	4.9	39.1	38.0	1.3	2.0	0.8

[a]Rank based on number of deaths.

[b]Multiple-race data were reported by 37 states and the District of Columbia in 2010.

Source: Murphy et al. [13].

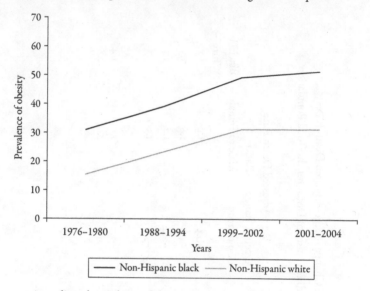

FIGURE 24.4 Age-adjusted prevalence of obesity among females age 20–74, 1976–2004. Created from table 74 of National Center for Health Statistics. Health, United States, 2007 With Chartbook on Trends in the Health of Americans. Hyattsville, MD; 2007 [8].

households in which the primary language is not English increase their risk of being unin-sured by at least twofold [22].

But there is another, more fundamental reason for health inequality in the United States—one that is linked to the deep and persistent economic inequalities that exist between groups.

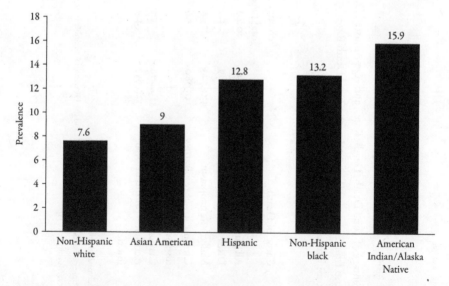

FIGURE 24.5 Age-adjusted prevalence of diagnosed diabetes among people 20 years old or older by race/ethnicity, 2010–2012. Centers for Disease Control and Prevention. National diabetes statistics report: Estimates of diabetes and its burden in the United States, 2014. Atlanta, GA: US Department of Health and Human Services; 2014 [14].

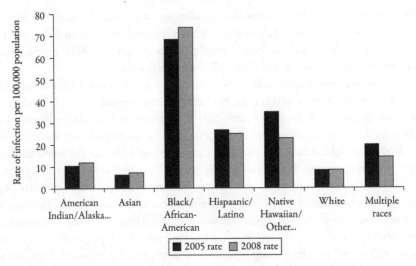

FIGURE 24.6 Estimated rate of HIV infection diagnoses among persons aged ≥13 years—CDC's national HIV surveillance system, 37 states, 2005 and 2008. Created from Table 1 of Hall HI, Hughes D, Dean HD, Mermin JH, Fenton KA. HIV Infection—United States, 2005 and 2008. Morbidity and Mortality Weekly Report (MMWR) [16].

In this country, adults living at or below the federal poverty level are more than five times more likely to say they are in poor or fair health [23]. The impact of economic disparities on health inequalities is pervasive, affecting access to opportunities—such as education—which, in turn, shape lifetime prospects for health. This deprivation extends not only to

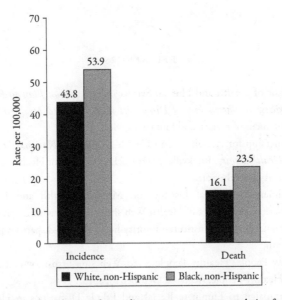

FIGURE 24.7 Age-adjusted incidence and mortality rates per 100,000 population from colorectal cancer by race/ethnicity, 2008. Steele CB, Rim SH, Joseph DA, King JB, Seeff LC. Colorectal cancer incidence and screening—United States, 2008 and 2010. Morbidity and Mortality Weekly Report (MMWR). 2013; 62(03): 53–60 [17].

differences between racial groups but also to differences within racial groups. For example, black women are much more likely to have a sexually transmitted infection if they also have a lower education status [24]. Without addressing the deeper problem of economic inequality, we cannot hope to narrow, and ultimately close, health gaps.

Widening our lens, it is possible to see what is perhaps the most critical determinant of all in the production of health gaps: the interplay of economic and social inequalities that create the conditions for poor health. Indeed, economic and social inequalities extend far beyond the "simple" remit of income as a means of acquiring salutary resources. They include the manifold, subtle, and pervasive challenges embedded in the wildly divergent geographic circumstances that characterize living conditions for different groups throughout the country. It is, at core, a matter of context. For example, low-income minority neighborhoods have more fast-food outlets, fewer grocery stores and recreational facilities, and are closer to sources of industrial pollution compared with more economically advantaged white neighborhoods [23]. At an even more complicated level, persistent interpersonal discrimination and structural marginalization of entire racial groups—perhaps brought most cruelly and nakedly to light in recent police shootings of unarmed black men—likely structure our entire range of social, economic, and health interactions [25]. This creates a near-insurmountable barrier to health equality that will require an honest and unstinting focus on the *conditions* that make us healthy, if we are to appropriately promote the health of all populations and narrow inequalities in health between groups in the United States. Is it possible to narrow health gaps without addressing these conditions? There is substantial theoretical and empiric argument to be made that it is not [26]. Going forward, then, the role of public health is clear: to address the social, economic, and environmental causes of health, not only to improve the overall well-being of populations but also as a means of narrowing the health divides that have created, tragically, a nation of "health haves and health have-nots."

REFERENCES

1. US Department of Health and Human Services. *HHS Action Plan to Reduce Racial and Ethnic Disparities: A Nation Free of Disparities in Health and Health Care.* Washington, DC: US Department of Health and Human Services; 2011.

2. National Partnership for Action to End Health Disparities. *National Stakeholder Strategy for Achieving Health Equity.* Rockville, MD: US Department of Health & Human Services, Office of Minority Health; 2011.

3. The NIH Almanac: National Institute on Minority Health and Health Disparities (NIMHD). National Institutes of Health Web site. https://www.nih.gov/about-nih/what-we-do/nih-almanac/national-institute-minority-health-health-disparities-nimhd. Accessed October 29, 2016.

4. About Healthy People. Healthy People 2020 Web site. https://www.healthypeople.gov/2020/About-Healthy-People. Accessed October 29, 2016.

5. California Campaign to Eliminate Racial and Ethnic Disparities in Health. Prevention Institute Web site. https://www.preventioninstitute.org/projects/california-campaign-eliminate-racial-and-ethnic-disparities-health. Accessed October 29, 2016.

6. About Health Centers. Bureau of Primary Health Care—HRSA Web site. http://bphc.hrsa.gov/about/index.html. Accessed October 29, 2016.

7. Walker AT, Smith PJ, Kolasa M. Reduction of racial/ethnic disparities in vaccination coverage, 1995–2011. *Morbidity and Mortality Weekly Report (MMWR)*. 2014; 63(1): 7–12.

8. National Center for Health Statistics. *Health, United States, 2007 with Chartbook on Trends in the Health of Americans*. Hyattsville, MD; 2007.

9. Benz JK, Espinosa O, Welsh V, Fontes A. Awareness of racial and ethnic health disparities has improved only modestly over a decade. *Health Affairs*. 2011; 30(10): 1860–867. doi:10.1377/hlthaff.2010.0702

10. National Center for Health Statistics. *Healthy People 2010 Final Review*. Hyattsville, MD: Author; 2012.

11. Harper S, Rushani D, Kaufman JS. Trends in the black–white life expectancy gap, 2003–2008. *JAMA: The Journal of the American Medical Association*. 2012; 307(21): 2257–9.

12. Deaths: Final Data for 2013; National Vital Statistics Reports. Centers for Disease Control and Prevention Web site. http://www.cdc.gov/nchs/data_access/Vitalstatsonline.htm. Accessed April 22, 2015.

13. Murphy SL, Xu J, Kochanek DK. Deaths: Final data for 2010. *National Vital Statistics Reports*. 2013; 61(4).

14. Centers for Disease Control and Prevention. *National Diabetes Statistics Report: Estimates of Diabetes and Its Burden in the United States, 2014*. Atlanta, GA: US Department of Health and Human Services; 2014.

15. Herbst JH, Painter TM, Tomlinson HL, Alvarez ME. Evidence-based HIV/STD prevention intervention for black men who have sex with men. *Morbidity and Mortality Weekly Report (MMWR)*. 2014; 63(1): 21–7.

16. Hall HI, Hughes D, Dean HD, Mermin JH, Fenton KA. HIV Infection—United States, 2005 and 2008. *Morbidity and Mortality Weekly Report (MMWR)*. 2011: 60(1); 87–9.

17. Steele CB, Rim SH, Joseph DA, King JB, Seeff LC. Colorectal cancer incidence and screening—United States, 2008 and 2010. *Morbidity and Mortality Weekly Report (MMWR)*. 2013; 62(3): 53–60.

18. Cunningham PJ, Hibbard J, Gibbons CB. Raising low "patient activation" rates among Hispanic immigrants may equal expanded coverage in reducing access disparities. *Health Affairs*. 2011; 30(10): 1888–94. doi:10.1377/hlthaff.2009.0805

19. Osborn CY, Paasche-Orlow MK, Davis TC, Wolf MS. Health literacy: An overlooked factor in understanding HIV health disparities. *American Journal of Preventive Medicine*. 2007; 33(5): 374–78.

20. Institute of Medicine. *Unequal Treatment: Confronting Racial and Ethnic Disparities in Health Care* (full printed version). Washington, DC: The National Academies Press; 2003.

21. Thrasher AD, Earp JA, Golin CE, Zimmer CR. Discrimination, distrust, and racial/ethnic disparities in antiretroviral therapy adherence among a national sample of HIV-infected patients. *Journal of Acquired Immune Deficiency Syndromes*. 2008; 49(1): 84–93. doi:10.1097/QAI.0b013e3181845589

22. Disparities in Health Care Quality Among Racial and Ethnic Minority Groups: Findings from the National Healthcare Quality and Disparities Reports, 2008. Agency for Healthcare Research and Quality Web site. https://archive.ahrq.gov/research/findings/nhqrdr/nhqrdr08/minority.html. Accessed October 29, 2016.

23. Health Policy Brief: Achieving equity in health. *Health Affairs.* 2011.

24. Annang L, Walsemann KM, Maitra D, Kerr JC. Does education matter? Examining racial differences in the association between education and STI diagnosis among black and white young adult females in the US. *Public Health Reports.* 2010; 125(Suppl 4): 110–121.

25. Schmidt MS, Apuzzo M. South Carolina officer is charged with murder of Walter Scott. *The New York Times.* April 7, 2015. http://www.nytimes.com/2015/04/08/us/south-carolina-officer-is-charged-with-murder-in-black-mans-death.html. Accessed October 29, 2016.

26. Phelan JC, Link BG, Diez-Roux A, Kawachi I, Levin B. "Fundamental causes" of social inequalities in mortality: A test of the theory. *Journal of Health and Social Behavior.* 2004; 45(3): 265–85.

25

Income and Health

IN THE SUMMER of 2015, the release of the US Census report on household income and poverty was an acute reminder of how income and poverty shape all our social structures [1]. That report clearly demonstrated that incomes were rising for many Americans in the middle of the income distribution and that the income gaps between the richest and the poorest quintiles, already dramatic, have continued to widen.

These findings have direct implications for population health, as economic conditions always do. Indeed, income is related to health on all axes, and it has been since time immemorial. William Farr, for example, found in his 1841 study of mortality in English asylums that death rates were higher among poor patients [2, 3]. Jumping to more recent circumstances, a 2016 UNICEF report found that, globally, children born into the poorest 20 percent of households are nearly twice as likely to die before reaching the age of 5 years than children born into the wealthiest 20 percent [4].

The foundational drivers of health, particularly forces that shape social divides, are inextricably linked to our understanding of health divides, and income is no exception. Previous chapters covered the depth of these health gaps; gaps in income—driving, as they do, disparities in health—are no less pronounced. In 2014, for example, the US Census Bureau reported the median household income as $53,657 [5]. However, that median was not the same for all populations. For Asians, the median household income was $74,297; for white non-Hispanics, it was $60,256; for Hispanics, it was $42,491; and for blacks, it was $35,398 [1]. These differences have proven to be stubbornly persistent [6]. With the exception of non-Hispanic white households, whose median income declined by 1.7 percent between 2013 and 2014, changes in income among racial groups during this same period were not statistically significant [7].

An examination of income in the United States also makes plain the existence of gender divides. The Census Bureau reported a gap between median yearly income for women and men, with women earning $39,621 in 2014 and men earning $50,383 [1]. This difference was reinforced by the female-to-male earnings ratio for that year: 0.79 [1]. The gender wage gap ties in with the larger picture of gender inequity, itself an enormously consequential determinant of well-being.

When we discuss income, it is key to note that we are also discussing wealth. Wealth, in many ways, compounds the effects of income, although it is important to distinguish between the two. Definitionally, income is simply a flow of money that is received by groups or individuals [8]. Wealth, on the other hand, is a stock of resources that people may draw on to support their livelihoods or, in the case of debt (i.e., negative wealth), use to pay down an expense, reducing the proportion of income that can be used for goods and services [9]. At a fundamental level, income delineates haves and have-nots in the United States, but its influence runs even deeper. This becomes apparent when we consider wealth and, specifically, wealth gaps—which are staggering. In *Trends in Family Wealth, 1989 to 2013*, the US Congressional Budget Office found the aggregate family wealth in this country to be $67 trillion in 2013, more than double the amount of family wealth in 1989 [10]. However, this growing increase has not been shared by all families equally. In 2013, 76 percent of all family wealth was held by families in the top 10 percent of the wealth distribution [10]. Furthermore, intergenerational transmission of wealth has led to large, persistent disparities between groups. In many respects, these disparities are a consequence of our country's history (of slavery, union busting, etc.), which now makes its mark on the present in the form of health gaps.

How, then, does income affect health? Given the ubiquity of income's influence, it might be simpler to ask how does it not. From the neighborhood we can afford to live in to the food we can afford to eat and to our opportunities for social and educational advancement, our income shapes our circumstances and the opportunities to which we have access. Income also, crucially, determines the quality of health care we can afford and the treatment possibilities available to us in the event of illness [11]. These factors all contribute to overall well-being, shaping health by shaping context. Low-income neighborhoods, for example, can be more polluted, more dangerous, and less food-secure than more affluent communities, with attendant health effects [12, 13, 14].

Like the air we breathe, the water we drink, and the political system under which we live, the very ubiquity of income's influence can make it easy to take for granted or even ignore. However, it is this very ubiquity that agitates for keeping a concern for the link between income and health at the center of our efforts. The key is a focus on scholarship that aims to understand the role of income, how best to mitigate the consequences of low income, and how to redistribute income *if* such redistribution can be shown to improve population health. For example, how will minimum wage regulations influence population health? Transfers such as the Earned Income Tax Credit (EITC)? Which educational interventions can most effectively break the cycle of poverty? How can we leverage affordable housing toward creating income-heterogeneous, urban neighborhoods? As we work to answer these questions, we must also play an active role in advocacy, striving to keep health at the center of the continuing conversation about income inequality. This means shifting the focus of the debate from the concentration of wealth at the top of the economic ladder to the conditions of poverty at the bottom [15].

I have increasingly come to believe that one of the hidden/unspoken challenges to our society—and one that is central to public health—is the circumstances of the bottom

50 percent of the population, who have no passports, abysmal incomes, and equally abysmal health indicators. These concerns are, in a larger sense, very much in keeping with the broader focus of public health. Modern public health has long been preoccupied with the poor and the social, environmental, and economic conditions that shape the lives of the less advantaged. In many respects, modern public health emerged in the mid-19th century as a direct consequence of the Industrial Revolution and the effect this changing world had on the lives and health of the poor [16]. As economies mechanized, widespread urbanization meant that the working classes often lived in close, unsanitary quarters, leading to the spread of infectious diseases such as cholera and tuberculosis [17]. To mitigate this problem in England, reformers passed the Public Health Act of 1848, which provided a framework for better sanitation and water quality, and established a Board of Health [18]. These measures, a public good benefitting all, were centrally motivated by the plight of the poor. Edwin Chadwick, one of the key architects of the Act, argued that if the poor were healthier, they would be less likely to seek government relief, saving money in the long term [19]. The circumstances surrounding the passage of the Act are one of the first examples of how the conditions of poverty, fueled by prevailing economic trends, can drive population health and the broader public health agenda. This same impulse should inform our present-day efforts.

How does our focus on poverty relate to our broader consideration of income inequality? Although there has been much discussion about inequality in recent years, the conversation has tended to focus more on the excesses of the rich and the decline of the middle class than it has on the poverty rate in this country—a rate that remains stubbornly high [15, 20, 21, 22, 23]. But our picture of the link between income and health would be incomplete without taking into account the many ways that poverty undermines the health of populations. Indeed, there is little doubt that poverty is inextricably linked to health. During the past 15 years, life expectancy in the United States has increased for middle- and upper-income Americans. However, top earners have gained relatively little ground against the median. This suggests that wealth, for all its benefits, makes little difference in improving health past a certain basic threshold of well-being. In sharp contrast, low-income Americans have seen little or no life expectancy increase, lagging ever further behind the rest of the population [24].

Another motive for public health's focus on the poor is that (in addition to the causal link between poverty and health) they are the most likely to face health expenditures that reduce their ability to meet life's other needs. These necessaries can include school fees, food, rent, or heat. The epidemic of medical bankruptcy in the United States is a salient indicator of this challenge [25]. Our society's failure to create a health system that protects people from disease-related financial ruin contributes to the vicious cycle of poverty and poor health in this country and represents an area in which public health should, consistent with its values, take the lead in creating change.

Next, I provide a few words on the scope of the problem of US poverty. The federal government's 2014 poverty guideline for a four-person household in the 48 contiguous states and the District of Columbia was an income of $23,850 per year [26]. According to the US Census Bureau, there were 46.7 million Americans living in poverty in 2014 [1]. This figure, representing 14.8 percent of the population, has remained fairly consistent in recent years. In fact, 2014 represented the fourth consecutive year of the national poverty rate remaining statistically the same [1]. In addition, these data made it clear just how many people poverty touches, even if it is only for a short time. Between 2009 and 2012, 34.5 percent of the population had at least one period of poverty lasting 2 or more months.

Perhaps the key takeaway from these data is that vast numbers of Americans live in an entirely different world than those at the top of the income ladder. Alarming as this difference is in purely economic terms, the startling racial gaps that exist within the overall poverty rate are, in their way, just as distressing as the widening gulf between the very rich and the very poor. Again, the numbers tell the tale. Among non-Hispanic whites, the poverty rate in 2014 was 10.1 percent (19.7 million people) [27]. Asians had a poverty rate of 12 percent (2.1 million people), Hispanics had a rate of 23.6 percent (13.1 million people), and black Americans had a rate of 26.2 percent (10.8 million people) [1]. These gaps are indicative of deeply entrenched, structural disparities that persist in this country, independent of macroeconomic trends. They are in many ways symptomatic of the foundational social, economic, and cultural forces—such as racism, mass incarceration, and the absence of affordable housing—that have allowed poverty to thrive on a grand scale in the wealthiest nation on earth [28].

But the effects of poverty, perhaps paradoxically, run far deeper than merely not meeting a certain financial benchmark. Although the rather narrow federal definition of poverty itself rests on a remarkably low income for a family of four, that figure barely begins to capture the true scope of this problem. To be poor is to be the victim of a complex interplay of harmful factors, with lack of income being just one of many. In their report *Five Evils: Multidimensional Poverty and Race in America*, Richard Reeves, Edward Rodrigue, and Elizabeth Kneebone identify five principal areas of vulnerability faced by people living in poverty: low income, lack of education, no health insurance, living in a poor area, and unemployment [29]. Nearly half of the adult population classified as poor suffers from at least one of these disadvantages, whereas 23 percent suffers from two or more, 9 percent suffers from at least three, and 2 percent suffers from at least four [29]. Racial disparities are, once again, troublingly apparent. Multidimensional poverty affects blacks and Hispanics far more than it does whites, with more than 3 million black and 5 million Hispanic adults experiencing a minimum of three disadvantages [29]. This combination of disadvantage likewise varies according to race, with some groups more likely to suffer from combined low income, lack of education, and health insurance, whereas others have a higher chance of experiencing, for example, the triple threat of low income, lack of health insurance, and unemployment [29]. Taken together, these disadvantages reflect a poverty not merely of income but also of opportunity, stability, hope, and health.

For these reasons, a concern for the conditions of poverty must remain at the heart of public health. It falls to us to make it clear that present-day poverty and the unfairness embedded therein are consequences of foundational inequalities that have long bedeviled our society, favoring certain racial groups over others even as the country overall remains a land of plenty. The role of public health, then, is to make poverty unignorable, through our scholarship and our advocacy, as we work to address the social, economic, and environmental conditions that allow the conditions of poverty—and attendant poor health—to persist.

REFERENCES

1. DeNavas-Walt C, Proctor BD. *Income and Poverty in the United States: 2014, Current Population Reports.* Washington, DC: US Census Bureau; 2015.

2. William Farr (1807–83). Science Museum, London Web site. http://www.sciencemuseum.org.uk/broughttolife/people/williamfarr. Accessed November 29, 2016.

3. Singer RB. The first mortality follow-up study: The 1841 report of William Farr (physician) on the mortality of lunatics. *Journal of Insurance Medicine.* 2001; 33(4): 298–309.

4. United Nations Children's Fund (UNICEF). *The State of the World's Children 2016: A Fair Chance for Every Child.* New York, NY: Author; 2016.

5. White GB. America's poverty problem hasn't changed. *The Atlantic.* September 16, 2015. http://www.theatlantic.com/business/archive/2015/09/americas-poverty-problem/405700. Accessed November 29, 2016.

6. Wilson V. New Census Data Show No Progress in Closing Stubborn Racial Income Gaps. Economic Policy Institute Web site. http://www.epi.org/blog/new-census-data-show-no-progress-in-closing-stubborn-racial-income-gaps. Published September 16, 2015. Accessed November 29, 2016.

7. Income, Poverty and Health Insurance Coverage in the United States: 2014. United States Census Bureau Web site. https://www.census.gov/newsroom/press-releases/2015/cb15-157.html. Published September 16, 2015. Accessed November 29, 2016.

8. Income (definition). Dictionary.com Web site. http://www.dictionary.com/browse/income. Accessed November 29, 2016.

9. Wealth (definition). Dictionary.com Web site. http://www.dictionary.com/browse/wealth?s=t. Accessed November 29, 2016.

10. Congress of the United States Congressional Budget Office. *Trends in Family Wealth, 1989 to 2013.* https://www.cbo.gov/publication/51846. Published August 18, 2016. Accessed November 29, 2016.

11. Schoen C, et al. *Health Care in the Two Americas: Findings from the Scorecard on State Health System Performance for Low-Income Populations, 2013.* New York, NY: The Commonwealth Fund; 2013.

12. Katz C. People in poor neighborhoods breathe more hazardous particles. *Scientific American.* November 1, 2012. https://www.scientificamerican.com/article/people-poor-neighborhoods-breate-more-hazardous-particles. Accessed November 29, 2016.

13. Pedestrian deaths in poorer neighborhoods report. *Governing.* http://www.governing.com/gov-data/pedestrian-deaths-poor-neighborhoods-report.html. Accessed November 29, 2016.

14. Food Deserts. Food Empowerment Project Web site. http://www.foodispower.org/food-deserts. Accessed November 29, 2016.

15. Appelbaum B. The millions of Americans Donald Trump and Hillary Clinton barely mention: The poor. *The New York Times.* August 11, 2016. http://www.nytimes.com/2016/08/12/us/politics/trump-clinton-poverty.html?_r=1&mtrref=undefined. Accessed November 30, 2016.

16. Effects of the Industrial Revolution. World History Textbook Web site. http://webs.bcp.org/sites/vcleary/ModernWorldHistoryTextbook/IndustrialRevolution/IREffects.html. Accessed November 30, 2016.

17. Trueman CN. Diseases in Industrial Cities in the Industrial Revolution. The History Learning Web site. http://www.historylearningsite.co.uk/britain-1700-to-1900/industrial-revolution/diseases-in-industrial-cities-in-the-industrial-revolution. Accessed November 30, 2016.

18. The 1848 Public Health Act. UK Parliament Web site. http://www.parliament.uk/about/living-heritage/transformingsociety/towncountry/towns/tyne-and-wear-case-study/about-the-group/public-administration/the-1848-public-health-act. Accessed November 30, 2016.

19. Edwin Chadwick (1800–90). Science Museum, London Web site. http://www.sciencemuseum.org.uk/broughttolife/people/edwinchadwick. Accessed November 30, 2016.

20. Guo J. Income inequality today may be higher today than in any other era. *The Washington Post.* https://www.washingtonpost.com/news/wonk/wp/2016/07/01/income-inequality-today-may-be-the-highest-since-the-nations-founding/?utm_term=.60c11244ec42. Accessed November 30, 2016.

21. The Atlantic Editors. 17 things we learned about income inequality in 2014. *The Atlantic.* December 23, 2014. http://www.theatlantic.com/business/archive/2014/12/17-things-we-learned-about-income-inequality-in-2014/383917. Accessed November 30, 2016.

22. Crash course. *The Economist.* September 7, 2013. http://www.economist.com/news/schoolsbrief/21584534-effects-financial-crisis-are-still-being-felt-five-years-article. Accessed November 30, 2016.

23. Fletcher MA. Income inequality has squeezed the middle class out of the majority. *The Washington Post.* December 9, 2015. https://www.washingtonpost.com/news/wonk/wp/2015/12/09/income-inequality-has-squeezed-the-middle-class-out-of-the-majority/?utm_term=.e85095e65b38. Accessed November 30, 2016.

24. National Academies of Sciences, Engineering, and Medicine. *The Growing Gap in Life Expectancy by Income: Implications for Federal Programs and Policy Responses.* Washington, DC: The National Academies Press; 2015.

25. Banegas MP, et al. For working-age cancer survivors, medical debt and bankruptcy create financial hardships. *Health Affairs.* 2016; 35(1): 54–61. doi:10.1377/hlthaff.2015.0830

26. 2014 Poverty Guidelines. Office of the Assistant Secretary for Planning and Evaluation Web site. https://aspe.hhs.gov/2014-poverty-guidelines. Published December 1, 2014. Accessed November 30, 2016.

27. New Census Report on Income and Poverty in the United States. National Low Income Housing Coalition Web site. http://nlihc.org/article/new-census-report-income-and-poverty-united-states. Published September 21, 2015. Accessed November 30, 2016.

28. Sherman E. America is the richest, and most unequal, country. *Fortune.* September 30, 2015. http://fortune.com/2015/09/30/america-wealth-inequality. Accessed November 30, 2016.

29. Reeves R, Rodrigue E, Kneebone E. *Five Evils: Multidimensional Poverty and Race in America.* Washington DC: Brookings Institution; 2016.

26

What Flint Teaches Us

EARLY 2016 SAW a torrent of articles written about the drinking water of Flint, Michigan. The root of the problem was the corrosion of water pipes, representative of an aging city infrastructure, which resulted in the contamination of the city's water supply [1]. This contamination was the product of a range of pathogens, notably lead [1]. The health danger was so great that former President Obama met with the mayor of Flint during a visit to Michigan and declared a state of emergency in the city [2].

The problem seems to have originated in 2011, when Flint, along with many other cities in the area, needed to cut costs in the face of a financial emergency. One solution was to stop paying the Detroit Water and Sewerage Department for water from Lake Huron and use a different supply line instead. Because this transition could not be made immediately, Flint started, as a temporary measure, to source water from the Flint River in April 2014. Soon after, residents began complaining about the taste, smell, and appearance of the water, and they voiced health concerns about problems such as skin rashes.

Despite growing public protests about the water problem, it was not until January 2015 that Flint sought an independent review of the water supply [3]. This review was prompted by concerns about high levels of trihalomethanes, a byproduct of disinfecting efforts [3]. By this time, protestors had started to bring samples of dirty and discolored water from their faucets to public meetings. The US Environmental Protection Agency (EPA) was engaged after protests by LeeAnne Walters, a mother of four, who persistently complained about the effects of the water on the health of her children [4]. Eventually, the water at her home was tested and found to contain alarmingly high levels of lead. Despite these findings, city officials continued to insist that the water supply was safe and that the problems in Walters' home may have been the result of plumbing issues. Dissatisfied with the response, Walters contacted the EPA.

Eventually, a research team led by Marc Edwards of Virginia Tech conducted a study of the water conditions in Flint. Edwards' report found that the Flint River water contained eight times the amount of chlorine as Lake Huron water and was highly corrosive [5]. This caused pipe corrosion, with dangerous levels of lead leaching into the water supply. While this was being established, research was being conducted on the health effects of this problem. Mona Hanna-Attisha, from the Hurley Children's Hospital in Flint, called attention to a significant increase in the blood lead levels of children and demonstrated that this increase in lead levels followed the change in the water supply source [1]. Lead is a potent neurotoxin, and lead toxicity can lead to developmental delay in children, as well as many other health challenges, including mood disorders, memory impairment, and miscarriages [6].

Flint would later reconnect to Detroit's water supply. In December 2015, the director of the Department of Environmental Quality resigned soon after the City of Flint declared an emergency. Following revelations that elected and appointed officials tried repeatedly to avoid dealing with the water issue, Michigan Governor Rick Snyder issued a very public apology, promising to fix the problem [7, 8].

A *New York Times* editorial about the Flint crisis expressed the view that "no Americans should have to live with poisoned water that is a direct result of the government's decisions and neglect" [9]. That in some ways is an important reiteration of resolution 64/292 passed by the United Nations General Assembly on July 28, 2010, which recognized that clean drinking water and sanitation are essential to the realization of all human rights [10]. This suggests that there is a consensus regarding what happened in Flint—namely that it should never have occurred. It certainly should never have occurred in the United States. And yet it did. Why did it happen, and what can the Flint events teach us about the role of public health in preventing similar catastrophes in the future?

First, it is important to note the wide range of factors that contributed to the problem during a period of almost two decades. Indeed, the core etiology of the Flint crisis dates back 18 years. Efforts were made to cut costs with the hope that these measures would not affect the health of the public. The Michigan Department of Environmental Quality never enforced the installation of corrosion control systems in accordance with the Federal Lead and Copper Rule of 1998 [11]. These actions set the stage for severe corrosion in the water pipes, which was then accelerated by the 2014 change in the water supply. Saving money again took precedence over safeguarding health, when a subsequent offer to revert to the original water supply from Detroit was rejected in January 2015 due to cost concerns. This happened despite the growing drumbeat of concerns about water quality in Flint.

This is not to suggest that cost-cutting measures are innately negative or anti-public health. Elected and appointed officials are charged with balancing budgets and with the responsible use of public resources in the face of multiple competing demands. However, it is clear that much of the trouble in Flint arose from the idea that short-term cost-saving measures can be applied to vital public health infrastructure without consequence. Historical examples have shown just how wrong this belief can be. For example, some years ago, my colleagues and I published an analysis of how the 1975 New York fiscal crisis affected the tuberculosis, HIV, and homicide epidemics in New York City [12]. We found that cuts to public infrastructure, and the diminution of public health resources, contributed to the amplification of these health challenges [12]. We also estimated that $10 billion in cuts to services were followed by costs exceeding $50 billion to then control the epidemics. This is not counting, of course, the human costs of these events. These numbers further highlight the folly of short-term cost-cutting that threatens public health.

A second notable feature of the tragedy in Flint is how preventable it was. As the story of the crisis developed, it became clear that there was, at several steps along the way, ample opportunity to reverse course, as locals raised the alarm about water quality in the city. These concerns were ignored, despite the fact that some of them were likely actionable. For example, the findings of Edwards and Hanna-Attisha were refuted and ignored until October 2015, when the US Department of Health and Human Services urged residents to stop drinking the water. This represents in many ways a failure of responsive governance. In hindsight, it is fairly obvious that elected and appointed officials in Flint considered public concerns to be, at best, a public relations problem and, at worst, something that could be ignored altogether. The consequences of this negligence speaks to the role of governance as a determinant of the health of populations [13]. This suggests we must view promoting good governance as central to our mission of promoting population health.

Third, the Flint crisis has laid bare the problem of racism—in this case, environmental racism—in the United States [14]. It has shown us how the concerns of a predominantly minority and marginalized community can go unheeded, with tragic results [14]. In this respect, Flint highlights yet another way that race, class, and power influence the health of the public, showing just how easy it can be for those in power to turn a deaf ear to the plight of those who are not. This reinforces both the role of power as a foundational cause of health and the responsibility of public health to remain alert to the challenges that are often faced by marginalized, frequently minority, populations [15].

Finally, the Flint issue brings to the fore the importance of values. Values inform what we do and why we find some circumstances unacceptable, even if they were formerly acceptable. They determine what we prioritize; when we prioritize saving money over potentially saving lives, for example, that is a values-driven decision. This underlines the responsibility of public health to be clear about the values that should animate public action, and it highlights the core role that the promotion of the public's health should play in discussions about the social, economic, cultural, and financial conditions that shape the cities in which we live, the air we breathe, and the water we drink.

REFERENCES

1. Hanna-Attisha M, LaChance J, Sadler RC, Champney Schnepp A. Elevated blood lead levels in children associated with the Flint drinking water crisis: A spatial analysis of risk and public health response. *American Journal of Public Health*. 2016; 106(2): 283–90. doi:10.2105/AJPH.2015.303003

2. McCaskill ND. Flint mayor meeting with Obama. *Politico*. January 19, 2016. http://www.politico.com/story/2016/01/flint-michigan-obama-water-217974. Accessed October 25, 2016.

3. Ketchum WE. People take to streets to protest Flint water quality. *MLive*. February 14, 2015. http://www.mlive.com/news/flint/index.ssf/2015/02/flint_residents_protest_citys.html. Accessed October 25, 2016.

4. Guyette C. Scary: Leaded water and one Flint family's toxic nightmare. *Deadline Detroit*. July 9, 2015. http://www.deadlinedetroit.com/articles/12697/scary_leaded_water_and_one_flint_family_s_toxic_nightmare#.WA_zvMo5h-J. Accessed October 25, 2016.

5. Edwards MA. Why is it possible that Flint River water cannot be treated to meet federal standards? *FlintWaterStudy.org.* 2015.

6. Diseases and Conditions: Lead poisoning. Mayo Clinic Web site. http://www.mayoclinic. org/diseases-conditions/lead-poisoning/basics/symptoms/con-20035487. Accessed October 25, 2016.

7. Pérez-Peña R. Michigan governor says race had no role in Flint water response. *The New York Times.* January 22, 2016. http://www.nytimes.com/2016/01/23/us/flint-water-crisis-michigan-governor-rick-snyder.html. Accessed October 25, 2016.

8. Bosman J, Smith M. Gov. Rick Snyder of Michigan apologizes in Flint water crisis. *The New York Times.* January 19, 2016. http://www.nytimes.com/2016/01/20/us/obama-set-to-meet-with-mayor-of-flint-about-water-crisis.html. Accessed October 25, 2016.

9. The New York Times Editorial Board. Fix Flint's water system, now. *The New York Times.* January 23, 2016. http://www.nytimes.com/2016/01/24/opinion/sunday/fix-flints-water-system-now.html. Accessed October 25, 2016.

10. The Human Right to Water and Sanitation. The United Nations Web site. http://www. un.org/waterforlifedecade/human_right_to_water.shtml. Accessed October 25, 2016.

11. Grevatt PC. Lead and copper rule requirements for optimal corrosion control treatment for large drinking water systems. Memorandum to EPA Regional Water Division Directors, Regions I–X. US Environmental Protection Agency, Washington, DC, November 3, 2015. Print.

12. Freudenberg N, Fahs M, Galea S, Greenberg A. The impact of New York City's 1975 fiscal crisis on the tuberculosis, HIV, and homicide syndemic. *American Journal of Public Health.* 2006; 96(3): 424–34.

13. Putnam S, Galea S. Epidemiology and the macrosocial determinants of health. *Journal of Public Health Policy.* 2008; 29(3): 275–89. doi:10.1057/jphp.2008.15

14. Eligon J. A question of environmental racism in Flint. *The New York Times.* January 21, 2016. http://www.nytimes.com/2016/01/22/us/a-question-of-environmental-racism-in-flint. html. Accessed October 25, 2016.

15. Link BG, Northridge ME, Phelan JC, Ganz ML. Social epidemiology and the fundamental cause concept: On the structuring of effective cancer screens by socioeconomic status. *Milbank Quarterly.* 1998; 76(3): 375–402, 304–5.

27

Gender Equity, Almost

IN A BOOK co-authored with my colleague Katherine Keyes, I define population health as "the study of the conditions that shape distributions of health within and across populations, and of the mechanisms through which these conditions manifest as the health of individuals" [1]. This definition is meant to reflect a concern both with improving overall population health and also with the distribution of health within populations. Concerning ourselves with this often unequal distribution can illuminate disparities in lived experience—disparities that can translate into health gaps. A discussion of gender equity is therefore necessary and very much in keeping with this focus, examining as it does the gap between two very large, significant populations—women and men.

It is important to mention at the outset of this discussion that comparisons in overall health between women and men provide a rather inadequate snapshot of gender health inequalities. Women have lower mortality rates than men on a broad range of causes of death, and life expectancy for women is higher than it is for men worldwide [2]. Conversely, women face higher rates of disability-adjusted life years relative to men due to several particular conditions, such as depression and anxiety disorders, breast cancer, and migraine [3].

A much more enlightening view considers health *equity*. A health equity focus is concerned with health gaps that develop as a consequence of social, economic, and cultural disparities between groups. As defined by Paula Braveman and Sofia Gruskin, "equity in health is the absence of systematic disparities in health (or in the major social determinants of health) between groups with different levels of underlying social advantage/disadvantage—that is, wealth, power, or prestige" [4].

To begin, the more fundamental and proximal factors that drive these inequities are discussed. In the report *Unequal, Unfair, Ineffective and Inefficient—Gender Inequity in Health: Why It Exists and How We Can Change It*, Gita Sen and colleagues discuss the concept of gender as a "social stratifier." They note, "Girls in some contexts are fed less, educated less, and more physically restricted; and women are typically employed and segregated in lower-paid, less secure, and 'informal' occupations" [5]. This statement captures the unfortunate reality that key determinants of health, such as education and employment, are unequally and disproportionately distributed between women and men worldwide [6]. There are many examples of the persistence of the gender wage gap in different countries, and there is equally abundant evidence about the relationship between income and a range of health indicators, from mental health to physical health [7, 8].

The Millennium Development Goals Report 2015, commenting on MDG goal 3—which aims to promote gender equality and empower women—shows how far we still have to go to achieve gender equity in education [9]. Gender parity has been achieved for primary education in two-thirds of low-income countries, whereas disparities in secondary and tertiary education persist more widely. In addition, roughly half of women participate in the global labor force, compared to 76 percent of men.

Access to appropriate health services, particularly specialized reproductive care, is another driver of women's health. The fifth Millennium Development Goal (MDG 5) aimed for the reduction of the maternal mortality ratio by 75 percent between 1990 and 2015 and universal access to reproductive health care by 2015 [10]. Although a 44 percent decrease in the maternal mortality ratio was seen globally, only nine countries met the 75-percent goal. And although we have achieved overall gains toward universal reproductive health, only about half of pregnant women in developing regions have appropriate access to reproductive care. Urban versus rural disparities further demonstrate the role of economic development and health equity [9]. Much work remains to be done on maternal and reproductive health throughout the world, particularly in low-income countries. However, it is worth noting that reproductive rights remain under assault in high-income countries, including the United States.

Moving further upstream, abundant evidence shows that macrosocial policies designed to support women and gender equity (e.g., policies that provide support for working mothers) are associated with better health and greater health equity [11, 12]. These social, structural, and economic policies shape both workplace conditions and the possibility for social and economic mobility [13].

Despite their enormous positive potential, policies that level the gender playing field are sorely lacking in many countries worldwide. They are particularly, and glaringly, missing in the United States [14]. A forward-looking approach to gender equity should therefore tackle the structural drivers of gender inequities in health at the macro level to advance the core aspirations of public health.

To influence future policy and practical action on gender equity, the World Health Organization (WHO) released a report titled *Roadmap for Action, 2014–2019: Integrating Equity, Gender, Human Rights and Social Determinants into the Work of WHO* [15]. The roadmap has three main directions to guide the trajectory of this mission. It suggests the need for elevating gender-responsive action that addresses the social determinants of health, as well as the collection of data that can adequately document health gaps to the end of correcting them, and the development of approaches that advance health equity within a human rights framework. Although these directions are intended for WHO organizations, they clearly have broad institutional relevance and might serve as a rallying cry for work in this area across multiple sectors.

Note that although gender equity shapes the health of women, it also shapes the well-being of their families, social networks, and children, resulting in intergenerational effects that have far-reaching health consequences [16].

Within the academic community, we clearly have a particular responsibility to tackle health inequity of all kinds. This means producing scholarship that documents both the maldistribution of health across genders and the mechanisms that drive gender inequities. It also means pushing for curricula that keeps gender inequities at the core of what we teach. And, finally, it necessitates a relentless effort to translate our science as we make the case, strongly and repeatedly, for the central role of equity in all public health considerations.

REFERENCES

1. Keyes K, Galea S. *Population Health Science*. New York, NY: Oxford University Press; 2016.

2. Yin S. Gender disparities in health and mortality. Population Reference Bureau Web site. http://www.prb.org/Publications/Articles/2007/genderdisparities.aspx. Published November 2007. Accessed July 26, 2016.

3. Social Determinants of Health: Women and Gender Equity. World Health Organization Web site. http://www.who.int/social_determinants/themes/womenandgender/en. Accessed July 26, 2016.

4. Braveman P, Gruskin S. Defining equity in health. *Journal of Epidemiology & Community Health*. 2003; 57(4): 254–8.

5. Sen G, et al. *Unequal, unfair, ineffective and inefficient—Gender inequity in health: Why it exists and how we can change it*. Final Report to the WHO Commission on Social Determinants of Health; September 2007.

6. Link BG, Phelan J. Social conditions as fundamental causes of disease. *Journal of Health and Social Behavior*. 1995; Spec No: 80–94.

7. Platt J, Prins S, Bates L, Keyes K. Unequal depression for equal work? How the wage gap explains gendered disparities in mood disorders. *Social Science & Medicine*. 2016; 149: 1–8. doi:10.1016/j.socscimed.2015.11.056

8. World Health Organization, Commission on Social Determinants of Health. *Closing the Gap in a Generation: Health Equity Through Action on the Social Determinants of Health*. Geneva, Switzerland: Author; 2008.

9. The Millennium Development Goals Report 2015. United Nations Development Programme Web site. http://www.undp.org/content/undp/en/home/librarypage/mdg/the-millennium-development-goals-report-2015.html. Accessed July 26, 2016.

10. We Can End Poverty: Millennium Development Goals and Beyond 2015. The United Nations Web site. http://www.un.org/millenniumgoals/maternal.shtml. Accessed July 26, 2016.

11. Borrell C, et al. Influence of macrosocial policies on women's health and gender inequalities in health. *Epidemiologic Reviews*. 2014; 36: 31–48. doi:10.1093/epirev/mxt002

12. Support for Paid Sick Leave and Family Leave Policies. American Public Health Association Web site. https://www.apha.org/policies-and-advocacy/public-health-policy-statements/policy-database/2014/07/16/11/05/support-for-paid-sick-leave-and-family-leave-policies. Accessed July 26, 2016.

13. Osypuk TL, Joshi P, Geronimo K, Acevedo-Garcia D. Do social and economic policies influence health? A review. *Current Epidemiology Reports.* 2014; 1(3): 149–64.

14. Kimitch R. America lacks support for working mothers. *Los Angeles Daily News.* May 10, 2014. http://www.dailynews.com/lifestyle/20140510/america-lacks-support-for-working-mothers. Accessed July 26, 2016.

15. World Health Organization. *Roadmap for Action, 2014–2019: Integrating Equity, Gender, Human Rights and Social Determinants into the Work of WHO.* Geneva, Switzerland: Author; 2015.

16. Aizer A, Currie J. The intergenerational transmission of inequality: Maternal disadvantage and health at birth. *Science.* 2014; 344(6186): 856–61. doi:10.1126/science.1251872

28

The Well-Being of Lesbian, Gay, Bisexual,

and Transgender Populations

ON JUNE 26, 2015, the US Supreme Court ruled, in *Obergefell v. Hodges*, that the 14th Amendment requires states to issue marriage licenses to same-sex couples and that it also requires states to recognize same-sex marriages performed in other states [1]. This decision addressed what has long been one of the central demands of the lesbian, gay, bisexual, and transgender (LGBT) community and of anyone with an interest in creating a more equal, less unfair country. Although marriage equality is just one civil right for a group that has long been marginalized—and other barriers to full equality for this group certainly exist—it is a step in the right direction, toward greater equality for all. It also stands to be a step toward improving the health of LGBT populations.

As encouraging as the *Obergefell* decision was in the area of civil rights, why is it also a step toward greater health? The answer emerges when we examine research on the health of LGBT populations. A growing body of work suggests that LGBT health is worse on multiple levels than the health of comparable majority populations and that this poor health affects all stages of the life course.

Two key indicators of poorer health among LGBT populations are their rates of HIV and suicide compared to those of heterosexual populations. In the United States, HIV disproportionally affects gay men, bisexual men, and transgender women [2, 3]. Making matters worse, only 51 percent of men who have sex with men who were diagnosed with HIV by 2010 stayed in treatment for an entire year [4]. In addition to the threat of HIV, LGBT people are also at higher risk for syphilis, human papillomavirus, and viral hepatitis [5, 6, 7].

The problem of suicide is also alarming. In the United States, population-based studies have found reported suicide attempt rates among LGBT-identifying adolescents to be two to seven times greater than those among heterosexual-identifying adolescents [8]. Sexual orientation may be a particularly strong predictor of suicide attempts among male adolescents [9].

The LGBT population also contends with a range of mental health challenges. A meta-analysis found a twofold excess in suicide attempts among LGBT individuals, a 1.5 times higher risk of anxiety and depression, and a 1.5 times higher risk of alcohol or substance dependence, which was even higher among lesbian and bisexual women [10]. This risk is present across genders and at different stages of the life course. In the Nurses' Health Study II, lesbian women were more likely to report depression and the use of antidepressants [11]. A study of middle-aged adults revealed that gay and bisexual men experienced more panic attacks and depression compared to heterosexual men, and it also found a higher prevalence of generalized anxiety disorder among lesbian/bisexual women than heterosexual women [12].

As discussed in the next chapter, transgender individuals, in particular, face many health challenges. Although these challenges have been less studied, we know that HIV, suicide, and abuse are worse for transgender individuals than they are for lesbian, gay, and bisexual individuals [13, 14, 15, 16].

Other studies have shown that LBGT populations are more likely than heterosexual populations to report a variety of health problems, including asthma, overweight, hypertension, diabetes, and physical disability [17, 18, 19]. The Nurses' Health Study II found that lesbian women had a higher prevalence of risk factors for cardiovascular disease, including higher body mass index, smoking, and greater alcohol consumption [11]. A study using the National Adult Tobacco Survey found that LGBT respondents had higher smoking rates compared to heterosexual adults, despite comparable exposure to tobacco cessation advertising and use of cessation methods [20].

Sexual minority women—defined as women who have sex with females only or both males and females—have been shown to have a higher lifetime breast cancer risk (although findings in this area have been mixed) [21, 22]. A state-level study found that among men, higher bisexual population density was associated with lower incidence of lung cancer and with higher incidence of colorectal cancer [23]. However, this study does not necessarily tell us about individual risk. Among women, lesbian population density was associated with lower incidence of lung and colorectal cancer and with higher incidence of breast cancer; however, bisexual population density was associated with higher incidence of lung and colorectal cancer and with lower incidence of breast cancer. Ulrike Boehmer's book, *Cancer and the LGBT Community*, eloquently presents the data about cancer disparities as they relate to LGBT populations [24].

Challenges are especially acute for LGBT youth, who are more likely to be homeless, engage in sex work, and be victims of abuse [25, 26].

These data suggest the need for a careful look at the health disparities between LGBT and heterosexual populations. Why should the health of the LGBT community be so different from the health of comparable majority populations? And how does marriage equality stand to make a difference toward improving the health of this population?

The answers to these questions are closely tied to the central challenges of discrimination and marginalization faced by LGBT populations. The harmful health effects of these challenges are well illustrated by the data. For example, a study using the 2004–2005 National Epidemiologic Survey on Alcohol and Related Conditions found that lesbian, gay, and bisexual individuals had high levels of past-year perceived discrimination and that this discrimination was associated with past-year mood, anxiety, and substance use disorders [27]. Similarly, the National Survey of Midlife Development data showed that LGBT individuals reported more lifetime and daily experiences of discrimination, with nearly half of these individuals attributing this discrimination to their sexual orientation [28]. Even when stratified by race, perceived discrimination due to LGBT status was associated with having a psychiatric disorder, and it has been found to interfere with living a full, productive life.

The ways that discrimination shapes the health of LGBT populations are complex and subject to a number of factors. The minority stress model posits that chronic stress may result from the interplay of stigmatization, prejudice, and discrimination [29]. The confluence of these factors creates a hostile social environment for minorities, undermining health [29]. A 2011 Institute of Medicine report emphasized the complex influences on LGBT health, including the minority stress model [30]. It also incorporated a life course perspective, an intersectionality perspective (which considers different aspects of an individual's multiple identities), and a social ecology perspective (which considers outside spheres of influence, including families, communities, and society at large) [30]. There is also the social ecology perspective. An example of this perspective considers individual experienced discrimination and societal discrimination within the context of access to health insurance, housing, marriage, employment, and retirement benefits [31]. Data suggest that improvement in these areas stands to improve health. For example, Mark Hatzenbuehler and colleagues compared US states that have protection against sexual orientation-based hate crimes and employment discrimination to states that do not, and they found that LGBT adults who live in states that lack these policies had a significantly higher prevalence of psychiatric disorders compared to both heterosexual adults living in the same states and LGBT adults living in states that did have protective laws [32].

LGBT populations may also have trouble accessing care, relative to heterosexual populations. This appears, in part, to be influenced by stigma around sexual orientation and gender identity and the distrust of authorities that this stigma can lead to. The National Health Interview Survey reported that women in same-sex relationships were less likely than women in heterosexual relationships to have health insurance or to have seen a medical provider in the past year, and they were more likely to have unmet medical needs [33]. When LGBT individuals do access care, they can face further difficulty, often reporting a lack of culturally competent health care providers. This is particularly the case with transgender individuals, who are liable to distrust the health care system due to stigma and lack of affordability [34, 35].

The problem of smoking among LGBT populations well encapsulates how stigma and marginalization can lead to poor health. It has been shown that although LGBT individuals do not desire to quit smoking cigarettes any less than their heterosexual counterparts, or are any less aware of quitting programs, the stress generated by facing discrimination as a sexual minority may contribute to elevated smoking rates in LGBT populations [36, 37].

The experience of being LGBT in today's society can affect health in different ways at different stages of life. Lack of acceptance among families of LGBT youth, for example, may result in isolation from families. The circumstances of this isolation can be harmful in a number of ways, particularly by contributing to the burden of homelessness and substance use among this population. At the other end of the life course, elderly LGBT people are less likely to have adult children help them with care and are more likely to live alone [38]. There are also distinct challenges for transgender individuals. One study of transgender adults and their nontransgender siblings found that the transgender siblings reported less perceived social support from the same families [39].

In summary, LGBT populations generally bear a greater burden of disease than their heterosexual counterparts, largely due to the consequences of stigma and discrimination. Marriage equality stands to provide a needed social "buffer" between LGBT populations and the worst of these effects. It brings with it the legal, financial, and social benefits that come from being a part of a fully recognized family unit. This extends to visitation rights at hospitals, rights to accessing information from physicians, and being able to add one's partner to one's employer's health care plan. These are all rights that many LGBT partners have long not enjoyed, and now they will. Marriage equality, then, is one small step toward full equality for LGBT populations. In addition to its legal benefits, it removes many of the structural differences that reinforce stigma and lead to marginalization. As a matter of health, and as a matter of justice, this is an encouraging development in our country.

REFERENCES

1. *Obergefell v. Hodges. Oyez.* Chicago-Kent College of Law at Illinois Tech Web site. https://www.oyez.org/cases/2014/14-556. Accessed October 31, 2016.

2. HIV Among Gay and Bisexual Men. Centers for Disease Control and Prevention Web site. https://www.cdc.gov/hiv/group/msm. Updated September 30, 2016. Accessed October 31, 2016.

3. HIV Among Transgender People. Centers for Disease Control and Prevention Web site. http://www.cdc.gov/hiv/group/gender/transgender. Updated April 18, 2016. Accessed October 31, 2016.

4. Singh S, et al. Men living with diagnosed HIV who have sex with men: Progress along the continuum of HIV care—United States, 2010. *Morbidity and Mortality Weekly Report (MMWR).* 2014; 63(38): 829–33.

5. Syphilis & MSM (Men Who Have Sex with Men)—CDC Fact Sheet. Centers for Disease Control and Prevention Web site. http://www.cdc.gov/std/Syphilis/STDFact-MSM-Syphilis.htm. Updated October 28, 2016. Accessed October 31, 2016.

6. HPV and Men—Fact Sheet. Centers for Disease Control and Prevention Web site. http://www.cdc.gov/std/HPV/STDFact-HPV-and-men.htm. Updated May 19, 2016. Accessed October 31, 2016.

7. Viral Hepatitis and Men Who Have Sex with Men. Centers for Disease Control and Prevention Web site. http://www.cdc.gov/hepatitis/Populations/MSM.htm. Updated May 31, 2015. Accessed October 31, 2016.

8. Haas AP, et al. Suicide and suicide risk in lesbian, gay, bisexual, and transgender populations: Review and recommendations. *Journal of Homosexuality.* 2011; 58(1): 10–51. doi:10.1080/00918369.2011.534038

9. Garofalo R, Wolf RC, Wissow LS, Woods ER, Goodman E. Sexual orientation and risk of suicide attempts among a representative sample of youth. *Archives of Pediatrics & Adolescent Medicine.* 1999; 153(5): 487–93.

10. King M, et al. A systematic review of mental disorder, suicide, and deliberate self harm in lesbian, gay and bisexual people. *BMC Psychiatry.* 2008; 8: 70. doi:10.1186/1471-244X-8-70

11. Case P, et al. Sexual orientation, health risk factors, and physical functioning in the Nurses' Health Study II. *Journal of Women's Health.* 2004; 13(9): 1033–47.

12. Cochran SD, Mays VM, Sullivan JG. Prevalence of mental disorders, psychological distress, and mental health services use among lesbian, gay, and bisexual adults in the United States. *Journal of Consulting and Clinical Psychology.* 2003; 71(1): 53–61.

13. Herbst JH, et al. Estimating HIV prevalence and risk behaviors of transgender persons in the United States: A systematic review. *AIDS and Behavior.* 2008; 12(1): 1–17.

14. Kenagy GP. HIV among transgendered people. *AIDS Care.* 2002; 14(1): 127–34.

15. Clements-Nolle K, Marx R, Katz M. Attempted suicide among transgender persons: The influence of gender-based discrimination and victimization. *Journal of Homosexuality.* 2006; 51(3): 53–69.

16. Kenagy GP. Transgender health: Findings from two needs assessment studies in Philadelphia. *Health & Social Work.* 2006; 30(1): 19–26.

17. Heck JE, Jacobson JS. Asthma diagnosis among individuals in same-sex relationships. *Journal of Asthma.* 2006; 43(8): 579–84.

18. Dilley JA, Simmons KW, Boysun MJ, Pizacani BA, Stark MJ. Demonstrating the importance and feasibility of including sexual orientation in public health surveys: Health disparities in the Pacific Northwest. *American Journal of Public Health.* 2010; 100(3): 460–7. doi:10.2105/AJPH.2007

19. Wallace SP, Cochran SD, Durazo EM, Ford CL. *The health of aging lesbian, gay and bisexual adults in California.* Policy brief, UCLA Center for Health Policy Research, 2011 (PB2011-2): 1–8.

20. Fallin A, Lee YO, Bennett K, Goodin A. Smoking cessation awareness and utilization among lesbian, gay, bisexual, and transgender adults: An analysis of the 2009–2010 National Adult Tobacco Survey. *Nicotine & Tobacco Research.* 18(4): 496–500. doi:10.1093/ntr/ntv103

21. Clavelle K, King D, Bazzi AR, Fein-Zachary V, Potter J. Breast cancer risk in sexual minority women during routine screening at an urban LGBT health center. *Women's Health Issues.* 2015; 25(4): 341–8. doi:10.1016/j.whi.2015.03.014

22. Meads C, Moore D. Breast cancer in lesbians and bisexual women: Systematic review of incidence, prevalence and risk studies. *BMC Public Health.* 2013; 13: 1127. doi:10.1186/1471-2458-13-1127

23. Boehmer U, Miao X, Maxwell NI, Ozonoff A. Sexual minority population density and incidence of lung, colorectal and female breast cancer in California. *BMJ Open.* 2014; 4(3): e004461. doi:10.1136/bmjopen-2013-004461

24. Boehmer U, Elk R, eds. *Cancer and the LGBT Community: Unique Perspectives from Risk to Survivorship.* New York, NY: Springer; 2015.

25. Kruks G. Gay and lesbian homeless/street youth: Special issues and concerns. *Journal of Adolescent Health.* 1991; 12(7): 515–8.

26. Saewyc EM, et al. Hazards of stigma: The sexual and physical abuse of gay, lesbian, and bisexual adolescents in the United States and Canada. *Child Welfare.* 2006; 85(2): 195–213.

27. McLaughlin KA, Hatzenbuehler ML, Keyes KM. Responses to discrimination and psychiatric disorders among black, Hispanic, female, and lesbian, gay, and bisexual individuals. *American Journal of Public Health.* 2010; 100(8): 1477–84. doi:10.2105/AJPH.2009.181586

28. Mays VM, Cochran SD. Mental health correlates of perceived discrimination among lesbian, gay, and bisexual adults in the United States. *American Journal of Public Health.* 2001; 91(11): 1869–76.

29. Meyer IH. Prejudice, social stress, and mental health in lesbian, gay, and bisexual populations: Conceptual issues and research evidence. *Psychological Bulletin*. 2003; 129(5): 674–97.

30. Institute of Medicine. *The Health of Lesbian, Gay, Bisexual, and Transgender People: Building a Foundation for Better Understanding*. Washington, DC: The National Academies Press; 2011.

31. Lesbian, Gay, Bisexual, and Transgender Health. Healthy People 2020 Web site. https://www. healthypeople.gov/2020/topics-objectives/topic/lesbian-gay-bisexual-and-transgender-health?topicid=25. Accessed November 1, 2016.

32. Hatzenbuehler ML, Keyes KM, Hasin DS. State-level policies and psychiatric morbidity in lesbian, gay, and bisexual populations. *American Journal of Public Health*. 2009; 99(12): 2275–81. doi:10.2105/AJPH.2008.153510

33. Heck JE, Sell RL, Gorin SS. Health care access among individuals involved in same-sex relationships. *American Journal of Public Health*. 2006; 96(6): 1111–8. doi:10.2105/AJPH.2005.062661

34. Hayhurst C. Managing patients who are transgender. *PT in Motion*. July 2016. http://www. apta.org/PTinMotion/2016/7/Feature/Transgender. Accessed November 1, 2016.

35. Sanchez NF, Sanchez JP, Danoff A. Health care utilization, barriers to care, and hormone usage among male-to-female transgender persons in New York City. *American Journal of Public Health*. 2009; 99(4): 713–9. doi:10.2105/AJPH.2007

36. Fallin A, Goodin A, Lee YO, Bennett K. Smoking characteristics among lesbian, gay, and bisexual adults. *Preventive Medicine*. 2015; 74: 123–30. doi:10.1016/j.ypmed.2014.11.026

37. Ryan H, Wortley PM, Easton A, Pederson L, Greenwood G. Smoking among lesbians, gays, and bisexuals: A review of the literature. *American Journal of Preventive Medicine*. 2001; 21(2): 142–9.

38. Lesbian, Gay, Bisexual and Transgender Aging. American Psychological Association Web site. http://www.apa.org/pi/lgbt/resources/aging.aspx. Accessed November 1, 2016.

39. Factor RJ, Rothblum ED. A study of transgender adults and their non-transgender siblings on demographic characteristics, social support, and experiences of violence. *Journal of LGBT Health Research*. 2007; 3(3): 11–30.

29

Transgender Today

⌒

IT IS DIFFICULT to arrive at a precise estimate of the disease burden borne by transgender, gay, lesbian, bisexual, or queer populations. This is because the Census, and many other official surveys, does not explicitly ask about sexual orientation and gender identity, as well as the fact that gender identity can be nonbinary [1]. There is also the problem of bias due to underreporting; one study found that 71 percent of transgender people have hidden their gender in order to avoid discrimination [2]. Finally, transgender people are sometimes "lumped in" with other populations. This has been the case with HIV studies that have characterized transgender women as "men who have sex with men" [3]. A 2011 Williams Institute analysis, compiling different databases, estimated that approximately 8 million American(3.5 percent) identify as gay, bisexual, or lesbian, with another 700,000 identifying as transgender [4].

The lesbian, gay, bisexual, and transgender (LGBT) population is, in many respects, a vulnerable group in terms of health. Discrimination and marginalization of this population are associated with a range of health conditions. These challenges include substance use, anxiety, and mood disorders [5]. In addition, LGBT individuals may suffer from lack of access to health care [6, 7]. More broadly, we know that the experience of discrimination is closely linked with negative health outcomes such as depression, heart disease, obesity, hypertension, and substance use; we need better data to determine how these and other health effects are tied to being transgender [8, 9]. When the American Civil Liberties Union made its case against a North Carolina law nullifying local antidiscrimination ordinances based on gender identity, it was supported by an expert declaration on transgender and intersex children from Deanna Adkins, who powerfully pointed out, "With the exception of some serious childhood cancers, gender dysphoria is the most fatal condition that I treat because of the harms that flow from not properly recognizing gender identity" [10, 11]. This lack of recognition and respect can follow transgender people throughout life. According to the Human Rights Campaign, for example, 20 to 57 percent of transgender individuals have some experience with workplace discrimination [12]. Globally, transgender women are nearly 50 times more likely to get HIV compared to the general population, and transgender individuals belonging to an ethnic or racial minority are at an even greater risk of discrimination and harassment [2, 13]. Finally, there is the matter of violence directed against this group. In 2015, the number of transgender and gender nonconforming people murdered in the United States was the highest on record; almost all of the victims were black or Latina women [14, 15]. In addition, at least 10 transgender/gender nonconforming people were murdered in the United States in 2016 [16].

With efforts to marginalize the transgender population gaining traction in states throughout the country, academic public health has a responsibility to protect the health and well-being of this group. There are three key ways we can do this.

As an academic community, we are charged with generating the knowledge that can guide public discussions and thinking about this issue and many others. This means that we have to do the intellectual work that elevates human dignity and human rights as a core mission of public health and to continually reaffirm how marginalization and structural discrimination of any group adversely affect that group's health. Moreover, we must make it clear that when one group suffers, it diminishes us all. It falls to us to communicate the direct link between greater social inclusion and better health. Any efforts that systematically marginalize particular groups are therefore inimical to the goals of public health. In making this moral appeal, we must also take care to support our argument with ever-better data [17].

Second, it is our job to educate students, shaping the next generation of thinkers, teachers, and doers in population health. This teaching must not stop with the canonical foundations of our field. Rather, it is important that we expose students to the issues that dominate the public conversation and stand to alter the social, economic, and cultural conditions that shape the health of populations, and vulnerable populations in particular.

Third, we must also act on our knowledge. To paraphrase Goethe's well-worn aphorism, adorning all National Academy of Medicine reports, knowing is not enough, we must do. This means tackling issues that represent a threat to population health and also partnering with organizations and advocates who are positioned to "move the needle" on these issues, always remaining open to outside-the-box partnerships and solutions.

We as a country have reached a crucial moment in the fight for transgender equality. We should capitalize on the gains that have already been made and continue to push for a more equitable society for this too-often marginalized group, embracing its struggle for recognition and respect as a key public health concern.

REFERENCES

1. Miller CC. The search for the best estimate of the transgender population. *The New York Times*. June 8, 2015. http://www.nytimes.com/2015/06/09/upshot/the-search-for-the-best-estimate-of-the-transgender-population.html. Accessed October 31, 2016.
2. Grant JM, et al. *Injustice at Every Turn: A Report of the National Transgender Discrimination Survey*. Washington, DC: National Center for Transgender Equality and National Gay and Lesbian Task Force; 2011.

3. Brydum S. Why transgender women have the country's highest HIV rates. *Plus*. April 2, 2015. http://www.hivplusmag.com/case-studies/2013/04/08/invisible-women-why-transgender-women-are-hit-so-hard-hiv. Accessed October 31, 2016.

4. Gates GJ. *How Many People Are Lesbian, Gay, Bisexual, and Transgender?* Los Angeles, CA: The Williams Institute, UCLA School of Law; 2011.

5. McLaughlin KA, Hatzenbuehler ML, Keyes KM. Responses to discrimination and psychiatric disorders among black, Hispanic, female, and lesbian, gay, and bisexual individuals. *American Journal of Public Health*. 2010; 100(8): 1477–1484. doi:10.2105/AJPH.2009.181586

6. Heck JE, Sell RL, Gorin SS. Health care access among individuals involved in same-sex relationships. *American Journal of Public Health*. 2006; 96(6): 1111–1118. doi:10.2105/AJPH.2005.062661

7. Safer JD, et al. Barriers to healthcare for transgender individuals. *Current Opinion in Endocrinology, Diabetes and Obesity*. 23(2): 168–171. doi:10.1097/MED.0000000000000227

8. Pascoe EA, Smart Richman L. Perceived discrimination and health: A meta-analytic review. *Psychological Bulletin*. 2009; 135(4): 531–554. doi:10.1037/a0016059

9. Williams DR, Neighbors HW, Jackson JS. Racial/ethnic discrimination and health: Findings from community studies. *American Journal of Public Health*. 2003; 93(2): 200–208.

10. Domonoske C. North Carolina passes law blocking measures to protect LGBT people. *NPR*. March 24, 2016. http://www.npr.org/sections/thetwo-way/2016/03/24/471700323/north-carolina-passes-law-blocking-measures-to-protect-lgbt-people. Accessed October 31, 2016.

11. Adkins D. *Expert Declaration of Deanna Adkins MD to United States District Court for the Middle District of North Carolina*. 2016. Print.

12. Discrimination Against Transgender Workers. Human Rights Campaign Web site. http://www.hrc.org/resources/discrimination-against-transgender-workers. Accessed October 31, 2016.

13. van Griensven F, Na Ayutthaya PP, Wilson E. HIV surveillance and prevention in transgender women. *The Lancet Infectious Diseases*. 2013; 13(3): 185–186.

14. Atkinson K. More transgender people reported killed in 2015 than in any other year. *MSNBC*. November 20, 2015. http://www.msnbc.com/msnbc/more-transgender-people-reported-killed-2015-any-other-year. Accessed October 31, 2016.

15. Starr TJ. 16 trans people (that we know of) have been murdered this year. *Alternet*. August 17, 2015. http://www.alternet.org/civil-liberties/16-trans-people-we-know-have-been-murdered-year. Accessed October 31, 2016.

16. Advocate.com Editors. These are the trans people killed in 2016. *Advocate*. http://www.advocate.com/transgender/2016/9/16/these-are-trans-people-killed-2016. Accessed October 31, 2016.

17. Grant JM, et al. *National Transgender Discrimination Survey Report on Health and Health Care*. Washington, DC: National Center for Transgender Equality and National Gay and Lesbian Task Force; 2010.

30

The Health of Immigrants

IN 2013, THERE were 232 million immigrants living worldwide, with approximately 2.4 million migrating across national borders each year [1, 2]. However, immigration is not limited to those who seek a better life abroad. It is estimated that 763 million people live within their country of birth but in a different region, having migrated within national borders [3]. This migration is driven by a range of economic, political, and social factors. Often, migration is the result of armed conflict that forces citizens from their native soil. Migrants who are forced to leave their country due to war or persecution are typically called refugees—globally, there were 19.5 million refugees at the end of 2014 [4]. Given the scale of mass migration, it is important to consider how this phenomenon affects the health of populations. I do so here, adopting life course and urban health frameworks to better explicate this influence.

Currently, the study of migrant health is characterized by ambiguity. It is not at all clear whether the health of migrants is better or worse than the well-being of counterparts who do not migrate or that of populations living in receiving countries. Some studies, such as one comparing cardiovascular risk factors among Portuguese who stayed in Portugal to those who migrated to Switzerland, find very few differences in health between migrants and those who do not leave their countries of origin [5]. Other studies have documented poorer outcomes among migrants. One study that examined the country of origin among people living in Italy found that citizens of countries with high migration pressure had a higher prevalence of diabetes [6]. This prevalence was observed mostly among immigrants from Southern Asia and Northern Africa, and especially among females [6]. This study also found that immigrants from these areas had a lower chance of being tested for glucose levels. One review that examined several European countries determined that the health effects of immigration vary across the continent [7]. The review found that immigrants, independent of country of origin, fared worse overall than natives in France, Belgium, and Spain, although immigrants fared better than natives in Italy, in contrast with results from the previously mentioned study.

In the context of this conflicting evidence, a life course perspective can be useful to help us understand the link between migration and health. This is because a life course perspective requires us to look at migration processes as they intersect with life experiences, including pre-migration, peri-migration, and post-migration circumstances. For example, a review of immigrant and refugee youth in Canada illustrated the influence of pre-migration experiences, including trauma, and post-migration family and school environments [8]. Multiple characteristics of the pre-migration experience, captured by migrant country of origin, have been shown to determine heterogeneity in immigrant health [9]. There is also ready evidence of the association between health and the migration experience itself—particularly with regard to the health of vulnerable populations—although the literature on this is sparser [10]. Regarding post-migration experiences, it is perhaps not surprising that the conditions experienced by migrants in their new countries appear to be strongly determinative of migrants' health. Examining cardiovascular disease outcomes in Denmark, for example, a study found that refugees were disadvantaged in terms of some outcomes and equal or better off than Danish-born citizens in others, but family-reunified immigrants had significantly lower across-the-board incidence of stroke, cardiovascular disease, and myocardial infarction [11].

Conditions of assimilation are also broadly associated with health. Legal status in the host country is associated with the use of a range of health services, which can improve the well-being of immigrant populations [12]. There is also the matter of immediate social context. Various studies have shown that residence in "ethnic enclaves" after immigration is associated with better health outcomes over time and can help mitigate unhealthy assimilation [13, 14, 15]. Finally, there are the intergenerational effects of migration. Extending the life course paradigm across generations, a study on rural-to-urban migrants in Bangladesh found that under-5 mortality was almost twice as high among children born to urban migrants compared to children born to lifelong urban natives, likely due to a disadvantaged economic status [16].

Examining how the migration experience intersects with life stages may also shed light on the dynamics that shape mental and physical health among migrants. A study of immigrants to the United States based on the National Comorbidity Study Replication found a higher risk of psychiatric disorder among immigrants to be associated with earlier age of immigration and longer duration of residence [17]. This could imply that any attempt to safeguard the mental health of immigrants in the United States is attenuated when immigrants experience a longer period of socialization. A similar effect was observed in Shenzhen, China, where pre-adulthood migration was a predictor of major depressive disorder [18]. We have also seen a change in obesity over time, where immigrants newly arrived to the United States had a significantly lower prevalence of obesity compared to US-born residents [19]. However, this prevalence dramatically increased over time, as more years passed since immigration [19].

Much of the literature on intranational migration has focused on rural-to-urban migration within a given country. A growing literature has studied this in China, informed by the country's rapid urbanization, which has been at work since the turn of the century [20, 21]. Rural-to-urban migrants in China generally have more communicable diseases and suffer from worse maternal and infant health [22, 23]. This population tends to be younger, male, and single, which may confound relationships between migration and health [24]. The issue is further complicated by the fact that migrants are often excluded from urban health services and insurance [24]. This exclusion can undermine both mental and physical health. One study in Beijing found perceived social inequity and the experience of discrimination to be linked with mental health challenges among rural migrant populations [25].

It is important to note that the migration experience is fluid and sometimes continual. Populations may migrate more than once in a lifetime, or temporarily migrate for occupational purposes, while remaining linked to a rural household [26, 27]. Several authors have studied these cycles of migration. Eric Nauman and colleagues used a longitudinal approach to follow migrants from rural western Thailand to urban destinations such as Bangkok and then assessed the migrants, return migrants, and rural counterparts who remained in origin villages [28]. Their findings supported the "healthy migrant" hypothesis: Migrants were physically healthier than nonmigrants both before and after moving. Migrants who stayed in urban destinations displayed an improvement in mental health, and return migrants fared worse on both physical and mental health indicators. This effect has also been observed globally. The World Health Organization's Study on Global AGEing and Adult Health (SAGE) compared behavioral risk factors for noncommunicable diseases across rural, urban, and migrant populations in several different countries, finding that—with some exceptions based on destination—alcohol consumption and occupational physical activity were lower in migrant and urban groups [29].

Locating the migrant experience within the context of the life course, the life stage at the time of migration, and the specificity of macro context (i.e., urban or not) all contribute to our understanding of the health of migrants. This suggests the utility of a life course perspective in organizing our thinking around how migration processes influence well-being, pointing us toward a fuller understanding of how moving between countries and cultures shapes the health of populations.

REFERENCES

1. Wallcharts. United Nations Department of Economic and Social Affairs, Population Division, International Migration Web site. http://www.un.org/en/development/desa/population/migration/publications/wallchart/index.shtml. Accessed October 13, 2016.

2. Immigration. Global Issues Web site. http://www.globalissues.org/article/537/immigration. Updated May 26, 2008. Accessed October 13, 2016.

3. Technical Paper Series. United Nations Department of Economic and Social Affairs, Population Division, International Migration Web site. http://www.un.org/en/development/desa/population/publications/technical/index.shtml. Accessed October 13, 2016.

4. United Nations High Commissioner for Refugees Web site. http://www.unhcr.org/uk. Accessed October 13, 2016.

5. Alves L, et al. Prevalence and management of cardiovascular risk factors in Portuguese living in Portugal and Portuguese who migrated to Switzerland. *BMC Public Health*. 2015; 15: 307. doi:10.1186/s12889-015-1659-8

6. Ballotari P, et al. Differences in diabetes prevalence and inequalities in disease management and glycaemic control by immigrant status: A population-based study (Italy). *BMC Public Health*. 2015; 15: 87. doi:10.1186/s12889-015-1403-4

7. Moullan Y, Jusot F. Why is the "healthy immigrant effect" different between European countries? *European Journal of Public Health*. 2014; 24(Suppl 1): 80–86. doi:10.1093/eurpub/cku112

8. Guruge S, Butt H. A scoping review of mental health issues and concerns among immigrant and refugee youth in Canada: Looking back, moving forward. *Canadian Journal of Public Health*. 2015; 106(2): e72–78. doi:10.17269/cjph.106.4588

9. Anderson KK, Cheng J, Susser E, McKenzie KJ, Kurdyak P. Incidence of psychotic disorders among first-generation immigrants and refugees in Ontario. *Canadian Medical Association Journal*. 2015; 187(9): E279–86. doi:10.1503/cmaj.141420

10. Kasl SV, Berkman L. Health consequences of the experience of migration. *Annual Review of Public Health*. 1983; 4: 69–90.

11. Byberg S, Agyemang C, Zwisler AD, Krasnik A, Norredam M. Cardiovascular disease incidence and survival: Are migrants always worse off? *European Journal of Epidemiology*. 2016; 31(7): 667–77. doi:10.1007/s10654-015-0024-7

12. Sousa E, et al. Immigration, work and health in Spain: The influence of legal status and employment contract on reported health indicators. *International Journal of Public Health*. 2010; 55(5): 443–51. doi:10.1007/s00038-010-0141-8

13. Glaser SL, et al. Hodgkin lymphoma incidence in ethnic enclaves in California. *Leukemia & Lymphoma*. 2015; 56(12): 3270–80. doi:10.3109/10428194.2015.1026815

14. Peak C, Weeks JR. Does community context influence reproductive outcomes of Mexican origin women in San Diego, California? *Journal of Immigrant and Minority Health*. 2002; 4(3): 125–36.

15. Park J, Myers D, Kao D, Min S. Immigrant obesity and unhealthy assimilation: Alternative estimates of convergence or divergence, 1995–2005. *Social Science & Medicine*. 2009; 69(11): 1625–33. doi:10.1016/j.socscimed.2009.09.008

16. Islam MM, Azad KM. Rural–urban migration and child survival in urban Bangladesh: Are the urban migrants and poor disadvantaged? *Journal of Biosocial Science*. 2008; 40(1): 83–96.

17. Breslau J, et al. Risk for psychiatric disorder among immigrants and their US-born descendants: Evidence from the National Comorbidity Survey Replication. *Journal of Nervous and Mental Disease*. 2007; 195(3): 189–95.

18. Zhong BL, et al. Prevalence and correlates of major depressive disorder among rural-to-urban migrant workers in Shenzhen, China. *Journal of Affective Disorders*. 2015; 183: 1–9. doi:10.1016/j.jad.2015.04.031

19. Singh GK, Siahpush M, Hiatt RA, Timsina LR. Dramatic increases in obesity and overweight prevalence and body mass index among ethnic-immigrant and social class groups in the United States, 1976–2008. *Journal of Community Health*. 2011; 36(1): 94–110. doi:10.1007/s10900-010-9287-9

20. Mou J, Griffiths SM, Fong H, Dawes MG. Health of China's rural–urban migrants and their families: A review of literature from 2000 to 2012. *British Medical Bulletin*. 2013; 106: 19–43. doi:10.1093/bmb/ldt016

21. Gong P, et al. Urbanisation and health in China. *The Lancet*. 2012; 379(9818): 843–52.

22. Zou X, et al. Rural-to-urban migrants are at high risk of sexually transmitted and viral hepatitis infections in China: A systematic review and meta-analysis. *BMC Infectious Diseases*. 2014; 14(1): 490. doi:10.1186/1471-2334-14-490

23. Yuan B, Qian X, Thomsen S. Disadvantaged populations in maternal health in China who and why? *Global Health Action.* 2013; 6: 19542. doi:10.3402/gha.v6i0.19542

24. Hu X, Cook S, Salazar MA. Internal migration and health in China. *The Lancet.* 2008; 372(9651): 1717–9. doi:10.1016/S0140-6736(08)61360-4

25. Lin D, et al. Discrimination, perceived social inequity, and mental health among rural-to-urban migrants in China. *Community Mental Health Journal.* 2011; 47(2): 171–80. doi:10.1007/s10597-009-9278-4

26. Yang H, et al. Health-related lifestyle behaviors among male and female rural-to-urban migrant workers in Shanghai, China. *PLoS One.* 2015; 10(2): e0117946. doi:10.1371/journal.pone.0117946

27. Collinson MA, et al. Migration and the epidemiological transition: Insights from the Agincourt sub-district of northeast South Africa. *Global Health Action.* 2014; 7:23514. doi:10.3402/gha.v7.23514

28. Nauman E, VanLandingham M, Anglewicz P, Patthavanit U, Punpuing S. Rural-to-urban migration and changes in health among young adults in Thailand. *Demography.* 2015; 52(1): 233–57. doi:10.1007/s13524-014-0365-y

29. Oyebode O, et al. Rural, urban and migrant differences in non-communicable disease risk-factors in middle income countries: A cross-sectional study of WHO-SAGE data. *PLoS One.* 2015; 10(4): e0122747. doi:10.1371/journal.pone.0122747

31

Caring for Refugees

THE UNITED NATIONS Refugee Agency (UNHCR) estimates that there are currently 59.5 million people forcibly displaced worldwide [1]. The reason is often war. Conflict and persecution force 42,500 persons per day to seek protection, either within their countries or abroad. As a consequence of this and other factors, there were, by the end of 2014, 19.5 million refugees throughout the world. This number is considerably higher than the previous 10 years, mostly due to the refugee crisis in Syria [2]. It is estimated that more than 4 million Syrians have been forced to leave their country [3]. These refugees most commonly settle in Turkey, making that country host to the largest number of refugees worldwide [3]. As of March 2015, more than half of all Syrians were forced to flee their homes, including 7.6 million people displaced internally in the country [4]. Iraq has also contributed to the refugee crisis, displacing more than 9 million people since the 1980s, with most leaving Baghdad and settling in Jordan and Syria [5]. Many refugees also come from Africa. According to the United Nations, 53% of worldwide refugees come from Somalia, Syria, and Afghanistan [6].

In 1951, UNHCR defined a refugee as someone who

owing to a well-founded fear of being persecuted for reasons of race, religion, nationality, membership of a particular social group or political opinion, is outside the country of his nationality, and is unable, or owing to such fear, is unwilling to avail himself of the protection of that country. [7]

Although substantial logistical challenges complicate investigations into the health of refugee populations, an empiric literature has emerged that documents refugee health. This literature has brought to light the substantial burden of noncommunicable and communicable diseases carried by refugees—diseases that characterize the health of vulnerable populations the world over.

Among Iraqi refugees, major disease burdens have been identified as diabetes, hypertension, and malnutrition [8]. Prevalence of malnutrition among refugee children in 2011 was 4.5 percent in Syria, and more than 90 percent of households reported food aid receipt [9]. Of the almost 12,000 adult refugees who were screened in International Organization for Migration clinics in Jordan, 38 percent were considered overweight, and 34 percent were obese [10]. Smoking levels are also very high among male refugees [10]. Additional health concerns include anemia: In 2012, 13 percent of Iraqi refugees who had lived in the United States for up to 3 years reported anemia among their household members [11]. In the same survey, 43 percent reported delaying or not seeking care for a problem in the past year, and 60 percent reported suffering from a chronic condition. Within refugee populations, certain groups are at particular risk. Domestic violence, for example, is a common threat faced by refugee women [12]. Women and girls escaping the Iraq war report rape by armed groups and civilians in Iraq—a problem that may be worse than we know because sexual violence is likely underreported due to cultural stigma and shame [12]. Many refugees are forced into sex work for financial support, although population-level estimates of refugees suffering this fate are difficult to obtain. Pregnant women are particularly vulnerable as international humanitarian funds run low and women are forced to give birth in unsafe conditions [13, 14].

Mental health among refugees has justifiably received much recent attention, especially in the Syrian context [15]. The International Rescue Committee reports a high prevalence of depression, anxiety, and post-traumatic stress disorder among refugee populations in general, and a 2012 Centers for Disease Control and Prevention survey of Iraqi refugees living in the United States found that half of participants reported anxiety, depression, and emotional distress [11, 16]. Fortunately, there is cause to hope that these health challenges might be prevented through attention to context. Fazel and colleagues reviewed available evidence on mental health in children who are displaced to high-income countries and found that social support and stable settlement in the host country have the potential to mitigate exposure to violence and exert a positive effect on psychological functioning [17]. This is consistent with evidence in non-refugee populations, and it shows, I think, the potential to ameliorate the often harmful effects of the refugee experience.

In contrast to the state of the data on Middle Eastern refugee populations, systematic data on the health of refugees from other areas of the world are sparse. We know that the burden of infectious disease has weighed heavily on refugees from the Central African Republic who settled in the Democratic Republic of Congo [18]. These populations have been forced to fight parasites, malaria, typhoid fever, and respiratory infections in a place where infections are easily spread through camps and makeshift housing that lacks sanitation infrastructure [18]. Central African refugees have also arrived in Cameroon extremely malnourished [19]. Despite gaps in our understanding, we do know that the scale of this problem is horrendous. Approximately 25 percent of the Central African Republic's population has also been internally displaced since 2013 [20].

The Refugee Health Technical Assistance Center organizes the refugee experience into three stages: preflight, flight, and resettlement [21]. Each of these stages involves unique hazards, manifesting as potentially traumatic exposures that are likely to be associated with health [21]. For example, preflight experiences in Iraq and Syria often involve violence, including air bombardments, shelling, shootings, harassment by militias, and the death of loved ones [22]. As a result, perhaps, of these highly dramatic circumstances, the conditions of flight in these countries have been harshly visible in the global press, casting a much-needed spotlight on the global refugee challenge [23]. But escape from war zones does not necessarily mean safety. Ongoing stressors can continue in settlement camps; these stressors can include uncertain access to food and water and poor living accommodation [24].

Once refugees have arrived in a new country, there remains the difficulty of ensuring that their often substantial health needs are met. The recent European refugee crisis has highlighted some of the challenges the world faces in attempting to address the resettlement needs of refugees. Encouragingly, there has been a shift in the past few years in policies related to international refugees, with recent policies advocating for the integration of refugees into the health systems of their host countries rather than the creation of parallel, often substandard systems. The UNHCR policy on alternatives to camps is a good example of this shift [25]. The initiative calls for policies that would enable refugees to live in communities lawfully and without harassment. Moreover, following the steady increase of the number of refugees in urban areas—where more than half of refugees live—UNHCR introduced a policy on refugee protection and solutions [26, 27]. This policy acknowledges that refugees in urban areas often lack even the community support offered to poor citizens and focuses on supporting existing systems rather than creating parallel ones. To this end, the policy entails working with authorities on behalf of refugees to provide health care freely or with a limited cost. It also involves monitoring the health status of refugees and augmenting existing service providers. Beyond this focus on cities, the shift to refugee integration has also been adopted on a country-wide scale. For example, the government of New Zealand has adopted a refugee resettlement strategy with maintaining the health and well-being of refugees as one of its main declared goals, toward the ultimate aim of refugee integration [28]. It is worth repeating, however, that the vast majority of the world's refugees live in low-income countries, many of which are struggling with the provision of sustainable and effective health systems for their own people. To these already strained infrastructures, an influx of refugees represents an additional challenge—one that does not lend itself to easy solutions.

Finally, climate change—the topic of Chapter 20—has emerged as a clear concern for those working to safeguard the health of refugees. In 2010, the United Nations Commissioner for Refugees, Antonio Guterres, now the United Nations Secretary General, addressed the link between climate change and forced displacement: "Today's challenges are interconnected and complex. Population growth, urbanization, climate change, water scarcity, and food and energy insecurity are exacerbating conflict and combining in other ways that oblige people to flee their countries" [29]. Other entities, such as Refugees International, have expressed worry about the potential of climate change to drive population displacement now and in the future [30]. This concern represents a growing understanding of the interlinked and complex forces that create the conditions for forced migration and add to the hazards of the already uncertain, perilous journey of refugees.

REFERENCES

1. United Nations High Commissioner for Refugees Web site. http://www.unhcr.org/uk. Accessed October 18, 2016.

2. Syria Regional Refugee Response: Inter-agency Information Sharing Portal. United Nations High Commissioner for Refugees—Emergencies Web site. http://data.unhcr.org/syrianrefugees/regional.php. Accessed October 18, 2016.

3. Cumming-Bruce N. Number of Syrian refugees climbs to more than 4 million. *The New York Times*. July 9, 2015. http://www.nytimes.com/2015/07/09/world/middleeast/number-of-syrian-refugees-climbs-to-more-than-4-million.html?em_pos=large&emc=edit_nn_20150709&nl=nytnow&nlid=469459838&_r=2&mtrref=undefined. Accessed October 18, 2016.

4. Crisis in Syria. United Nations Population Fund Web site. http://www.unfpa.org/emergencies/crisis-syria. Accessed October 18, 2016.

5. Iraqi Refugee Health Profile; Background. Centers for Disease Control and Prevention Web site. http://www.cdc.gov/immigrantrefugeehealth/profiles/iraqi/background/index.html. Updated December 15, 2014. Accessed October 18, 2016.

6. Figures at a Glance. United Nations High Commissioner for Refugees Web site. http://www.unhcr.org/en-us/figures-at-a-glance.html. Accessed February 11, 2017.

7. Refugees. United Nations High Commissioner for Refugees Web site. http://www.unhcr.org/pages/49c3646c125.html Accessed October 18, 2016.

8. Iraqi Refugee Health Profile. Centers for Disease Control and Prevention Web site. http://www.cdc.gov/immigrantrefugeehealth/profiles/iraqi/index.html. Accessed October 18, 2016.

9. Doocy S, et al. Food security and humanitarian assistance among displaced Iraqi populations in Jordan and Syria. *Social Science & Medicine*. 2011; 72(2): 273–782. doi:10.1016/j.socscimed.2010.10.023

10. Iraqi Refugee Health Profile; Non-communicable Disease. Centers for Disease Control and Prevention Web site. http://www.cdc.gov/immigrantrefugeehealth/profiles/iraqi/health-information/non-communicable-disease.html. Updated December 19, 2014. Accessed October 18, 2016.

11. Taylor EM, et al. Physical and mental health status of Iraqi refugees resettled in the United States. *Journal of Immigrant and Minority Health*. 2014; 16(6): 1130–7.

12. Chynoweth SK. The need for priority reproductive health services for displaced Iraqi women and girls. *Reproductive Health Matters*. 2008; 16(31): 93–102. doi:10.1016/S0968-8080(08)31348-2

13. Shortage in Funding Threatens Care for Pregnant Syrian Refugees. United Nations Population Fund Web site. http://www.unfpa.org/news/shortage-funding-threatens-care-pregnant-syrian-refugees. Published June 25, 2015. Accessed October 18, 2016.

14. Syrian refugees in Lebanon face health care crisis—Amnesty. *BBC News*. May 21, 2014. http://www.bbc.com/news/world-middle-east-27496889. Accessed October 18, 2016.

15. Leigh K. Syria's mental health crisis. *The New York Times*. August 1, 2014. http://kristof.blogs.nytimes.com/2014/08/01/syrias-mental-health-crisis/?_r=2&mtrref=undefined&assetType=opinion. Accessed October 18, 2016.

16. Millions Uprooted; Iraq. International Rescue Committee Web site. https://www.rescue.org/country/iraq. Accessed October 18, 2016.

17. Fazel M, Reed RV, Panter-Brick C, Stein A. Mental health of displaced and refugee children resettled in high-income countries: Risk and protective factors. *The Lancet*. 2012; 379(9812): 266–82. doi:http://dx.doi.org/10.1016/S0140-6736(11)60051-2

18. Mueller K. Health concerns for thousands of refugees from Central African Republic in makeshift camps. International Federation of Red Cross and Red Crescent Societies Web site. http://www.ifrc.org/en/news-and-media/news-stories/africa/central-african-republic/health-concerns-for-thousands-of-refugees-from-central-african-republic-in-makeshift-camps-61188. Published April 5, 2013. Accessed October 18, 2016.

19. Mbaiorem D. UNHCR addresses alarming health situation of refugees in Cameroon. United Nations High Commissioner for Refugees Web site. http://www.unhcr.org/5322e2582.html. Published March 14, 2014. Accessed October 18, 2016.

20. Central African Republic. United Nations High Commissioner for Refugees Web site. http://www.unhcr.org/pages/49e45c156.html. Accessed October 18, 2016.

21. Mental Health. Refugee Health Technical Assistance Center Web site. http://refugeehealthta.org/physical-mental-health/mental-health. Accessed October 18, 2016.

22. Iraqi Refugee Health Profile; Mental Health. Centers for Disease Control and Prevention Web site. http://www.cdc.gov/immigrantrefugeehealth/profiles/iraqi/health-information/mental-health.html#six. Updated December 19, 2014. Accessed October 18, 2016.

23. Peçanha S, Wallace T. The flight of refugees around the globe. *The New York Times.* June 20, 2015. http://www.nytimes.com/interactive/2015/06/21/world/map-flow-desperate-migration-refugee-crisis.html?_r=0. Accessed October 18, 2016.

24. Module 2: Mental Health in Refugee Camps and Settlements. Unite for Sight Web site. http://www.uniteforsight.org/refugee-health/module2. Accessed October 18, 2016.

25. Alternatives to Camps. United Nations High Commissioner for Refugees Web site. http://www.unhcr.org/pages/54d9c7686.html Accessed October 18, 2016.

26. Urban Refugees. United Nations High Commissioner for Refugees Web site. http://www.unhcr.org/pages/4b0e4cba6.html. Accessed October 18, 2016.

27. UN High Commissioner for Refugees (UNHCR). *UNHCR Policy on Refugee Protection and Solutions in Urban Areas.* 2009. http://www.unhcr.org/cgi-bin/texis/vtx/search?page=search&docid=4ab356ab6&query=urban%20refugees. Accessed October 18, 2016.

28. Marlowe J, Elliott S. Global trends and refugee settlement in New Zealand. *Kōtuitui: New Zealand Journal of Social Sciences Online.* 2014; 9(2): 43–9.

29. Guterres A. *High Commissioner's opening remarks; 2010 dialogue on protection gaps and responses.* 2010.

30. Gabaudan M. Blog Post: Confronting the Impacts of Climate Change. Refugees International Web site. http://www.refugeesinternational.org/blog/2016/5/3/climate. Published May 3, 2016. Accessed October 18, 2016.

SECTION 4

The Challenges Faced by Public Health

32

Population Health Science—Are We Doing It Wrong?

IN 2015, THE *New York Times* published an editorial by Nina Teicholz titled "The Government's Bad Diet Advice" [1]. In the piece, Teicholz takes issue with dietary guidelines, many of which are based on nutritional epidemiology studies that have been reconsidered in the 2015 Dietary Guidelines Advisory Committee recommendations [2]. Teicholz suggests that "the primary problem is that nutrition policy has long relied on a very weak kind of science: epidemiological, or 'observational,' studies in which researchers follow large groups of people over many years." I side with Teicholz in her lament. When policies turn out to be wrong, it is a challenge for both politics and public health. I disagree, however, with her diagnosis of the problem. By blaming observational epidemiology for the fruits of bad policy, she is taking a rather narrow view of what is, in fact, a complex set of problems.

Most striking about the article, perhaps, is that Teicholz pointed her finger at our quantitative methods in an op-ed page in a "newspaper of record." Such a prominent placement suggests that the opinion expressed is, to some extent, received wisdom, an expression, indeed, of "the Establishment." How, then, are we to respond to this kind of challenge, one that "calls out" the foundations of our work—the quantitative methods of population health science? More disquietingly, could it be that Teicholz is right, or is she wildly off the mark? Finally, what has brought us to a place where we are seeing such high-profile skepticism of our core methodologies?

There are several approaches to these questions. The easiest might be a reflexive dismissal of Teicholz's comments. More productive, and more difficult, would be to acknowledge them as real and valid concerns and to meet the very public challenge they present. This requires us to both defend the foundational approaches we take in population health science and, at a deeper level, consider what it is we are doing that creates the perception of our work that we see reflected in Teicholz's piece. I suggest that there are five misdirections in population health that contribute, at least in part, to the perception of population health science as being unhelpful in its contributions to an improved health landscape.

A FOCUS ON INDIVIDUAL PREDICTION

As a society, we overwhelmingly prioritize, and invest in, improving individual health [3]. This is reflected in our focus on developing approaches and initiatives to improve the health of the individual [3]. This disproportionate investment is, in some ways, typical of our politics. The challenge of determining spending priorities reflects a larger challenge of resource allocation at the federal level. However, our fascination with individual health is also accompanied by a growing confidence in our capacity to improve and, ultimately, to predict it. That is, of course, the underlying principle behind the dietary recommendations that are targeted by Teicholz, which suggest that if I, the individual, can eat less of X and more of Y, I can improve my health by an appreciable Z increment. This belief is also the foundation of a plethora of risk prediction calculators, starting with the Friedewald formula, which had much to do with putting dietary cholesterol "on the map" [4, 5]. This appetite for prediction has reached a kind of peak in the surge of interest in personalized/precision medicine, a field that stands to shape much of federal health research in the coming decades [6]. The problem with this approach is that our capacity to predict the health of individuals is nowhere near as evolved as the hype would have it. The data that inform risk prediction models come from population-based studies; these data are indeed useful for models fit to population-level inference. However, they fall dramatically short when it comes to individual-level prediction. Although the guidelines are now catching up to this, these limitations have long been recognized. We have known for some time, for example, that although cholesterol intake at the population level is associated with higher cardiovascular disease, knowing someone's cholesterol level does very little to predict whether she will have heart disease or not [7].

What accounts for this limitation? In many ways, it is a mathematical extension of the fact that relative measures of association derived from population-level data have very limited discriminant ability to identify to which population—one with disease, one without—any individual with a particular characteristic belongs [8]. This creates problems for individual prediction. It also explains our frequent failure to provide useful estimates of individual health linked to particular exposures, which is what Teicholz faults us for. The argument could be made, then, for a renewed focus on our methods in order to find better predictive approaches than our current models. I endorse that. But, absent such methods, we need to make sure that we are clear in our own minds about what we are actually able to predict, given our current limitations. We must also take care that our efforts are informed by suitable humility about the the present state of our science and its predictive capacity. In this context, I worry most about the ascent of precision medicine and its dominance of the biomedical research agenda, predicated on an individual prediction focus. Absent an appreciation of our limits on this front, we are, societally, investing in an approach that, although compelling, is not grounded in methods that can deliver on its promise.

WHAT MATTERS AND WHY

During the past 30 years, population health science has been centrally concerned with understanding the association between particular determinants and the health of populations so that we may minimize the influence of these determinants when they cause harm. These efforts have animated the corpus of nutritional epidemiology—the same body of work challenged by Teicholz [9]. A focus on the fundamental causes of health has also informed much of quantitative population health science during the past several decades, yielding many public health successes [9]. It is important to add, however, that this approach has also resulted in a baffling array of suggestions about what may or may not be harmful or helpful to health. For example: is butter good or bad for you? One can find evidence that points in both directions [10, 11]. Does green tea prevent stomach cancer, or does it not [12]? The list of similar questions could go on and on. Why does our science point in so many different directions? Part of the answer rests on the very nature of science itself: We learn through trial and error, moving forward in one direction before realizing we are wrong and correcting ourselves. I also suggest that much of the challenge lies in our methods and approaches.

We owe this particular pickle in no small part to a "risk factor" approach to etiologic thinking in population health science. This approach has arisen as we have, for the past several decades, worked ever harder to isolate the causes of disease in order to intervene. Our efforts in this area have driven our attempts to create ever better methods of controlling extraneous influences so that we may identify and isolate single causes. In doing so, we have drifted away from the recognition that rather than thinking primarily about lone causes, we should be thinking about relative weights of health influencers so that we might take action *where it matters most.*

How do we determine what matters most? The key is context. The import of any given population health factor is dependent as much on that factor itself as it is on the prevalence of those other factors that interact with it. This might not matter very much if we believed that any one cause works in isolation. But, apart from a few rare genetic germline mutations (e.g., cystic fibrosis), vanishingly few causes do so. For our interventions to be most effective, they must therefore take into account not only causes but also the *interplay* of causes and how that interplay shapes population health. This is the perspective that needs to inform our efforts going forward. Recognizing that the causation of complex diseases rests on a complex network of co-occurring causes necessitates an approach that considers these other factors if we are to determine the relative weights to give our actions.

This is particularly resonant in population health science. We are by definition concerned with the determination of the health of populations—a determination that is ineluctably linked to context. If we are to understand what matters most, we must understand how a particular factor matters within the broader context in which it appears. This will require a dramatically different causal inferential approach, as well as a mathematical appreciation of the role of context in the production of population health. It also means that we must better appreciate that there are mathematical limits to how much any single cause can matter. This explains why, for example, the import of butter or fat to individual diet is inconsistent across studies, given that studies vary across contexts. It also suggests why authors such as Teicholz might bemoan the perceived shortcomings of population health science.

THREE ADDITIONAL MISDIRECTIONS

Economists consider fundamental attribution error to be "our tendency to ignore context and attribute an individual's success or failure solely to inherent qualities" [13]. We see this error at work in our daily lives. A parent-friendly example, by way of illustration: When my son's soccer team won a game, he once attributed this success to the fact that he played very well and scored two goals. It was my unfortunate duty to inform him that this was not entirely so. Certainly his performance contributed to his team's victory, yet the team still would not have won had he scored his two goals in isolation. He won because *they* won, and "they" is a more difficult concept to understand than "I."

By way of further illustration, consider popular health books. If you browse any online bookseller for books on health, you will find an array of literature telling you how you can improve your health by exercising more, eating less, and generally taking better care of yourself. All these books are based on the idea that if you behave better, you will be healthier. This lifestyle focus was reflected on an even larger scale by former First Lady Michelle Obama's "Let's Move!" project, which aimed to fight childhood obesity through an emphasis on exercise and nutrition [14].

But would this approach work at the population level? Will encouraging exercise in a population reduce the overall risk of obesity in that population? The perhaps counterintuitive answer is "no." More exercise does not necessarily mean less obesity; indeed, exercise is not particularly relevant to obesity rates at all. It is impossible to predict which populations are going to develop obesity without taking into account the environmental factors that allow the condition to flourish. This underlies the core fundamental attribution error in our society's concept of health. Health is a function of our behavior and our environment. Attention to the latter stands to shift the health of populations, whereas emphasis on the former is less likely to do so. We are likelier to be much more successful attributing health to environments and focusing population health thinking on those factors that shape health in populations [15].

COMPELLING IDEAS, DOUBT, AND CERTITUDE

Population health is a pragmatic science. Our work is motivated by a desire to find actionable solutions to improve the health of populations. It is therefore not surprising that we work hard to identify opportunities for active intervention. We encounter difficulties, however, in the moments when we are swept away by compelling ideas, despite limited evidence. This can lead to us adopt those ideas without due skepticism, investing them with a certitude that is not yet justified by the data.

Nina Teicholz's core argument is with policy decisions that rest on research that does not stand up to scrutiny. Population health, unfortunately, is rife with examples in which this is the case—where compelling ideas push us beyond the scope of our present data and cause us to take positions that do not stand the test of time. As Teicholz's rebuke of the field proves, these episodes of overreach are not cost-free.

I have been engaged around issues similar to the ones raised by Teicholz, principally around the controversy over salt. Starting in the late 1960s, a sometimes furious battle has raged among scientists over the extent to which elevated salt consumption has adverse implications for population health and contributes to deaths from stroke and cardiovascular disease. This conflict has been exacerbated by conflicting results produced by various studies and trials. Despite "the jury being out" on dietary salt and its role in causing disease, public health leaders at local, national, and international levels have pressed the case for salt reduction at the population level. The director of the Centers for Disease Control and Prevention asserted that 100,000 deaths a year could be attributed to excess sodium, and many public health agencies launched efforts to reduce sodium intake in populations [16]. These actions have created the appearance of a consensus where, in fact, none exists. In an article in *Health Affairs*, my colleagues and I explored the development of this controversy [17]. We found that science has invested substantial energy in trying to find an "answer" before the data were able to justify such a conclusion. A subsequent Institute of Medicine report affirmed this observation [18, 19].

I suggest that the salt controversy adds to the body of cases in which we have based policy on compelling, though flawed, ideas. This begs the question: Why do these ideas gain such currency so fast, compelling action? The *Oxford American Dictionary* defines "compelling" as "evoking interest, attention, or admiration in a powerfully irresistible way; not able to be refuted; inspiring conviction" [20]. It is this conviction—and a dash of what can only be called wishful thinking—that gets us into trouble. It would be nice, for example, to believe that by reducing cholesterol in populations, we can reduce cardiovascular disease in these groups. But the fact remains that we probably cannot do so because individual dietary cholesterol is a poor predictor of an individual's likelihood of having heart disease [7].

This has led to our current dilemma about dietary recommendations. The trouble is that, on the surface, the false consensus about the dangers of salt seems to make sense. More than that, it comes off as actionable, leading to public health efforts to lower salt consumption. But if less salt consumption in populations is not associated with better population health (or in fact is potentially associated with *worse* health), then we are tethering ourselves to ideas that are not based on data [21]. This potentially compromises both our standing as population health scientists and our ability to improve the health of populations, our core purpose. To avoid this pitfall, we must insist, always, on a rigorous standard of proof for all ideas, including and especially ones we may consider, on an intuitive level, to be correct. This can be easier said than done. Christopher Martyn notes, "No matter how hard you try to guard against it, there is always a tendency to require a higher standard for evidence that challenges your prejudices than for evidence that supports them" [22]. This suggests that we need to hold ourselves to a higher standard of skepticism about our data, to make sure that we are not propelled by compelling ideas that mislead us, and the public, undermining our credibility and utility.

ATTRIBUTING CAUSES

The fifth misdirection, building on the previous four, rests on our attribution of the production of health to causes we understand and think we can act on. This challenge is as old, perhaps, as public health itself. In a fascinating paper, Christopher Hamlin tells the tale of a mid-19th-century argument between two of the founders of modern public health—Edwin Chadwick and William Farr—about whether starvation was a "cause" of death in England at the time [23]. Farr argued that it was, whereas Chadwick argued that it was not. Chadwick "won," largely because the politics of the time did not allow for the notion that an "advanced" society such as mid-19th-century England could countenance starva-tion killing its citizens. At heart, Chadwick and Farr's arguments were arguments about causal architecture—about the network of causes that influences health—and about which of these causes death can be attributed to. Although I have elsewhere in this chapter talked about causal attribution as a mathematical, perhaps near abstract concern, attribution of causes has real political import. Insofar as politics are about the allocation of resources, we as a society allocate resources to address what we think poses the major threat to our health. If we view heart disease, for example, as an immediate threat, we will likely invest in the study of heart disease. This investment may, in turn, lead to endless studies searching for genes that cause the condition. On the other hand, if we think that the cause of heart disease is smoking, we may invest in the study of smoking. If we think that the cause of heart disease is poverty, we may devote resources to studying and acting on poverty. Clearly, a sophisticated reader recognizes that these causes are all interrelated and are all component causes of heart disease. Despite this reality, policy decisions are often made based on simple and focused approaches, not on complex causal diagrams. This suggests that those of us in population health science need to focus on clearly attributing causes to the factors that mat-ter most while at the same time communicating the importance of context and complexity. How may we best do so? An example of a potential way forward rests in the agenda-setting work of J. Michael McGinnis and William Foege in the mid-1990s—work that suggested that the "actual causes of death" in the United States were behavioral, including such factors as smoking and dietary intake (this work was replicated in the mid-2000s by Ali Mokdad and colleagues) [24]. Our research group's work used these same methods to show, through similar logic, that in the year 2000, approximately 245,000 deaths in the United States were attributable to low education, 176,000 deaths were attributable to racial segregation, 162,000 deaths were attributable to low social support, 133,000 deaths were attributable to individual-level poverty, 119,000 deaths were attributable to income inequality, and 39,000 deaths were attributable to area-level poverty. These numbers are roughly equivalent to the deaths attributed to acute myocardial infarction, stroke, lung cancer, chronic lower respira-tory disease, unintentional injury, and renal failure, respectively. Framed this way, the link between health and the broader social, economic, and environmental context becomes stark and unignorable.

At the end of the day, do these distinctions matter? Does it matter if we think that death is caused by myocardial infarction, smoking, or low income and low education? It cer-tainly does. It determines what we prioritize—how we allocate resources toward what we think must be addressed to keep our society healthy. The Estimates of Funding for Various Research, Condition, and Disease Categories (RCDC) report shows that approximately $320 million was spent by the federal government on "smoking and health" in fiscal year 2014 [25]. Approximately $3.6 billion was spent in the same period on research on "behavioral and social sciences." None of the funded work in the database has the word "income" in the title. It matters, therefore, that we point to a causal attribution that will shift resources in the direction of what matters most to population health. This means promoting policies that are based on evidence that stands to improve the health of populations and deemphasizing ideas that may be compelling but built on shaky data.

CONCLUSION

Let us return to the piece by Nina Teicholz. Unfortunately, Teicholz does little to rise above the fray on the particular issue she engages, concluding essentially that we should go back to "what worked better for previous generations." This suggests that it may be best to simply embrace practices that are based on no data at all. Although this prescription is somewhat simplistic, it does speak to a frustration among the general public with the state of population health scholarship. This frustration is not unreasonable. The points enumerated in this chapter provide plenty of motivation for such feelings, demonstrating the harm that population health misdirections can cause. When our science goes down the wrong path, it risks losing the confidence of the public—confidence that is difficult to earn back. Doing so will require a thoughtful re-examination of our methods and the way we present, and act on, our findings. Going forward, we need to temper our enthusiasm for compelling solutions with the patience necessary to fully investigate them. We need to distinguish between the urgent and the important. This was well expressed by McGinnis and Foege, who argued that "one of [our] most difficult challenges is to ensure that the urgent does not crowd out the important. In health the challenge is especially difficult because urgent matters can be so riveting" [26]. I agree. To improve the health of populations, we must minimize misdirections in order to retain the efficacy of our work and the confidence of the public we serve.

REFERENCES

1. Teicholz N. The government's bad diet advice. *The New York Times*. February 20, 2015. http://www.nytimes.com/2015/02/21/opinion/when-the-government-tells-you-what-to-eat.html?_r=1. Accessed November 1, 2016.

2. 2015 Dietary Guidelines Advisory Committee. Health.gov. https://health.gov/dietaryguidelines/committee/ Accessed November 1, 2016.

3. Bayer R, Galea S. Public health in the precision-medicine era. *The New England Journal of Medicine*. 2015; 373(6): 499–501. doi:10.1056/NEJMp1506241

4. New Online Calculator Estimates Cardiovascular Disease Risk. Harvard T.H. Chan School of Public Health Web site. https://www.hsph.harvard.edu/news/press-releases/new-online-calculator-estimates-cardiovascular-disease-risk. Accessed November 1, 2016.

5. Martin SS, et al. Comparison of a novel method vs. the Friedewald equation for estimating low-density lipoprotein cholesterol levels from the standard lipid profile. *JAMA: The Journal of the American Medical Association*. 2013; 310(19): 2061–8. doi:10.1001/jama.2013.280532

6. Collins FS, Varmus H. A new initiative on precision medicine. *The New England Journal of Medicine*. 2015; 372(9): 793–5. doi:10.1056/NEJMp1500523

7. Rose G. Sick individuals and sick populations. *International Journal of Epidemiology*. 1985; 14(1): 32–8.

8. Pepe MS, Janes H, Longton G, Leisenring W, Newcomb P. Limitations of the odds ratio in gauging the performance of a diagnostic, prognostic, or screening marker. *American Journal of Epidemiology*. 2004; 159(9): 882–90.

9. Domestic Public Health Achievements Team, CDC. Koppaka R. Ten great public health achievements—United States, 2001–2010. *Morbidity and Mortality Weekly Report (MMWR)*. 2011; 60(19): 619–23.

10. Kromhout D, Geleijnse JM, Menotti A, Jacobs DR Jr. The confusion about dietary fatty acids recommendations for CHD prevention. *British Journal of Nutrition*. 2011; 106(5): 627–32. doi:10.1017/S0007114511002236

11. Chowdhury R, et al. Association of dietary, circulating, and supplement fatty acids with coronary risk: A systematic review and meta-analysis. *Annals of Internal Medicine*. 2014; 160(6): 398–406. doi:10.7326/M13-1788

12. Hamajima N, et al. Tea polyphenol intake and changes in serum pepsinogen levels. *Japanese Journal of Cancer Research*. 1999; 90(2): 136–43.

13. Surowiecki J. The turnaround trap. *The New Yorker*. March 25, 2013. http://www.newyorker.com/magazine/2013/03/25/the-turnaround-trap. Accessed November 1, 2016.

14. Let's Move! Web site. http://www.letsmove.gov. Accessed November 1, 2016.

15. Keyes KM, Smith GD, Koenen KC, Galea S. The mathematical limits of genetic prediction for complex chronic disease. *Journal of Epidemiology and Community Health*. 2015; 69(6): 574–9. doi:10.1136/jech-2014-204983

16. Frieden TR, Briss PA. We can reduce dietary sodium, save money, and save lives. *Annals of Internal Medicine*. 2010; 152(8): 526–7, W182. doi:10.7326/0003-4819-152-8-201004200-00214

17. Bayer R, Johns DM, Galea S. Salt and public health: Contested science and the challenge of evidence-based decision making. *Health Affairs*. 2012; 31(12): 2738–46. doi:10.1377/hlthaff.2012.0554

18. Institute of Medicine. *Sodium intake in populations: Assessment of evidence*. Washington, DC: The National Academies Press; 2013.

19. Johns DM, Bayer R, Galea S. Controversial salt report peppered with uncertainty. *Science*. 2013; 341(6150): 1063–4. doi:10.1126/science.341.6150.1063

20. Stevenson A, Lindberg CA, eds. *New Oxford American Dictionary* (3rd ed.). New York, NY: Oxford University Press; 2010.

21. Jürgens G, Graudal NA. Effects of low sodium diet versus high sodium diet on blood pressure, renin, aldosterone, catecholamines, cholesterols, and triglyceride. *Cochrane Database of Systematic Reviews*. 2003; (1): CD004022.

22. Martyn C. Politics as a determinant of health. *The BMJ*. 2004; 329(7480): 1423–4.

23. Hamlin C. Could you starve to death in England in 1839? The Chadwick–Farr controversy and the loss of the "social" in public health. *American Journal of Public Health*. 1995; 85(6): 856–66.

24. Mokdad AH, Marks JS, Stroup DF, Gerberding JL. Actual causes of death in the United States, 2000. *JAMA: The Journal of the American Medical Association*. 2004; 291(10): 1238–45. doi:10.1001/jama.291.10.1238

25. Estimates of Funding for Various Research, Condition, and Disease Categories (RCDC). NIH Research Portfolio Online Reporting Tools (RePORT) Web site. https://report.nih.gov/categorical_spending.aspx. Published February 10, 2016. Accessed November 1, 2016.

26. McGinnis JM, Foege WH. The immediate vs. the important. *JAMA: The Journal of the American Medical Association*. 2004; 291(10): 1263–4.

33

To Screen, or Not to Screen

THE GOAL OF public health has historically been to prevent disease and promote health. Given this objective, screening, with its ability to detect early markers of pathology and prevent disease, stands to be a great asset to our work. However, the promise of screening rests on the core concept that underlies it: that we can detect pathology early, so that we may alter the progression of disease. The reliability of this premise, however, is not unshakable, particularly in the case of pathologies we do not yet fully understand, making it less clear how effectively screening can safeguard population health.

In October 2015, *Time* magazine ran a cover story, "Why Doctors Are Rethinking Breast Cancer Treatment" [1]. The patient at the center of this story, Desiree Basila, was diagnosed with ductal carcinoma in situ (DCIS) at age 52 years [2]. Her surgeon asked her what she wanted to do about the 5-cm-long, 2.5-cm-wide tumor found in her right breast and told her a slot for a mastectomy was open the following week. She responded, "What if I just do nothing?" At the time of her diagnosis, nearly a decade ago, Desiree, by choosing hormone therapy and close surveillance over surgery, was making an unorthodox choice. Now, however, her decision appears to be empirically supported. Recent epidemiologic data on breast cancer screening and survival rates in women suggest that overdiagnosis represents one-fourth to one-third of cases identified [3, 4]. Overdiagnosis, in this case, may be defined as the identification of tumors that would not actually have led to clinical symptoms. Indeed, a diagnosis of DCIS has been associated with a 3.3 percent mortality rate, comparable to the mortality rate from breast cancer in the general population [5, 6]. Among those who received lumpectomy, radiotherapy was not associated with breast cancer-specific mortality at 10 years, which suggests that the procedure may not be as beneficial as popularly assumed. As stated in a *JAMA Oncology* editorial, "Given the low breast cancer mortality risk, we should stop telling women that DCIS is an emergency and that they should schedule definitive surgery within 2 weeks of diagnosis" [6].

The emerging evidence that suggests we should rethink our understanding of DCIS is mirrored by new findings casting doubt on the benefits of mammography itself.

According to a large-scale US study, since the introduction of breast cancer screening mammography more than 30 years ago, the rate of early stage detection has doubled (112 to 234 cases per 100,000), whereas the rate of late-stage identification has decreased by only 8 percent (102 to 94 cases per 100,000) [4]. The authors of the study suggest that in 2008, overdiagnosis accounted for 70,000 cases, or 31 percent of all breast cancers diagnosed; they estimate that 1.3 million US women have been overdiagnosed in the past 39 years. Published at approximately the same time, an independent UK review on breast cancer came to similar conclusions, estimating that for each prevented breast cancer case, three cases are overdiagnosed [3]. These data clearly suggest limitations in our use of screening to detect disease early enough to intervene and that screening may even result in more harm, rather than less. Why is this?

SCREENING, CUT-OFFS, AND THE HEART OF THE TRADE-OFF

Screening procedures such as mammography are the process of using a test or set of tests to determine whether an individual likely has, or will likely develop, a given disease or health indicator [7]. These tests are based on prior data produced by comparisons of a screening tool against a gold-standard measure. Broadly speaking, screening measures aim to maximize sensitivity and specificity [8]. Critically, the cut-off choice for a given measure depends on a value judgment regarding the cost of false positives versus false negatives. In the case of HIV, for example, favoring sensitivity (i.e., minimizing false negatives) over specificity (i.e., minimizing false positives) is a good strategy given the transmissibility of the disease. Conversely, if the follow-up procedures and treatments are highly expensive and invasive, as in the case of Pap smears for cervical cancer, a higher false-negative rate may be permissible. It is important to note that sensitivity and specificity are characteristics of a test in a particular context. In the case of breast cancer, mammography is frequently a highly sensitive procedure, readily detecting breast tissue irregularities, but has limited specificity—it is quite poor at identifying whether these irregularities represent genuine pathology. This can result in significant overdiagnosis, which can create challenges. By detecting irregularities that would, if left untouched, do no harm, screening can lead to further testing, with the costs and risks falling on patients.

WHY CONTEXT MATTERS: HOW POPULATION PREVALENCE DETERMINES THE UTILITY OF A TEST

Another way to understand screening test performance is through positive predictive value (PPV) and negative predictive value (NPV). In contrast to sensitivity and specificity, PPV and NPV are characteristics that pertain to individuals. PPV is the probability of truly having a disease after screening positive, whereas NPV is the probability of truly not having a disease after screening negative. As the prevalence of a given health indicator increases, PPV rises; as the prevalence declines, PPV drops, even as sensitivity and specificity remain stable.

In the case of breast cancer, the relatively low prevalence of the condition among 40- to 49-year-old women, and the accompanying low PPV, has helped drive the argument that mammography screening should be implemented at age 50 years and not at age 40 years. The case that the frequency of false positives among this age group cannot justify the risks of testing was among those made in the controversial 2009 US Preventive Services Task Force recommendation statement on breast cancer screening; notably, this recommendation was not extended to women with a family history of breast cancer, who have a higher prevalence than those without such history [9].

FIRST DO NO HARM: THE UNINTENDED CONSEQUENCES OF UNNECESSARY SCREENING

Given the uncertainty of the procedure, why screen, and when? My colleague and I cover this topic in our textbook, *Epidemiology Matters*, in which we note that screening measures should be implemented when the health indicator in question is "an important determinant of population health"; when "it can be detected before signs and symptoms appear"; and when the process of screening, early detection, and treatment results in improvements in morbidity or mortality at the level of populations [7]. Pap smear for cervical cancer is one example of a screening test that meets all these criteria, whereas breast cancer screening illustrates an area in which such tests may be less beneficial. Although breast cancer remains an important determinant of population health, and may indeed be detected before signs and symptoms of the disease appear, it is not clear among certain subgroups of women that early detection and treatment result in improvements in morbidity and mortality among populations. Simply stated, we should only screen when screening can make a difference. We should not screen when doing so will likely not alter the course of a disease in populations. To screen under these circumstances would be to introduce the risk of substantial false positives, including attendant morbidity and potentially iatrogenic mortality. This rationale was well expressed by Biller-Andorno and Jüni, who stated, "From an ethical perspective, a public health program that does not clearly produce more benefits than harms is hard to justify" [10].

Screening is a sensitive issue, and an argument against screening in all cases can be a difficult one to make. Such tests, after all, appear to be a compelling social good. In addition, the endorsement of these procedures by celebrities has further increased widespread acceptance of across-the-board screening. This has led to phenomena such as "the Katie Couric effect," which came about when the celebrity journalist's endorsement of colonoscopies led to a temporary increase in colonoscopy rates [11].

In some ways, it is far easier to argue that "everyone should get screened" for any number of diseases. We hear this argument not infrequently, particularly when it is in favor of testing for breast and prostate cancer. Unfortunately, screening for these diseases runs the risk of false positives and negatives; this is caused by the limitations of the tests themselves. We should therefore weigh the potential effects of both of these outcomes before recommending screening for particular populations, and we should reconsider generalizations about screening in all cases. Going forward, it is important for us to accept that we simply do not know enough about whether to screen or not at some ages and in the case of certain diseases.

This strikes me as a suitably humble approach to data—one that is reflective of the need to embrace complexity in our attitude to screening and its potential to improve population health while first doing no harm.

REFERENCES

1. O'Connor S. Why doctors are rethinking breast-cancer treatment. *TIME*. October 1, 2015. http://time.com/4057310/breast-cancer-overtreatment. Accessed November 1, 2016.

2. NCI Dictionary of Cancer Terms: Ductal Carcinoma in Situ (definition). National Cancer Institute Web site. https://www.cancer.gov/publications/dictionaries/cancer-terms?cdrid=45674. Accessed November 1, 2016.

3. Independent UK Panel on Breast Cancer Screening. The benefits and harms of breast cancer screening: An independent review. *The Lancet*. 2012; 380(9855): 1778-86. doi:10.1016/S0140-6736(12)61611-0

4. Bleyer A, Welch HG. Effect of three decades of screening mammography on breast-cancer incidence. *The New England Journal of Medicine*. 2012; 367(21): 1998-2005. doi:10.1056/NEJMoa1206809

5. Narod SA, Iqbal J, Giannakeas V, Sopik V, Sun P. Breast cancer mortality after a diagnosis of ductal carcinoma in situ. *JAMA Oncology*. 2015; 1(7): 888-96. doi:10.1001/jamaoncol.2015.2510

6. Esserman L, Yau C. Rethinking the standard for ductal carcinoma in situ treatment. *JAMA Oncology*. 2015; 1(7):881-3. doi:10.1001/jamaoncol.2015.2607

7. Keyes KM, Galea S. *Epidemiology Matters: A New Introduction to Methodological Foundations*. New York, NY: Oxford University Press; 2014.

8. Fletcher RH, Fletcher SW, Fletcher GS. *Clinical Epidemiology: The Essentials* (5th Edition). Baltimore, MD: Lippincott Williams & Wilkins; 2014.

9. US Preventive Services Task Force. Screening for breast cancer: US Preventive Services Task Force recommendation statement. *Annals of Internal Medicine*. 2009; 151(10): 716-26, W-236. doi:10.7326/0003-4819-151-10-200911170-00008

10. Biller-Andorno N, Jüni P. Abolishing mammography screening programs? A view from the Swiss Medical Board. *The New England Journal of Medicine*. 2014; 370(21): 1965-67. doi:10.1056/NEJMp1401875

11. Cram P, et al. The impact of a celebrity promotional campaign on the use of colon cancer screening: The Katie Couric effect. *Archives of Internal Medicine*. 2003; 163(13): 1601-5.

34

Knowledge and Values

THE CHALLENGES THAT undermine population health can often seem immutable. Obesity rates rise. The opioid epidemic rages. And tens of thousands of people are killed every year by guns [1, 2, 3]. Why is this the case? There are many reasons. Data are unclear, or clear data are ignored; policies are proposed and then rejected or overturned; and "ideological walls" make solutions difficult to come by. With this in mind, it is not unreasonable for us to sometimes question why we do what we do or to be frustrated by the deaf ears on which our findings sometimes fall. Why, then, is the gap between science and action so wide? Why does science not result in clearer action, particularly when the way forward is often so well supported by the data?

The central challenge of the evidence-to-practice gap rests, to my mind, around the intersection of two areas: our knowledge and our values—that is, what we know and what we hold to be important. Our knowledge anchors our aspirations in the realm of the possible—what we can appreciably *do* at a given time, informed by what we know. Our values shape the direction we would like to move toward as a community, the issues we would like to advance, and, indeed, our priorities. It is important to note that it is not always necessary that our knowledge and our values intersect in order to produce effective action. We are certainly able to act, and to succeed, without full knowledge; likewise, we have sometimes acted with imperfect knowledge when we have felt that the occasion required it. However, I argue that public health is at its strongest when we provide data that point to clarity of action, while also working to create a social context that is welcoming of these data.

To begin, I present some thoughts on the nature of knowledge. How do we generate knowledge? What does it really mean to "know" something? These questions fall within the realm of epistemology—the study of knowledge [4]. A traditional epistemological approach holds that there are three components to knowledge: truth, belief, and justification [4].

"Truth" simply means that something must be true for it to be considered genuine knowledge. This was famously expressed by Aristotle in his *Metaphysics*:

> To say of something which is that it is not, or to say of something which is not that it is, is false. However, to say of something which is that it is, or of something which is not that it is not, is true. [5, 6]

Compared to this somewhat oblique formulation, the importance of "belief" is fairly straightforward, as it would be contradictory to claim to both know something and not believe in it [7]. "Justification" is less clear-cut. In Plato's *Theaetetus*, Socrates considers that knowledge might be defined as "true belief with an account" [8]. This suggests that knowledge is not merely belief in a true proposition but, rather, true belief that is supported by some sort of evidence—true belief that has been properly accounted for. This process of justification, of accounting for what we believe to be true, is a key function of academic public health. To say that we "know" something, within the context of our field, is the result of countless hours of research, writing, and debate. The scientific method and the rigor of peer review exist to provide a framework for this work of justification. This process is neither simple nor quick. Yet for us to call "knowledge" what may have started as an idea, a hunch, means we must engage with each step along the road from supposition to proof to, ultimately, consensus around a given issue.

Then there is the matter of values. Values are what we choose to focus on, in a world of limited time and resources. This choice is both necessary—we must set priorities if we are to get anything done—and deeply revealing. Indeed, the philosopher José Ortega y Gasset once wrote, "Tell me to what you pay attention and I will tell you who you are" [9]. The branch of ethics that assigns moral value to actions is called *normative ethics* [10]. Normative ethics puts forth three types of ethical theories to inform action: virtue, deontology, and consequentialism [10]. The first, virtue ethics, is concerned with the moral character of the person or people performing an action—that is, are they good people acting in good faith? Within this framework, an ethical action does not necessarily have to produce positive results, as long as it is performed by virtuous people. Deontology is concerned with the action itself—that is, is it the right step to take? Is it being performed correctly? Under this system, intrinsically bad actions should be avoided, even if these actions may lead to positive results. Consequentialism is concerned with outcomes—that is, what did this action, in the end, actually do? In all of these cases, values are defined by their relationship to what we do. I have argued in other writings that consequentialism should play a role in informing population health science. That is because I see consequentialism as speaking to a fundamental truth about values—that they tend to catalyze action [11]. When we genuinely care about something, it is difficult to remain a spectator, or to simply accumulate knowledge for its own sake. Our values push us to mobilize what we know, in pursuit of healthier populations.

To illustrate the intersection, and occasional gulf, between our knowledge and our values, I propose a two-by-two grid (Figure 34.1) inspired by Donald Stokes and his Pasteur's quadrant, which I cited in Chapter 5 [12].

Represented at the top right of the table shown in Figure 34.1 are issues for which we know what to do—for which public consensus, informed by values, is aligned with a definite course of action. At the bottom left, we encounter cases for which the way forward is more

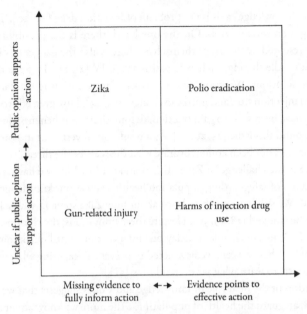

FIGURE 34.1 X axis represents the degree of evidence informing a particular action; y axis represents the degree to which public opinion supports a particular action.

ambiguous—for which our data are incomplete and our actions not yet bolstered by public opinion. In between fall cases for which we may have a value-informed consensus on the need for action but not yet enough data to inform that action and, vice versa, for which we have sufficient data but no clear mandate from the public to support our efforts. To illustrate this framework, consider the following four examples.

At the confluence of knowledge and values is the worldwide fight against polio in the 20th century. Today, polio is on the brink of global eradication [13]. This achievement is due to a combination of good data, well-tested methods, and the values-driven decision of governments and public health professionals to prioritize putting an end to this disease [13]. Humanity's long history with polio, and the game-changing development of a vaccine, has placed public health efforts against the disease in the strongest possible position [14, 15]. These efforts have been helped by a coming together of governments and nongovernmental organizations, which have mobilized resources in order to wipe out polio. Even better, the aims of the scientific community have dovetailed with the will of the public, further supporting this work.

Opposite the example of polio is that of gun-related injury. Gun violence is a clear public health threat. In 2016, there were more than 8,000 gun deaths and more than 17,000 gun-related injuries in the United States [16]. Unfortunately, our efforts to reduce these numbers are not yet supported by all the necessary data. Interest group success at blocking federal funding for gun violence research means that we do not yet know everything we should about the epidemiology of this problem, hindering our progress on this issue [17, 18]. The gun lobby has also succeeded at generating support by framing its case as a matter of values, whereas our efforts, although certainly motivated by our values, have been hindered by a lack of broad, organized public backing [19].

Closer to the "knowledge" axis is the problem of injection drug use [20]. This issue poses health challenges on several levels. On the one hand, there is the possibility of addiction and overdose presented by the drugs themselves; there is also the danger of diseases that are associated with needle sharing, such as hepatitis and HIV [21, 22]. Large as these problems loom, there are solutions. We know that the risks of injection drug use can be mitigated with supervised injection sites and needle exchanges [23, 24]. However, efforts to implement these measures have been slow to gain traction, despite their clear benefits, due largely to the social stigma around this issue [25, 26, 27]. As a result, our investment in potentially lifesaving interventions has not been commensurate with the scale of the threat.

Finally, there is the challenge of Zika. This is an area in which we have had to act decisively on our values of safeguarding population health, even as our knowledge of the disease remains limited. We still have much to learn about how Zika spreads, where it comes from, and how it can be stopped [28, 29, 30]. Despite these limitations, the risk posed by the virus means that we have not been able to delay our interventions until our knowledge is more fully formed [31]. As best we can, we have acted to prevent Zika, using what we know, while working assiduously to learn what we do not know [32].

An appreciation of the dual role of knowledge and values suggests that we need to work on both axes to safeguard the health of populations. The more we know about a problem, the more options we are able to apply toward solving it. Yet this knowledge is unlikely to result in action without a broad, value-informed consensus around the need for movement on a given issue. For our work to be at its most effective, it should aspire toward a balance of knowledge and values, proceeding on the basis of good data and an informed, supportive public.

REFERENCES

1. Griffin RM. Obesity epidemic "astronomical." WebMD Web site. http://www.webmd.com/diet/obesity/features/obesity-epidemic-astronomical#1. Accessed November 2, 2016.

2. Wade L. How America is battling its horrific opioid epidemic. *Wired*. October 3, 2016. https://www.wired.com/2016/10/america-battling-horrific-opioid-epidemic. Accessed November 2, 2016.

3. Key Gun Violence Statistics. Brady Campaign to Prevent Gun Violence Web site. http://www.bradycampaign.org/key-gun-violence-statistics. Accessed November 2, 2016.

4. The Analysis of Knowledge. Stanford Encyclopedia of Philosophy Web site. http://plato.stanford.edu/entries/knowledge-analysis/#BelCon. Updated November 15, 2012. Accessed November 2, 2016.

5. Epistemology definition. AskDefine Web site. http://epistemology.askdefinebeta.com. Accessed November 2, 2016.

6. Truth (Aristotle). The Logic Museum Web site. http://www.logicmuseum.com/wiki/Truth_%28Aristotle%29. Updated April 11, 2016. Accessed November 2, 2016.

7. Epistemology. The Basics of Philosophy Web site. http://www.philosophybasics.com/branch_epistemology.html. Accessed November 2, 2016.

8. Plato on Knowledge in the *Theaetetus*. Stanford Encyclopedia of Philosophy Web site. http://plato.stanford.edu/entries/plato-theaetetus. Accessed November 2, 2016.

9. José Ortega y Gasset. Wikiquote Web site. https://en.wikiquote.org/wiki/Jos%C3%A9_Ortega_y_Gasset#Man_and_Crisis_.281962.29. Updated October 4, 2016. Accessed November 2, 2016.

10. Normative Ethics. Moral Philosophy Web site. http://moralphilosophy.info/normative-ethics. Accessed November 2, 2016.

11. Galea S. An argument for a consequentialist epidemiology. *American Journal of Epidemiology.* 2013; 178(8): 1185-91. doi:10.1093/aje/kwt172

12. Stokes DE. *Pasteur's Quadrant: Basic Science and Technological Innovation.* Washington, DC: Brookings Institution; 1997.

13. Crowley P. Polio on the brink of eradication. *Devex.* October 27, 2015. https://www.devex.com/news/polio-on-the-brink-of-eradication-87156. Accessed November 2, 2016.

14. History of Polio (Poliomyelitis). The History of Vaccines Web site. http://www.historyofvaccines.org/content/articles/history-polio-poliomyelitis. Accessed November 2, 2016.

15. A Science Odyssey: Salk Produces Polio Vaccine 1952. Public Broadcasting Service Web site. http://www.pbs.org/wgbh/aso/databank/entries/dm52sa.html. Accessed November 2, 2016.

16. Galea S. Getting smarter about guns, one state at a time. *The Boston Globe.* August 9, 2016. https://www.bostonglobe.com/opinion/2016/08/09/getting-smarter-about-guns-one-state-time/68YctBIyldI9zDOo2lIxeO/story.html. Accessed November 2, 2016.

17. Galea S. Too many dead: The need to reframe gun violence as a public health issue. *WBUR.* June 3, 2016. http://www.wbur.org/cognoscenti/2016/06/03/gun-violence-as-a-public-health-issue-sandro-galea. Accessed November 2, 2016

18. Foran C. The missing data on gun violence. *The Atlantic.* January 21, 2016. http://www.theatlantic.com/politics/archive/2016/01/gun-control-laws-research/424956. Accessed November 2, 2016

19. Second Amendment. National Rifle Association Institute for Legislative Action Web site. https://www.nraila.org/second-amendment. Accessed November 2, 2016

20. Persons Who Use Drugs (PWUD). Centers for Disease Control and Prevention Web site. http://www.cdc.gov/pwud. Updated April 27, 2016. Accessed November 2, 2016.

21. Viral Hepatitis—CDC Recommendations for Specific Populations and Settings. Centers for Disease Control and Prevention Web site. http://www.cdc.gov/hepatitis/populations/idu.htm. Updated March 29, 2016. Accessed November 2, 2016.

22. People Who Inject Drugs, HIV and AIDS. AVERT Web site. http://www.avert.org/professionals/hiv-social-issues/key-affected-populations/people-inject-drugs. Updated October 20, 2016. Accessed November 2, 2016.

23. Zielinski A. Could heroin injection sites revolutionize the drug addiction crisis? *ThinkProgress.* March 15, 2016. https://thinkprogress.org/could-heroin-injection-sites-revolutionize-the-drug-addiction-crisis-b79d0fe7c62f#.04creh863. Accessed November 2, 2016.

24. D Vlahov, B Junge. The role of needle exchange programs in HIV prevention. *Public Health Reports.* 1998; 113(Suppl 1): 75–80.

25. Almendrala A. Needle exchanges are vital, but there's a major stigma around them. Here's why. *The Huffington Post.* March 27, 2015. http://www.huffingtonpost.com/2015/03/27/needle-exchanges-indiana_n_6949734.html. Accessed November 2, 2016.

26. Morris M. A controversial response to heroin epidemic: Supervised injections. *US News & World Report.* April 20, 2016. http://www.usnews.com/news/articles/

2016-04-20/a-controversial-response-to-heroin-epidemic-supervised-injections. Accessed November 2, 2016.

27. Foderaro LW. Ithaca's anti-heroin plan: Open a site to shoot heroin. *The New York Times*. http://www.nytimes.com/2016/03/23/nyregion/fighting-heroin-ithaca-looks-to-injection-centers.html?_r=0. Accessed November 2, 2016.

28. Maron DF. Zika mystery case raises questions about new transmission route. *Scientific American*. July 18, 2016. https://www.scientificamerican.com/article/zika-mystery-case-raises-questions-about-new-transmission-route. Accessed November 2, 2016.

29. Wright C. Even in the place where Zika virus was first discovered, its true origin is a mystery. *Quartz*. May 5, 2016. http://qz.com/635161/even-in-the-place-where-zika-virus-was-first-discovered-its-true-origin-is-a-mystery. Accessed November 2, 2016.

30. Mukherjee S. The government just launched its first Zika vaccine trial in humans. *Fortune*. August 3, 2016. http://fortune.com/2016/08/03/nih-launches-zika-vaccine-trial. Accessed November 2, 2016.

31. Herrera C, Dahlberg N, Nehamas N. Zika takes bite out of Miami–Dade economy—How bad will it get? *Miami Herald*. September 9, 2016. http://www.miamiherald.com/news/business/tourism-cruises/article100848577.html. Accessed November 2, 2016.

32. Zika Virus: Prevention. Centers for Disease Control and Prevention Web site. https://www.cdc.gov/zika/prevention. Updated August 31, 2016. Accessed November 2, 2016.

35

A Step Backwards on Vaccines

BY THE END of January 2015, there were 102 measles cases reported in the United States [1]. This figure is striking, in that it exceeded the yearly measles totals for nine of the proceeding 14 years [1]. These cases were reported in 14 states, mostly arising as a result of a December 2014 outbreak at Disneyland/Disney California Adventure Park. Secondary cases were also reported as part of this ongoing outbreak, and the California Department of Public Health noted that infectious cases visited Disney theme parks in January 2015 [2]. It is important to note that most of the people who contracted measles during this outbreak were reportedly unvaccinated.

It was somewhat strange to hear of so many measles cases in the United States—the disease had been declared eliminated in this country in 2000 [3]. This is not to say, of course, that it never appears here. Given that measles is still endemic throughout the world, travelers may bring the disease into the United States and transmit it among pockets of communities that are unvaccinated or undervaccinated [3]. The initial source of the 2015 outbreak is unclear, but as of January 29, 2015, the Centers for Disease Control and Prevention (CDC) reported that links to travel history in Dubai, India, and Indonesia were being investigated [4]. The 2015 outbreak was not the only recent case in which measles has recrudesced in the United States. In 2014, there was an enormous uptick in the incidence of the disease, with the largest outbreak (383 cases) occurring among unvaccinated Amish communities in Ohio [1]. Overall, in 2014, 644 cases of measles were reported, approximately seven times the mean number reported between 2001 and 2013 (89 cases) and approximately three times as many as were reported in 2011 (220 cases), which had the next highest number of annual cases during that period. Many of the 2014 cases were thought to be associated with a large outbreak in the Philippines [1]. Again, the common denominator between many of these US cases appears to be a lack of vaccination.

SORTING THROUGH THE NOISE

The outbreak traced to Disneyland parks in California sparked a number of news stories on measles, vaccines, and the now roundly discredited "link" between the measles, mumps, and rubella (MMR) vaccine and autism. Concerns continued to mount in the days after the disease appeared. As the Super Bowl approached, public health officials in Arizona were wary of a potential outbreak [5]. Arizona's Department of Health Services' Director Will Humble was quoted as saying, "This is a critical point in this outbreak. If the public health system and medical community are able to identify every single susceptible case and get them into isolation, we have a chance of stopping this outbreak here." Amid these worries, focus, and no small measure of opprobrium, was directed at parents who chose not to vaccinate their children. *USA Today* published an editorial on January 28 titled "Jail 'anti-vax' parents," and the satirical website *The Onion* published a piece titled "I Don't Vaccinate My Child Because It's My Right to Decide What Eliminated Diseases Come Roaring Back" [6, 7]. As covered by ABC News, infectious disease experts suggested that "for measles to become permanent—that is, become 'endemic'—again to the US, measles immunizations would have to drop below 90 percent" [8]. Hovering close to that threshold, the rate of measles immunization in the United States in 2013 was estimated to be 91 percent by the World Health Organization [9]. This is a worrying development.

The rise in the number of children not being vaccinated is, in some ways, difficult to understand, given the amply demonstrated health benefits of vaccination. Indeed, justifications for the choice not to vaccinate can sometimes be contradictory and not always in line with available evidence. An interview with Dan Olmstead, editor of the website Age of Autism, "the Daily Web Newspaper of the Autism Epidemic," is illuminating on this point [10, 11]. The expressed purpose of the site is "to give voice to those who believe autism is an environmentally induced illness," but much of the site's content is dedicated to the—again, roundly discredited—association between the MMR vaccine and autism. This internal incoherence is typical of the scientifically unsound basis on which the anti-vaccine argument often rests. The belief that the MMR vaccine causes autism stems from a now retracted article in *The Lancet* by Andrew Wakefield, and it persists despite a formal retraction grounded in evidence of academic dishonesty, financial conflicts of interest, and non-replicability [12]. The anti-vaccine cause, however, was given a boost in recent years with the release of recorded conversations with a CDC researcher named William Thompson, in which he states that a 2004 article published by CDC authors withheld the finding of a positive association between MMR vaccine timing and autism in a subgroup of African American boys [13, 14]. The recordings were released by Brian S. Hooker, who also published a reanalysis of the data used in the 2004 CDC study, which reported the very subgroup finding that Thompson said was suppressed [15]. The Hooker article has since been retracted by the editors due to "undeclared competing interests" and "concerns about the validity of the methods and statistical analysis" [16]. Despite all of this, the belief that the MMR vaccine causes autism persists in the face of an ever-growing mountain of evidence to the contrary [17]. How are we to account for this phenomenon? In a sense, it falls into the category of what Paul Krugman calls "zombie ideas"—"policy ideas that keep being killed by evidence, but nonetheless shamble relentlessly forward, essentially because they suit a political agenda" [18]. Interestingly, findings from a 2014 study suggest that current public health communication strategies aimed at decreasing vaccine misperceptions and increasing intent to vaccinate may not only be ineffective but also be counterproductive [19].

THE PUBLIC HEALTH RESPONSE

The stubbornness of anti-vaccine arguments—their persistence in the face of the data—brings those of us in public health to an odd impasse. Simply stated, what are we to do when evidence does not change people's minds? How are we to contend with scientifically unfounded claims that, nevertheless, will not go away? Three core observations emerge that suggest lessons that can be learned from the measles outbreak and subsequent vaccination debate.

First, general public understanding of health is frequently limited and can be ill-informed. This creates an opportunity for false ideas to take hold, particularly if they are grounded in seemingly compelling notions (i.e., vaccines may precede autism) or if they are touted by apparently credentialed experts (i.e., CDC scientists). This speaks to an unfortunate lack of health literacy among the US population. Although early universal education in primary and secondary schools has, in recent years, promoted an understanding of individual health, there is no comparable educational effort that encompasses the work of public health. This creates knowledge gaps around the production of health in populations—gaps that can then be filled with all manner of bad science or half-baked argument.

Second, there is the challenge of the Internet. Although the growing democratization of digital information has brought many positive changes, much of this information is chaotic and, frankly, not particularly informative, beyond providing a ready sound bite or a compelling data point (which may or may not be based on solid evidence). Rather than illuminate understanding, such "information" will, more often than not, only obscure it, muddying the waters of constructive discourse.

Finally, we come to the role of academic public health in this debate. We have, it seems to me, a central role to play, both in educating the public about the actual causes of health and disease in populations and in ensuring that people are able to recognize a bad argument when they hear or read one. It has long been canonical in schools of medicine that a role of the physician is to educate the patient about her health. Public health is concerned with the health of populations; our concern is therefore the education of the public. If we do not educate the populations we serve, many far less qualified individuals are clearly ready to do so in our stead. More than providing a counterbalance to their efforts, we must be persistent, clear, and, at times, forceful to ensure that no false equivalence is ever maintained between fact and factual-seeming fiction.

REFERENCES

1. Measles Cases and Outbreaks. Centers for Disease Control and Prevention Web site. http://www.cdc.gov/measles/cases-outbreaks.html. Updated October 18, 2016. Accessed November 3, 2016.

2. California Department of Public Health Confirms 59 Cases of Measles. California Department of Public Health Web site. http://www.cdph.ca.gov/Pages/NR15-008.aspx. Accessed November 3, 2016.

3. Frequently Asked Questions About Measles in the US. Centers for Disease Control and Prevention Web site. http://www.cdc.gov/measles/about/faqs.html#measles-elimination. Updated June 17, 2016. Accessed November 3, 2016.

4. Transcript for CDC Telebriefing: Measles in the United States, 2015. Centers for Disease Control and Prevention Web site. http://www.cdc.gov/media/releases/2015/t0129-measles-in-us.html. Updated January 29, 2015. Accessed November 3, 2016.

5. Mohney G. Super Bowl 2015: Officials on alert for measles during big game. *ABC News.* January 30, 2015. http://abcnews.go.com/Health/super-bowl-2015-officials-alert-measles-big-game/story?id=28605315. Accessed November 3, 2016.

6. Berezow A. Jail "anti-vax" parents: Column. *USA Today.* January 28, 2015. http://www.usatoday.com/story/opinion/2015/01/27/jail-anti-vax-parents-vaccines-cdc-measles-disney-world-california-column/22420771. Accessed November 3, 2016.

7. Martin A. I don't vaccinate my child because it's my right to decide what eliminated diseases come roaring back. *The Onion.* January 23, 2015. http://www.theonion.com/blogpost/i-dont-vaccinate-my-child-because-its-my-right-to--37839. Accessed November 3, 2016.

8. Mohney G. What would it take for measles to return permanently to the US. *ABC News.* February 4, 2015. http://abcnews.go.com/Health/measles-return-permanently-us/story?id=28699739. Accessed November 3, 2016.

9. Immunization Surveillance, Assessment and Monitoring. World Health Organization Global Health Observatory Map Gallery Web site. http://gamapserver.who.int/gho/interactive_charts/immunization/mcv/atlas.html. Accessed November 3, 2016.

10. Lopez G. Understanding the fear of vaccines: An activist explains why he buys a debunked idea. *Vox.* February 4, 2015. http://www.vox.com/2015/2/4/7972335/dan-olmsted-anti-vaxxers. Accessed November 3, 2016.

11. Age of Autism Web site. http://www.ageofautism.com. Accessed November 3, 2016.

12. Wakefield AJ, et al. RETRACTED: Ileal-lymphoid-nodular hyperplasia, non-specific colitis, and pervasive developmental disorder in children. *The Lancet.* 1998; 351(9103): 637-41.

13. Goldschmidt D. Journal questions validity of autism and vaccine study. *CNN.* August 28, 2014. http://www.cnn.com/2014/08/27/health/irpt-cdc-autism-vaccine-study. Accessed November 3, 2016.

14. DeStefano F, Bhasin TK, Thompson WW, Yeargin-Allsopp M, Boyle C. Age at first measles–mumps–rubella vaccination in children with autism and school-matched control subjects: A population-based study in metropolitan Atlanta. *Pediatrics.* 2004; 113(2): 259-66.

15. Hooker BS. Measles–mumps–rubella vaccination timing and autism among young African American boys: A reanalysis of CDC data. *Translational Neurodegeneration.* 2014; 3: 16. doi:10.1186/2047-9158-3-16

16. Hooker BS. Retraction note: Measles–mumps–rubella vaccination timing and autism among young African American boys: A reanalysis of CDC data. *Translational Neurodegeneration.* 2014; 3: 22. doi:10.1186/2047-9158-3-22

17. Institute of Medicine. *Adverse Effects of Vaccines: Evidence and Causality*. Washington, DC: The National Academies Press; 2012.

18. Krugman P. The ultimate zombie idea. *The New York Times*. November 3, 2012. http://krugman.blogs.nytimes.com/2012/11/03/the-ultimate-zombie-idea. Accessed November 3, 2016.

19. Nyhan B, Reifler J, Richey S, Freed GL. Effective messages in vaccine promotion: A randomized trial. *Pediatrics*. 2014; 133(4): e835-e842.

36

Living with Complexity

POPULATION HEALTH IS concerned with studying health outcomes across and within groups. Our dominant methodological approach in public health—reducing systems to their simplest components and applying principally linear methods to understand the relation between potential causal factors and health indicators—has yielded substantial public health success [1]. However, there are also challenges to this thinking. These challenges have come about as we have increasingly moved away from simpler unicausal disorders to complex disorders with multiple causes that have proven to be resistant to the identification of simple causes, or simple solutions. This speaks to the importance of complexity in our work, which I examine in this chapter.

By way of illustrating the role of complexity, take obesity. Obesity is associated with some of the most common preventable causes of death, including diabetes, coronary heart disease, and some types of cancers [2]. In 2008, an estimated $147 billion was spent on obesity in the United States alone [3]. The advance of obesity—truly a global epidemic—suggests that despite widespread investment in research and public health campaigns, standard public health approaches have not yielded effective interventions [4]. This is because they fail, in large part, to address the complexity at the heart of this epidemic. Obesity is the result of a range of social, economic, and environmental causes; it is not merely a matter of poor diet or lack of exercise. This has been well stated by other authors. In the conclusion of "Changing the Future of Obesity: Science Policy and Action," the authors write, "The obesity epidemics in countries throughout the world are driven by complex forces that require systems thinking to conceptualise the causes and to organise evidence needed for action" [5].

The importance of complexity has been recognized across many disciplines. Complex systems approaches have been widely used in the fields of engineering, biology, and economics [6, 7]. They have also been used within public health to model infectious disease transmission [6, 7]. The public health application of complex systems thinking rests on the recognition that populations display many properties of complex systems, including heterogeneity of agents; nonlinear dynamics (e.g., the link between income and mortality); social network organization and influences (e.g., the spread of obesity through social networks); sensitivity to feedback, adaptation, learning, and evolution; stochasticity (e.g., the seasonality of influenza epidemics); trade-offs (e.g., equity vs. efficiency in the provision of health care); dependence on historical contingencies (e.g., implicit bias against African American patients); separation of cause and effect by time and space (e.g., fetal undernutrition and adult coronary heart disease); and emergence (e.g., the bystander effect, wherein diffusion of personal responsibility occurs at the group level) [8, 9, 10, 11, 12, 13, 14].

It is becoming increasingly clear that these approaches have a place in public health thinking. Not only do they stand to improve our understanding of the origin and transmission of disease but also systems thinking can aid quantitative public health analysis for conditions that extend well beyond infectious disease. This includes health challenges—such as obesity—that have displayed classic hallmarks of complex conditions that are resistant to simple analytic and policy approaches centered around a more linear methodology.

The importance of complex systems thinking is reflected by the UK government's foresight project, which published a strategic plan for responding to obesity in the UK during a 40-year period [15]. In applying this approach to the problem, the researchers modeled the "central engine" of obesity as a function of four key variables: level of primary appetite control, force of dietary habits, level of physical activity, and level of psychological ambivalence. These four variables and their subcomponents represent a complex system of causal influences [15]. Yet even this interplay exists within a larger web of causality. The central engine defined by the researchers is but a small subset of a much larger complex system, which includes such disparate domains as social psychology, food production, and activity environment [16]. This approach, founded on an acknowledgment of complexity, has led to novel insights regarding the determination of obesity and also a growing focus on the contextual conditions that produce obesity, including walkability of neighborhoods and availability of healthy foods.

Beyond obesity, there is a role for complex systems approaches in solving many other public health challenges. Such approaches are becoming ever more necessary, as we deepen our understanding of various health threats. For example, efforts at cutting cigarette nicotine levels can lead to compensatory smoking, illustrating the unanticipated consequences of particular system perturbations if we do not fully consider the system's dimensions and interrelations [17]. Complexity is also a factor when we consider the role of antiretroviral therapy in prolonging the lives of HIV carriers while at the same time potentially causing HIV to spread due to lower risk perception [18]. Further examples include antibiotic overuse worsening pathogen resistance, antilock brakes leading to riskier driving, and the use of protective headgear failing to decrease football concussion due to risk compensation [19, 20, 21].

Fundamentally, complex systems thinking stands to enhance public health through an appreciation of the interconnectedness of the elements of population systems that both determine and are determined by health indicators. A number of methods can be applied to the analysis of complex systems. One key method is agent-based modeling. Agent-based modeling has gained traction during the past decade; such models are coming into greater use in epidemiology and public health [22, 23]. Returning to the problem of obesity, the following is an example of an agent-based modeling approach: The effect of policy measures on changes in body mass index (BMI) over time was simulated in relation to strength of social

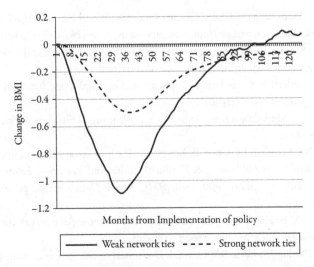

FIGURE 36.1 Agent-based-modeling simulation of population changes in BMI subsequent to the implementation of a policy to attract better food stores to local neighborhoods, stratified by populations characterized by strong and weak network ties. Galea S, Riddle M, Kaplan GA. Causal thinking and complex system approaches in epidemiology. *International Journal of Epidemiology*. 2010; 39(1): 97–106. doi: 10.1093/ije/dyp296 [24]

network ties (Figure 36.1) [24]. In the context of weak network ties, policy intervention had a more rapid, and greater, maximum impact, whereas in the context of strong network ties the impact of policy intervention on BMI was more persistent. This simulation demonstrates how complex systems approaches can capture the dynamic interrelations among causal influences, at multiple levels, over a period of time.

In summary, a complex systems approach is built on a recognition of the tremendous nuance inherent in the study of population health. Well-being, at the level of societies, is the product of a complex system of interrelated factors that produce health through dynamic processes characterized by interrelations, nonlinearity, reciprocity, and emergence. To be at our most effective, we must take all of these factors into account. Although system simplification can yield important insights that can inform public health efforts, we must recognize—and we increasingly are recognizing—the unintended consequences of oversimplification of complex systems. A complex systems conceptual lens, perhaps supplemented by complex systems analytic approaches, can therefore be a useful part of our armamentarium.

REFERENCES

1. Achievements in Public Health, 1900—1999: Control of Infectious Diseases. *Morbidity and Mortality Weekly Report (MMWR)*. 1999; 48(29): 621-9.

2. Adult Obesity Facts. Centers for Disease Control and Prevention Web site. http://www.cdc.gov/obesity/data/adult.html. Updated September 1, 2016. Accessed November 3, 2016.

3. Finkelstein EA, Trogdon JG, Cohen JW, Dietz W. Annual medical spending attributable to obesity: Payer- and service-specific estimates. *Health Affairs*. 2009; 28(5): w822-31. doi:10.1377/hlthaff.28.5.w822

4. Nutrition: Controlling the Global Obesity Epidemic. World Health Organization Web site. http://www.who.int/nutrition/topics/obesity/en. Accessed November 3, 2016.

5. Gortmaker SL, et al. Changing the future of obesity: Science, policy, and action. *The Lancet.* 2011; 378(9793): 838-47. doi:10.1016/S0140-6736(11)60815-5

6. Pearce N, Merletti F. Complexity, simplicity, and epidemiology. *International Journal of Epidemiology.* 2006; 35(3): 515-9.

7. Eubank S, et al. Modelling disease outbreaks in realistic urban social networks. *Nature.* 2004; 429(6988): 180-4.

8. Rehkopf DH, Berkman LF, Coull B, Krieger N. The non-linear risk of mortality by income level in a healthy population: US National Health and Nutrition Examination Survey mortality follow-up cohort, 1988-2001. *BMC Public Health.* 2008; 8: 383. doi:10.1186/1471-2458-8-383

9. Christakis NA, Fowler JH. The spread of obesity in a large social network over 32 years. *The New England Journal of Medicine.* 2007; 357(4): 370-9.

10. Dushoff J, Plotkin JB, Levin SA, Earn DJ. Dynamical resonance can account for seasonality of influenza epidemics. *Proceedings of the National Academy of Sciences of the United States of America.* 2004; 101(48): 16915-6.

11. Sassi F, Le Grand J, Archard L. Equity versus efficiency: A dilemma for the NHS. If the NHS is serious about equity it must offer guidance when principles conflict. *The BMJ.* 2001; 323(7316): 762-3.

12. Chapman EN, Kaatz A, Carnes M. Physicians and implicit bias: How doctors may unwittingly perpetuate health care disparities. *Journal of General Internal Medicine.* 2013; 28(11): 1504-10. doi:10.1007/s11606-013-2441-1

13. Barker DJ, Eriksson JG, Forsén T, Osmond C. Fetal origins of adult disease: Strength of effects and biological basis. *International Journal of Epidemiology.* 2002; 31(6): 1235-9.

14. Fischer P, et al. The bystander effect: A meta-analytic review on bystander intervention in dangerous and non-dangerous emergencies. *Psychological Bulletin.* 2011; 137(4): 517-37. doi:10.1037/a0023304

15. Tackling Obesities: Future Choices. GOV.UK Web site. https://www.gov.uk/government/collections/tackling-obesities-future-choices. Published October 17, 2007. Accessed November 3, 2016.

16. ShiftN Obesity System Influence Diagram. ShiftN Web site. http://www.shiftn.com/obesity/Full-Map.html. Accessed November 3, 2016.

17. US National Cancer Institute. *Risks Associated with Smoking Cigarettes with Low Machine-Measured Yields of Tar and Nicotine : Smoking and Tobacco Control Monograph No. 13.* Bethesda, MD: National Cancer Institute; 2001.

18. Cassell MM, Halperin DT, Shelton JD, Stanton D. Risk compensation: The Achilles' heel of innovations in HIV prevention? *The BMJ.* 2006; 332(7541): 605-7.

19. Antibiotic/Antimicrobial Resistance. Centers for Disease Control and Prevention Web site. http://www.cdc.gov/drugresistance. Updated August 17, 2016. Accessed November 4, 2016.

20. Winston C, Maheshri V, Mannering F. An exploration of the offset hypothesis using disaggregate data: The case of airbags and antilock brakes. *Journal of Risk and Uncertainty.* 2006; 32(2): 83-99.

21. Daneshvar DH, et al. Helmets and mouth guards: The role of personal equipment in preventing sport-related concussions. *Clinics in Sports Medicine*. 2011; 30(1): 145-63, x. doi:10.1016/j.csm.2010.09.006

22. Marshall BD, Galea S. Formalizing the role of agent-based modeling in causal inference and epidemiology. *American Journal of Epidemiology*. 2015; 181(2): 92-9. doi:10.1093/aje/kwu274

23. Maglio PP, Mabry PL. Agent-based models and systems science approaches to public health. *American Journal of Preventive Medicine*. 2011; 40(3): 392-4. doi:10.1016/j.amepre.2010.11.010

24. Galea S, Riddle M, Kaplan GA. Causal thinking and complex system approaches in epidemiology. *International Journal of Epidemiology*. 2010; 39(1): 97-106. doi:10.1093/ije/dyp296

37

Moving Beyond "Lifestyle"

‿ _____

THE NOTION THAT lifestyle is central to health is a relatively old one. It dates back more than 50 years, as studies such as Framingham and Alameda County in the United States and the World Health Organization (WHO)-led MONICA project in Europe focused primarily on identifying particular behavioral risk factors that have a significant effect on mortality and morbidity—risk factors such as smoking and physical inactivity [1, 2, 3, 4].

The link between lifestyle and health solidified in the public consciousness in the 1970s. Around this time, focus in the United States began to shift from infectious to chronic disease; this created increased interest in determining which risk factors predict chronic conditions. Consider the Nurses' Health Study [5]. Begun in 1976, it is one of the longest-running and most influential studies of health determination, and it has since produced voluminous findings on the role that lifestyle and behaviors play in health promotion [5]. This focus on lifestyle is not limited to the United States. In 1974, a report published by the Public Health Agency of Canada introduced a four-field framework proposing to shift the focus of health policy to include four key areas: lifestyle, environment, human biology, and health care environment [6]. One of the main positions in the report suggests that individuals are responsible for their health through their choice of lifestyles. This position was echoed in the United Kingdom, in 1976, in "Prevention and Health, Everybody's Business" [7, 8].

In 1985, the landmark "Report of the Secretary's Task Force on Black and Minority Health," also known as the Heckler Report, discussed lifestyle in the context of minority health disparities [9]. Although the report was comprehensive in its focus on cultural and other macro determinants of health, it also suggested the influence of lifestyle in a number of areas. According to the report, lifestyle influences homicide ("The high homicide rate can be related to . . . lifestyle, or individual and group ways of life") and differences among groups ("Differences in socioeconomic status, culture, and lifestyle are hypothesized to explain the lower relative mortality of Asian/Pacific Islanders in the United States"); the report also provides recommendations for improved health in general ("Health education activities should foster the development of lifestyles that maintain and enhance the state of health and well-being").

The United Nations has also drawn attention to lifestyle. It has referred to chronic conditions as "lifestyle diseases" [10]. WHO, for its part, has produced a podcast titled "Do Lifestyle Changes Improve Health?" [11].

It is important to stress that there is nothing inherently wrong with these efforts. Indeed, there is ample evidence that adverse population health behavior influences the well-being of those populations. The question here is one of emphasis. I argue that our, frankly, indiscriminate use of the word "lifestyle" is problematic. Worse, it may even set back our cause— improving the health of populations—and set it back further than we might think. Why? I offer four reasons.

First, there is the term "lifestyle" itself. It is often used vaguely, without reflection on its meaning, and without grounding in the "social and cultural location of health behaviors" [12]. This has not always been the case, of course. Sophisticated writers who use the term "lifestyle" situate it within its relevant cultural context. For example, the Heckler Report, mentioned previously, also notes that homicide "can be related to . . . external environment including physical, historical–cultural, social, educational, and economic environments" [9]. However, in the broader conversation about health, this nuance is often lost. The media-friendly appeal of lifestyle makes for its ready acceptance as a central determinant of disease over and above other drivers of health. This can mean that many factors of equal or greater importance, such as differences in life opportunities, can be ignored [13]. There is ample historical precedent that such misemphases are quite likely to result in attendant shifts in resources dedicated to solving a particular problem at the expense of other areas of intervention that may be likelier to find success [14].

Second, there is the question of efficacy. Simply stated, do changes in lifestyle produce changes in health? To answer by way of illustration: Whereas the American College of Gastroenterology suggests that lifestyle modifications (diet, body position, tobacco, alcohol, and obesity) are the first-line therapy for gastroesophageal reflux disease (GERD), a systematic review of relevant literature published between 1975 and 2004 concluded that evidence to support lifestyle modification recommendations has not been well established [15, 16, 17]. Although weight loss and head position improved the pH profile and symptoms, other lifestyle changes had no evident effect on substantiated GERD. Another study analyzed two Cochrane systematic reviews to assess the efficacy and safety of lifestyle interventions for the treatment of acute and chronic gout [18, 19]. The analysis concluded that although there is observational evidence linking lifestyle risk factors to the development of gout, there are no high-quality trials to either support or refute the effectiveness of lifestyle interventions in the treatment of acute or chronic gout. The unreliability of lifestyle interventions also extends into the area of diabetes care. A trial initiated in 2001 by the National Institutes of Health, called Look Action for Health in Diabetes, followed more than 5,000 diabetic adults for 11 years and randomly assigned them to an "intensive lifestyle intervention" [20]. As with the previous examples, the results were disappointing. The trial ended earlier than expected when there were no significant differences in cardiovascular disease rates between the different groups, despite reductions in body weight and other risk factors [20].

Third, a lifestyle emphasis suggests that we can not only improve health through a focus on individual risk factors but also predict disease in individuals in order to stop it. Unfortunately, it is well established that action on individual behavior will do little to solve large-scale, population-level problems such as obesity, absent attention to the social, economic, and environmental context that allows such conditions to flourish [21]. We also know that our capacity to predict health in individuals, characterized by any single risk factor, is extraordinarily limited [22]. This is because the production of disease is, in a word, complex. A lifestyle focus reduces this complexity to a series of individual choices, when in fact such choices are far less relevant to the production of health, and the prevention of disease, than the lifestyle hype would suggest.

Finally, the concept of "lifestyle" as a primary driver of health is in many ways a victim of its own seductiveness. It provides a media-friendly hook for popularizing health risks at the expense of more difficult to synthesize, but more accurate, pictures of disease causation. Worse, the word is sometimes applied by media commentators to research where it does not actually belong. In a telling illustration, the Centers for Disease Control and Prevention published a report titled "Potentially Preventable Deaths from the Five Leading Causes of Death—United States, 2008–2010" that did not mention the word "lifestyle," but several articles referring to the report called out "lifestyles" in the headline, including those in *TIME* magazine and on the American Cancer Society Web site [23, 24, 25]. Such misapplication of the word speaks to how ubiquitous "lifestyle" has become in the national conversation around health.

In summary, our overreliance on "lifestyle" has limited utility for promoting health. It tips our lens of focus to an individual locus of control—a set of psychological, internal stimuli that motivate individual choice. This almost inevitably leads to the stigmatizing of unhealthy individuals, as in the case of obese populations, shifting the blame for disease away from the foundational drivers of health and toward a mere lack of willpower [26]. This is counterproductive on two fronts, making it less likely that people will get well and less likely that we will turn our attention toward creating a society in which they do not get sick in the first place. It is probably time that we stop talking about "lifestyle."

REFERENCES

1. Watson J, Platt S, eds. *Researching Health Promotion*. London: Routledge; 2000.
2. History of the Framingham Heart Study. Framingham Heart Study Web site. https://www.framinghamheartstudy.org/about-fhs/history.php. Accessed November 4, 2016.
3. Alameda County Study. University of Minnesota School of Public Health Web site. http://www.epi.umn.edu/cvdepi/study-synopsis/alameda-county-study. Accessed November 4, 2016.
4. The WHO MONICA Project. Terveyden ja hyvinvoinnin laitos Web site. http://www.thl.fi/monica. Accessed November 4, 2016.
5. Nurses' Health Study Web site. http://www.nurseshealthstudy.org. Accessed November 4, 2016.
6. Lalonde M. *A New Perspective on the Health of Canadians: A Working Document*. Ottawa: Government of Canada; 1974.

7. Macintyre S. The Black Report and beyond: What are the issues? *Social Science & Medicine*. 1997; 44(6): 723-45.

8. UK Department of Health. *Prevention and Health: Everybody's Business—A Reassessment of Public and Personal Health*. London: Her Majesty's Stationery Office; 1976.

9. Heckler MM. *Report of the Secretary's Task Force Report on Black and Minority Health*. Washington, DC: US Department of Health and Human Services; 1985.

10. Al-Maskari F. Lifestyle diseases: An economic burden on the health services. *UN Chronicle*. July 2010. https://unchronicle.un.org/article/lifestyle-diseases-economic-burden-health-services. Accessed November 4, 2016.

11. World Health Organization. Do lifestyle changes improve health? *WHO podcast*. January 9, 2009. http://www.who.int/mediacentre/multimedia/podcasts/2009/lifestyle-interventions-20090109/en. Accessed November 4, 2016.

12. Backett KC, Davison C. Life-course and lifestyle: The social and cultural location of health behaviours. *Social Science & Medicine*. 1995; 40(5): 629-38.

13. Link BG, Phelan J. Social conditions as fundamental causes of disease. *Journal of Health and Social Behavior*. 1995; Spec No: 80-94.

14. Hamlin C. Could you starve to death in England in 1839? The Chadwick–Farr controversy and the loss of the "social" in public health. *American Journal of Public Health*. 1995; 85(6): 856-66.

15. Katz PO, Gerson LB, Vela MF. Guidelines for the diagnosis and management of gastroesophageal reflux disease. *The American Journal of Gastroenterology*. 2013; 108(3): 308-328; quiz 329. doi:10.1038/ajg.2012.444

16. Gastroesophageal Reflux Disease (GERD). WebMD Web site. http://www.webmd.com/heartburn-gerd/guide/reflux-disease-gerd-1#1. Accessed November 4, 2016.

17. Kaltenbach T, Crockett S, Gerson LB. Are lifestyle measures effective in patients with gastroesophageal reflux disease? An evidence-based approach. *Archives of Internal Medicine*. 2006; 166(9): 965-71. doi:10.1001/archinte.166.9.965

18. Moi JHY, et al. Lifestyle interventions for the treatment of gout: A summary of 2 Cochrane Systematic Reviews. *The Journal of Rheumatology*. 2014; 92: 26-32.

19. Gout—Topic Overview. WebMD Web site. http://www.webmd.com/arthritis/tc/gout-topic-overview#1. Accessed November 4, 2016.

20. Kwok CF, Ho LT. Look Action for Health in Diabetes trial: What we have learned in terms of real world practice and clinical trials. *Journal of Diabetes Investigation*. 2014; 5(6): 637-8. doi:10.1111/jdi.12231

21. Keyes KM, Smith GD, Koenen KC, Galea S. The mathematical limits of genetic prediction for complex chronic disease. *Journal of Epidemiology and Community Health*. 2015; 69(6): 574-9. doi:10.1136/jech-2014-204983

22. Pepe MS, Janes H, Longton G, Leisenring W, Newcomb P. Limitations of the odds ratio in gauging the performance of a diagnostic, prognostic, or screening marker. *American Journal of Epidemiology*. 2004; 159(9): 882-90.

23. Yoon PW, Bastian B, Anderson RN, Collins JL, Jaffe HW. Potentially preventable deaths from the five leading causes of death—United States, 2008-2010. *Morbidity and Mortality Weekly Report (MMWR)*. 2014; 63(17): 369-74.

24. Park A. Nearly half of US deaths can be prevented with lifestyle changes. *TIME*. May 1, 2014. http://time.com/84514/nearly-half-of-us-deaths-can-be-prevented-with-lifestyle-changes. Accessed November 4, 2016.

25. Simon S. CDC: Lifestyle changes can reduce death from top 5 causes. American Cancer Society Web site. http://www.cancer.org/cancer/news/news/cdc-lifestyle-changes-can-reduce-death-from-top-5-causes. Published June 24, 2014. Accessed November 4, 2016.

26. Papadopoulos S, Brennan L. Correlates of weight stigma in adults with overweight and obesity: A systematic literature review. *Obesity*. 2015; 23(9): 1743-60. doi:10.1002/oby.21187

38

On Ignorance

<hr>

PROFESSOR MICHAEL SMITHSON, who has long written on the topic of agnotology—the study of ignorance—describes the experience of ignorance using the very helpful metaphor of a "knowledge island" [1]. The more we know, the bigger the island; the bigger the island, the longer the island's shores. We are most comfortable at the center of the island of knowledge, where we know what we know. But how do we handle the uncomfortable fact that, as a consequence of our work, we may need to spend much of our time on the island's beaches, where the limits of our knowledge lie?

I have found this thinking helpful to a consideration of how we, in population health scholarship, operate. We aspire to improve the health of populations and to produce science and scholarship that help us understand how we may do so ever better. This rests on the production of knowledge—on getting ourselves to the center of the island so we may then think of actions we can take to promote population health. For example, a large body of scholarship convinces us that smoking is associated with a variety of pathologies; we then use this information to agitate for the introduction of measures that curb smoking, thereby improving population health [2]. Or consider efforts to stop drunk driving. Population health science evidence demonstrates that driving while under the influence of alcohol is associated with substantial vehicular morbidity and mortality; this results in the development of an action plan, the implementation of which creates a country-wide decrease in drunk driving and its harmful consequences [3, 4].

But what about cases in which the causes are not so clear—when our efforts are shrouded in ignorance and we walk on the shores of the islands of knowledge? This is far from uncommon. In fact, I suggest that this is probably the case more frequently than we are willing to admit.

Let us take one particularly contentious current issue: e-cigarettes. The central question here is whether electronic cigarettes—well accepted to be less harmful than regular cigarettes—are a "slippery slope" and might become a "gateway" to the use of regular cigarettes, thereby re-normalizing smoking and potentially chipping away at decades of hard-won gains against an unhealthy practice. Or do e-cigarettes represent a useful harm-reduction opportunity, providing a new tool in the public health armamentarium to decrease cigarette smoking in populations? A study from Los Angeles found that adolescents who used e-cigarettes were more likely than non-users to report subsequent initiation of combustible tobacco [5]. By contrast, a UK government independent review found no evidence that e-cigarettes represent a path to smoking for nonsmokers [6]. Several commentaries have dissected the evidence; some have urged action, concluding that the threats of e-cigarettes are real, whereas others have taken a more nuanced view [7, 8].

It is not my purpose here to review the e-cigarette literature—I leave that to others who are experts in the field. I simply raise the debate as a particularly interesting area of current contention in public health. Clearly, the e-cigarette industry is big business, and this introduces a new element into an area we thought we had a good grip on. But, just as clearly, the data are not at all conclusive, and relatively sober analysts are, on reviewing these data, reaching different, sometimes contradictory conclusions.

So what are we to do with ignorance? What are we to do with uncertainty and ambiguity? As members of an academic community, we have the extraordinary privilege of luxuriating in the expansion of the shores of the knowledge island. The fact that there may be ambiguity about e-cigarettes should therefore be cause for celebration. There are interesting questions to address, interesting studies to conduct, interesting answers to discover. What could be more engaging for those of us charged with generating knowledge as our core, foundational identity? But we are compelled to tackle these questions by more than just academic interest. We wish to generate knowledge so that we can transmit that knowledge to those who are in a position to improve the well-being of populations. To add further tension to this, our cause is so pressing—the health of many—that questions cry out for rapid answers. If e-cigarettes are emerging quickly, surely we should know quickly what effect they might have so that we may act with alacrity to save lives?

With these questions in mind, I suggest five thoughts that might help us cope with ignorance and ambiguity in population health scholarship.

First, we must recognize that ignorance is an inevitable part of what we do. Not knowing is not anomalous; it is, in many ways, normative. An embrace of ignorance can help recalibrate our expectations. We should expect not to know if e-cigarettes can help or hurt our progress against combustible tobacco. We should accept a degree of ignorance in other health areas too—in the area of cancer prevention, for example, we should accept that a substantial proportion of cancers are stochastically determined [9]. And we should recognize that this ambiguity is inevitable when dealing with complex, multiscale processes that evolve over time. This frees us to be clear when we do not know something and, likewise, to be clear when we determine it is time to act. It also means we must prepare our students to deal with ambiguity, to be comfortable with gray areas, and to understand that public health remains a pragmatic discipline, even in the face of uncertainty.

Second, we need to recognize that public health action does not necessarily need to follow causal certainty and that we can, and not infrequently *should*, act even when we do not know all the answers. Action can be predicated on values, on analogy, on anticipation of future trends, or on causal links built on a hard-won understanding of the likely consequences of omission of action. However, if we do act, we should not do so on false data pretexts, invoking knowledge and clarity when little exists. We must act with transparent honesty about the attendant uncertainties, allowing us the option of changing course when some of our ignorance falls away.

Third, we must recognize that false certitude is not without consequence. The obvious unintended outcome of false certitude is taking action that turns out to be inadvertently harmful. But other costs of false certitude are, if less direct, just as important, including losing the trust of the public and misdirecting resources from areas of scholarship and action that could be promising, as we put all our eggs in the wrong basket [10].

Fourth, we must carefully separate genuine ignorance from manufactured ambiguity. There is ample precedent of particular special interests working to generate doubt about the state of the science when, in fact, the scientific facts were clear. The classic example of this involves industry efforts to repudiate findings about lead poisoning [11]. Sometimes we *do* know the answer. We *do* know that combustible tobacco is deadly. We *do* know that seat belts save lives. In these cases, the role of public health is easier. We must muster as much creativity and communications savvy as possible to promote the health of the public, even if special interests (perhaps with commercial motivations) are aligned against our efforts.

Fifth, we need to remember that our capacity for individual prediction remains tremendously limited. Most of our understanding of the production of health comes from population-level data, making individual prediction on the basis of these data difficult.

By training our emerging scholars to expect that they will likely face ever-expanding shores of ignorance, and that much of their careers will involve action in the midst of uncertainty, we stand to help a new generation see the role of public health differently. Likewise, by fostering an academic culture that is comfortable with ignorance, we push ourselves to grapple with the role, constraints, and possibilities of public health action even when confronted with ambiguity and doubt.

REFERENCES

1. Prof Mike Smithson FASSA (faculty profile). Australian National University Web site. http://psychology.anu.edu.au/about-us/people/mike-smithson. Updated July 27, 2016. Accessed July 27, 2016.

2. The Health Consequences of Smoking—50 Years of Progress: A Report of the Surgeon General, 2014. The US Surgeon General Web site. http://www.surgeongeneral.gov/index.html. Accessed July 26, 2016.

3. US Department of Health and Human Services. *Surgeon General's Workshop on Drunk Driving: Proceedings.* Public Health Service, Office of the Surgeon General, Rockville, MD; December 14-16, 1988.

4. What Caused the Decrease? National Highway Traffic Safety Administration Web site. http://www.nhtsa.gov/people/injury/research/FewerYoungDrivers/iv__what_caused.htm. Accessed July 26, 2016.

5. Leventhal A, et al. Association of electronic cigarette use with initiation of combustible tobacco product smoking in early adolescence. *JAMA: The Journal of the American Medical Association.* 2015; 314(7): 700-707. doi:10.1001/jama.2015.8950

6. E-cigarettes: An Evidence Update. Gov.uk Web site https://www.gov.uk/government/publications/e-cigarettes-an-evidence-update. Published August 19, 2015. Updated August 28, 2015. Accessed July 26, 2016.

7. Chang A, Barry M. The global health implications of e-cigarettes. *JAMA: The Journal of the American Medical Association*. 2016; 314(7): 663-4. doi:10.1001/jama.2015.8676

8. Chaloupka FJ, Sweanor D, Warner KE. Differential taxes for differential risks—Toward reduced harm from nicotine-yielding products. *New England Journal of Medicine*. 2015; 373(7): 594-7. doi:10.1056/NEJMp1505710

9. Tomasetti C, Vogelstein B. Cancer etiology: Variation in cancer risk among tissues can be explained by the number of stem cell divisions. *Science*. 2015; 347(6217): 78-81. doi:10.1126/science.1260825

10. Hunter DJ, D'Agostino RB Sr. Let's not put all our eggs in one basket. *New England Journal of Medicine*. 2016; 373(8): 691-3. doi:10.1056/NEJMp1508144

11. Markowitz G, Rosner D. "Cater to the children": The role of the lead industry in a public health tragedy, 1900-1955. *American Journal of Public Health*. 2000; 90(1): 36-46.

39

Acknowledging Luck

WE ARE, IN our scholarship, largely in the business of population health science, an enterprise that is geared toward a "study of the conditions that shape distributions of health within and across populations, and of the mechanisms through which these conditions manifest as the health of individuals" [1]. Through our concern with these conditions, we seek to improve our understanding of what causes disease in populations so that we may more effectively intervene. Implicit in this goal is the assumption that we can, in fact, understand; that we can identify causes and anatomize their influence, until each element of their complexity is laid bare. This is what our field, at its best, does. There is, however, one element of population health that can prove elusive—luck; or, stated more traditionally, chance, randomness. Although we frequently take luck for granted, or ignore its influence altogether, I suggest that it is nevertheless central to the health of populations and needs to be part of our empirical and moral calculus as we attempt to improve population health.

Luck begins shaping health at the moment of birth. In the United States, for example, our well-being is closely linked to the socioeconomic status into which we are born. The more economically advantaged a person is, the longer that person is likely to live; the richest American men live a full 15 years longer than the poorest, and the richest American women live 10 years longer than the poorest [2].

The link between income, wealth, and health is well understood. Less appreciated is the degree to which income is linked to luck. Luck determines whether we are born rich or born poor, with all the attendant health effects of either socioeconomic circumstance. In some ways, the downplaying of luck is a consequence of cultural norms in the United States. Although the American dream is built on the myth of the capacity we all have to transcend the circumstances of our birth—the Horatio Alger story of self-made success—the data suggest that this is not so [3, 4, 5, 6]. A child born to parents in a lower income quintile is more than 10 times likelier to remain in that quintile in adulthood (Figure 39.1) [5]. Conversely, a

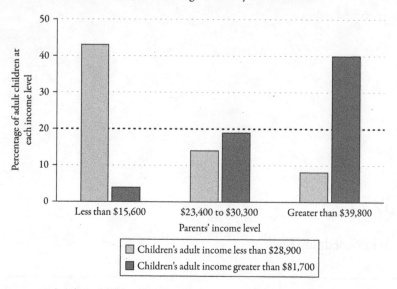

FIGURE 39.1 Probability of children's income level, given parents' income level. Children born into low-income families are likely to remain at the low end of the income distribution as adults. Greenstone M, Looney A, Patashnik J, Yu M. Thirteen Economic Facts about Social Mobility and the Role of Education. Washington, DC: Brookings Institution; 2013 [5].

child born to parents in a higher income quintile is 5 times likelier to maintain that privileged economic status in adulthood [5].

However much we may value individual self-determination, it remains a fact that luck decides whether we are born rich or poor, and we generally stay much as we were born. With income and wealth both strongly linked to health throughout life, it is clear that by determining our early economic status, luck shapes the trajectory of our health.

How, then, should we in public health account for the influence of luck? I argue that luck, as it relates to population health, is best viewed from a moral/philosophical perspective. The degree to which certain populations are more vulnerable than others to bad luck is a preoccupation of luck egalitarianism—a philosophical viewpoint concerned with the distribution of "brute luck and option luck" [7, 8]. The former characterizes the influence of what can only be described as fate—for example, the military coup that leads to the sudden withdrawal of government funding for a particular health intervention. The latter characterizes the risk inherent in a deliberate course of action a person or group decides upon—for example, the initial choice to establish a health intervention in an unstable area of the world. The distinction between option luck and brute luck can play an important role in public health thinking, as we seek to mitigate the influence of both and create a more level health playing field for all.

This is well illustrated by the challenge of obesity. The present paradigm suggests two ways a population can become obese: through the influence of brute luck and through the influence of option luck. This paradigm affords us some perspective on the causes of obesity—causes that can be easy to mischaracterize or distort. Where some may observe obesity in low-income neighborhoods and ascribe it to laziness or bad choices, we are able to perceive the underlying structural determinants, the brute luck, conspiring to make healthy eating difficult in these areas [9]. This is not to discount the role of personal responsibility in spreading obesity. Consumers choose what they buy and what they eat, even when their choices are limited. It follows that the resulting health outcomes would thus be a consequence of option luck. But individual decisions are by no means the decisive factor here. When food choices are limited and nutritious food is scarce, the influence of option luck is marginal, at best. If a store only carries processed foods and sugary drinks, and that store is the only food source a less advantaged family can conveniently access, then the circumstances of birth and income remain the major factors in determining that family's diet, leaving the family open to the influence of brute luck.

In many ways, the task of public health—indeed, the task of anyone looking to create positive change in the world—is to overcome the influence of brute luck. This task is deeply tied to our focus on equity and social justice. When one group, or multiple groups, within a society is burdened with near permanent, structured, often intergenerational bad luck while the population as a whole enjoys fairer prospects, then that society is not just, and the work of public health is not done. Rather, we must strive for redistributive justice, guided by a recognition that health should not be a matter of chance. To do so, we need to engage with the social, economic, and environmental conditions, many of them imposed by luck, that drive inequality within populations. Ultimately, this will strengthen the significance of option luck in decision-making, giving individuals more latitude in choosing the trajectory of their own well-being.

REFERENCES

1. Keyes KM, Galea S. *Population Health Science*. New York, NY: Oxford University Press; 2016.
2. How Can We Reduce Disparities in Health? The Health Inequality Project Web site. https://healthinequality.org. Accessed November 4, 2016.
3. Kraus MW, Tan JJX. Americans overestimate social class mobility. *Journal of Experimental Social Psychology*. 2015; 58: 101-11.
4. Horatio Alger, Jr. The Horatio Alger Society Web site. http://www.horatioalgersociety.net/100_biography.html. Accessed November 4, 2016.
5. Greenstone M, Looney A, Patashnik J, Yu M. *Thirteen Economic Facts About Social Mobility and the Role of Education*. Washington, DC: Brookings Institution; 2013.
6. Pinsker J. America is even less socially mobile than most economists thought. *The Atlantic*. July 23, 2015. http://www.theatlantic.com/business/archive/2015/07/america-social-mobility-parents-income/399311. Accessed November 4, 2016.
7. Mason A. Equality of opportunity. Encyclopedia Britannica Web site. https://www.britannica.com/topic/equality-of-opportunity#ref1187627. Accessed November 4, 2016.
8. Justice and Bad Luck. Stanford Encyclopedia of Philosophy Web site. http://plato.stanford.edu/entries/justice-bad-luck/#7. Published June 20, 2005. Updated April 11, 2014. Accessed November 4, 2016
9. Puhl RM, Heuer CA. Obesity stigma: Important considerations for public health. *American Journal of Public Health*. 2010; 100(6): 1019-28. doi:10.2105/AJPH.2009.159491

SECTION 5

Toward a Healthier World

40

Aging Healthy

WHEN JEANNE CALMENT was 90 years old, she sold her apartment to a lawyer named Andre-Francois Raffray on a contingency contract [1]. The arrangement was that Raffray would pay Calment each month a sum of 2,500 francs (approximately $400) until her death, whereupon the apartment would become his. This would have been an advantageous deal for Raffray were it not for the fact that Calment lived for another 32 years. She would eventually pass away at the age of 122 years, making hers the longest human life on record. When she died, Raffray's family was still paying for the apartment.

Although Calment's degree of longevity is uncommon, she is not the only person to live longer in recent decades. According to projections, between 1950 and 2050, the global population of those aged 65 years or older will have increased by a factor of 10, and it will triple between now and 2050 [2]. Population aging will not be evenly distributed throughout the world: In 2050, the proportion of people older than age 60 years is projected to be higher in high-income countries [3]. However, the older adult population is also growing faster in low-income areas of the globe [3]. By 2050, four of five older adults are expected to live in low-income countries [3]. This demographic shift is in many ways a positive development. Increased longevity is the happy result of the higher standards of living many of these countries are beginning to enjoy [4]. Globally, these changes are a consequence of falling birth rates and rising life expectancy [5].

As Calment's story illustrates, when people live longer, there are often costs involved. These costs can be both expected and unexpected. The way we manage these costs will affect the opportunities that we can create for ever-larger numbers of people to live healthier lives. Two key costs we must contend with are disability and disease. Currently, disability among older adults contributes to 23 percent of the global burden of disease; it contributes to half of the burden of disease in high-income countries and 20 percent of the burden in low-income countries [6]. Cardiovascular disease and cancer are the leading contributors to this burden [6]. Estimates of changes in Disability-adjusted life years

(DALYs) among seniors between 2004 and 2030 suggest that the DALYs for all causes will increase by 55.2 percent [6]. DALYs attributable to communicable, maternal, perinatal, and nutritional conditions will decrease by 18.7 percent, whereas those attributable to non-communicable diseases will increase by 61.3 percent and those attributable to injuries will increase by 78 percent. Specific diseases expected to rise most precipitously include diabetes (+95.7 percent), chronic obstructive pulmonary disease (+88.7 percent), dementia (+82.6 per cent), vision impairment (+86.3 percent), and hearing impairment (+70.6 percent). Cardiovascular disease and cancer are also projected to increase by 40.6 percent and 69.2 percent respectively. Countries that recently experienced an epidemiologic transition should expect sharper rises in the burden of disease due to these conditions. While the burden of chronic disease will increase most rapidly in low-income countries, high-income countries are more likely to see more cases of dementia, including Alzheimer's disease. This increase will be significant. Whereas in 2006, the number of worldwide Alzheimer's disease cases was 26.6 million, that figure is projected to quadruple by 2050, leaving 1 in 85 people in the world with this condition [7].

Bearing in mind these challenges, what are some approaches we could take to support populations as they age? A public health framework for healthy aging, as developed by the World Health Organization, is presented in Figure 40.1 [5].

This approach focuses on the promotion of functional ability, defined as "health-related attributes that enable people to be and to do what they have reason to value," and intrinsic

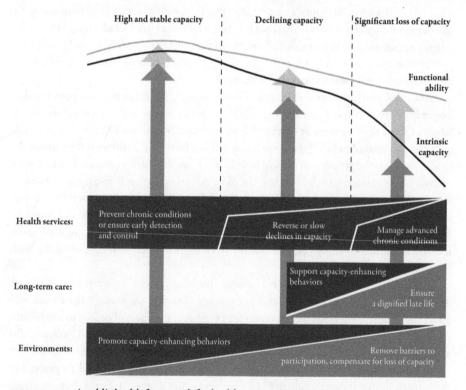

FIGURE 40.1 A public health framework for healthy aging. World Health Organization. World Report on Ageing and Health. Geneva, Switzerland: WHO Press; 2015 [5].

capacity, defined as "the composite of all the physical and mental capacities of an individual" [5]. Simply stated, this framework emphasizes enabling people to continue to perform the activities that they would like to do, longer. This means making sure that they are healthy enough to do so. Accordingly, the promotion of healthy aging aims to facilitate functional ability through "supporting the building and maintenance of intrinsic capacity" and also by "enabling those with a decrement in their functional capacity to do the things that are important to them" [5]. There are, of course, a number of variables at play in implementing this strategy. The application of this approach, and the effectiveness with which it can be adopted globally, depends very much on geography and economic status. Culture, too, plays an important role. In many low-income countries, for example, older adults have historically been cared for by families, a result of both necessity and social norms. However, as populations age, birth rates decline, and social norms change, this model becomes an increasingly less reliable means of providing stable, long-term care [8].

This speaks to a need for structural changes aimed at promoting healthy aging at all levels of society. Public systems, for example, might step into the role once played by families to ensure that older populations are cared for regardless of circumstance. At a perhaps deeper level, societies must become more welcoming of seniors to ensure the full participation of citizens of all ages. This welcome could be expressed in a number of ways. From advocating for more accessible built environments in cities and towns to pushing for more volunteer opportunities for older adults and—at the political level—making sure that the needs of this population (particularly the homebound) are not forgotten, we have a chance to redefine what aging looks like in the decades to come [9, 10, 11].

It is easy to think that the difficulties of aging are universal; this is perhaps true, but only up to a point. It remains a fact, however, that certain groups face their own particular challenges. It is therefore the job of public health to work to mitigate the health gaps that exist among aging populations [12, 13]. Race, for example, remains a persistent factor in determining health outcomes at all stages of life. The aging lesbian, gay, bisexual, and transgender population also faces a distinct set of issues, with socioeconomic status remaining central to the determination of health gaps for this population, as for all others. I discussed income inequality in Chapter 25; its influence is no less acute for older adults than for the young. Although increased total mortality among seniors can make the effects of income inequality more difficult to measure among older populations, economic resources remain a fundamental determinant of health in old age [14]. Perhaps the most obvious effect of income is in determining the kinds of medication seniors can afford to take. As drug prices continue to rise, a public health strategy of prevention, implemented throughout the life course, can ease the burden of the chronic and acute diseases that afflict older adults and reduce the need for prohibitively expensive medication [15, 16].

Despite the challenges of global aging, it also presents many opportunities for innovation. Broadening our scope beyond the prevention of disease, we find ever-more areas in which an engaged, creative public health approach can make a difference in the lives of older populations [17]. This means helping people live not only longer lives but also better ones. From exercise programs that facilitate greater mobility to home visits aimed at reducing isolation and mentoring partnerships that give seniors a chance to pass on what they have learned to younger generations, there are many opportunities for structured intervention [18, 19, 20]. Indeed, there are a variety of public health initiatives already in place that are doing good work in these areas. Such initiatives include community-based comprehensive models such as the PACE program (Program of All-Inclusive Care for the Elderly), which provides medical and social services to older adults in need [21].

To continue to advance healthy aging, then, we need to change the way that aging is viewed. This will allow us to better promote health at all stages of the life course. A change in perspective—from a focus on decreasing functional disability to one of prevention and increasing functional ability—opens up novel avenues in promoting the health of older adults, as we consider the coming large-scale population changes. We must continue to build on the successes of public health in this area, keeping our core focus on prevention and the maintenance of functionality. Rather than remain associated with decline, a person's later years might be viewed as a period of continual growth and improvement. This is a view that resonates well with public health and is consistent with our effort to ensure we maximize opportunities for all people so they can live longer, better lives.

REFERENCES

1. Whitney CR. Jeanne Calment, world's elder, dies at 122. *The New York Times*. August 5, 1997. http://www.nytimes.com/1997/08/05/world/jeanne-calment-world-s-elder-dies-at-122.html. Accessed November 14, 2016.

2. Haub C. World population aging: Clocks illustrate growth in population under age 5 and over age 65. Population Reference Bureau Web site. http://www.prb.org/Publications/Articles/2011/agingpopulationclocks.aspx. Accessed November 14, 2016.

3. United Nations, Department of Economic and Social Affairs, Population Division. *World Population Ageing 2013*. New York, NY: United Nation; 2013.

4. Ageing. United Nations Population Fund Web site. http://www.unfpa.org/ageing. Accessed November 27, 2016.

5. World Health Organization. *World Report on Ageing and Health*. Geneva, Switzerland: Author; 2015.

6. Prince MJ, et al. The burden of disease in older people and implications for health policy and practice. *The Lancet*. 2015; 385(9967): 549-62. doi:10.1016/S0140-6736(14)61347-7

7. Brookmeyer R, Johnson E, Ziegler-Graham K, Arrighi HM. Forecasting the global burden of Alzheimer's disease. *Alzheimer's & Dementia: Journal of the Alzheimer's Association*. 2007; 3(3): 186-91. doi:10.1016/j.jalz.2007.04.381

8. Kaneda T. A critical window for policymaking on population aging in developing countries. Population Reference Bureau Web site. http://www.prb.org/Publications/Articles/2006/ACriticalWindowforPolicymakingonPopulationAginginDevelopingCountries.aspx. Accessed November 27, 2016.

9. Healthy Aging & the Built Environment. Centers for Disease Control and Prevention Web site. http://www.cdc.gov/healthyplaces/healthtopics/healthyaging.htm. Updated September 21, 2016. Accessed November 27, 2016.

10. What Are the Public Health Implications of Global Ageing? World Health Organization Web site. http://www.who.int/features/qa/42/en. Accessed November 27, 2016.

11. Qiu WQ, et al. Physical and mental health of homebound older adults: An overlooked population. *Journal of the American Geriatrics Society*. 2010; 58(12): 2423-8. doi:10.1111/j.1532-5415.2010.03161.x

12. Artazcoz L, Rueda S. Social inequalities in health among the elderly: A challenge for public health research. *Journal of Epidemiology & Community Health*. 2007; 61(6): 466-7.

13. Battling Health Disparities: Closing the Gaps. Alliance for Aging Research Web site. https://www.agingresearch.org/newsletters/view/40. Published July 1, 2009. Accessed November 27, 2016.

14. Wallace SP. Equity and social determinants of health among older adults. *Generations: Journal of the American Society on Aging*. February 17, 2015. http://www.asaging.org/blog/equity-and-social-determinants-health-among-older-adults. Accessed November 27, 2016.

15. Jaret P. Prices spike for some generic drugs. *AARP Bulletin*. July/August 2015. http://www.aarp.org/health/drugs-supplements/info-2015/prices-spike-for-generic-drugs.html. Accessed November 27, 2016.

16. Caspersen CJ, Thomas GD, Boseman LA, Beckles GL, Albright AL. Aging, diabetes, and the public health system in the United States. *American Journal of Public Health*. 2012; 102(8): 1482-97. doi:10.2105/AJPH.2011.300616

17. Anderson LA, Goodman RA, Holtzman D, Posner SF, Northridge ME. Aging in the United States: Opportunities and challenges for public health. *American Journal of Public Health*. 2012; 102(3): 393-5. doi:10.2105/AJPH.2011.300617

18. Exercise Programs That Promote Senior Fitness. National Council on Aging Web site. https://www.ncoa.org/center-for-healthy-aging/physical-activity/physical-activity-programs-for-older-adults. Accessed November 27, 2016.

19. Dickens AP, Richards SH, Greaves CJ, Campbell JL. Interventions targeting social isolation in older people: A systematic review. *BMC Public Health*. 2011; 11: 647. doi:10.1186/1471-2458-11-647

20. Senior–Youth Mentoring Programs. TODAY Show Web site. http://www.today.com/id/6082216/ns/today-today_weekend_edition/t/senior-youth-mentoring-programs/#.WDtQ3MdlnVp. Updated September 23, 2004. Accessed November 27, 2016.

21. Program of All-Inclusive Care for the Elderly. Medicaid Web site. https://www.medicaid.gov/medicaid/ltss/pace/index.html. Accessed November 27, 2016.

41

In the Heart of the City, Health

HEALTH AND THE CITY

Urbanization, along with the aging of populations, is the most consequential global demographic shift to take place during the past 200 years. The evidence for the rapid pace of urbanization is unquestionable. In 2014, approximately 54 percent of the world's population was living in urban areas, compared to only 35 percent in 1960 and 5 percent in 1800 [1]. Just since 2000, more than 1 billion people have been added to urban areas, raising the proportion of urban dwellers to more than 80 percent in 64 different countries [2]. By 2010, there was roughly the same number of people living in urban areas as there were in the entire world in 1950 [3]. Where is this urban growth occurring? Defying conventional and perhaps media-driven images of cities and urban dwellers, the most rapidly growing cities today are in low- and middle-income countries [4]. The two cities with the highest average annual growth rate between 2006 and 2020 are expected to be Beihai in southern China and Ghaziabad in India, with other fast-growing cities in Nigeria, Mali, and Bangladesh [5]. The world's largest cities today probably are Karachi, Shanghai, Mumbai, Beijing, and Delhi, with New York City being one of the world's largest metropolitan areas, although the cross-country heterogeneity of what constitutes city boundaries makes such definitions challenging [6].

URBAN HEALTH

As the pace of urbanization increased, the field of urban health emerged around the turn of the 21st century [7]. This new field seeks to understand how, and why, cities influence the well-being of their inhabitants [7]. This focus is in keeping with larger trends in the study of the health of populations. An appreciation of how cities shape health reflects growing scholarship around the role of context as an inextricable determinant of health [8]. It is, in many respects, intuitive that cities would shape well-being. Cities influence the food we eat, the water we drink, and the air we breathe. Urban living can affect everything from available food to walkability and the spread of infectious diseases [9, 10, 11].

THE DETERMINANTS OF HEALTH IN CITIES

Three particular factors stand out as drivers of health in cities: the physical environment, the social environment, and access to health and social services [12]. There are many examples of how these factors wield their influence. Among the most studied determinants of urban health is the physical environment. One Boston-based study found a link between traffic-related air pollutants and impaired glucose tolerance during pregnancy [13]. The World Health Organization has linked 7 million premature deaths globally to air pollution [14]. Brian Saelens and colleagues found that children in Seattle and San Diego who lived in neighborhoods with more access to healthy foods and a better "physical activity environment" were, after adjusting for individual, family, and neighborhood-level demographics, less likely to be obese [15]. With respect to the social environment, Mahasin Mujahid and colleagues found that people were less likely to have hypertension when they lived in neighborhoods with higher social cohesion [16]. Less studied is the challenge of service access in urban areas, although some work has focused on access to services among urban subgroups such as immigrants and homeless youth [17, 18]. One study found that low-income and racial minority communities in Los Angeles had limited access to integrated mental health care in Los Angeles County [19]. Although work in this area is still very much a burgeoning field, there are many opportunities for development. Urban health has readily become transdisciplinary, and researchers are capitalizing on new technology and big data that target the drivers of health in cities, both domestically and globally [20, 21, 22, 23].

HEALTH AND BOSTON

Perhaps the abstraction of "urban health" is brought home more acutely when one considers a specific example. In this case, let us focus on the city of Boston. Boston is characterized by dramatic heterogeneity in health, with many health "haves and have-nots." Life expectancy in this relatively small city varies by as much as 33 years between neighborhoods that are only a couple of miles away from each other, with a high of 91.9 years in Back Bay and a low of 58.9 years in Roxbury [24]. Comparably, Jarvis Chen and colleagues examined premature mortality rates across neighborhoods in Boston and found that Roxbury and South Boston had by far the highest rates, and the wealthier Back Bay/Beacon Hill area had the lowest [25].

How do urban characteristics shape the health of Boston's residents? A spatial study by Dustin Duncan and colleagues examined this question, comparing open recreational space to neighborhood characteristics [26]. They found that neighborhoods with a high proportion of non-Hispanic black residents had significantly less open space, increasing the risk of obesity due to lack of physical activity [26]. Another study used the 2008 Boston Youth Survey to show a relationship between high neighborhood social fragmentation and lower physical activity among adolescents [27]. Consistent with research in other cities, study after study show that many of the indictors that are associated with poor health cluster together.

This is no less true in Boston, where the lowest-income neighborhoods coincide with those that have less open green space and worse health outcomes. In many studies, area-level poverty serves as a ready marker for the accumulation of factors that adversely affect health in urban areas. For example, in the aforementioned Boston study, Chen and colleagues found that the incidence of premature mortality rates was 1.4 times higher in the most economically deprived census tracts compared to those in the least impoverished tracts [25]. They also found an attributable fraction of 25 to 30 percent excess deaths due to living in high-poverty census tracts. These census tracts with the highest poverty have also consistently been found to have the highest proportion of black residents and the lowest levels of education [28].

OPPORTUNITIES IN URBAN HEALTH

In many ways, the study of health in cities presents a tremendous opportunity, both for a multilevel understanding of population health and for academic public health to find a focus for scholarship and action. Clearly, factors at the political, structural, social, and service delivery levels are jointly responsible for the health of urban residents, and an understanding of the dynamics that knit together this causal web presents opportunities for both knowledge and, potentially, intervention. There is growing interest in creating healthier cities and the potential for real movement in this area. This is particularly true as emerging municipal efforts aim to capitalize on the growing political latitude that cities are enjoying toward the development of innovative, health-promoting approaches [29]. Urbanization represents a chance for us to integrate many of the core concerns of public health—especially our focus on environmental context and the social determinants of disease—into advancing progress on this issue. Scholarship that aims to understand how cities influence health, and how the urban environment "gets under the skin," can be interesting, formative, and productive [30]. As cities evolve, public health must evolve with them to safeguard the well-being of the new urban majorities now and in the future.

REFERENCES

1. Urban Population Growth. World Health Organization Web site. http://www.who.int/gho/urban_health/situation_trends/urban_population_growth/en. Accessed November 28, 2016.

2. Urban Health. World Health Organization Web site. http://www.who.int/gho/urban_health/en. Accessed November 28, 2016.

3. McClean D, ed. *World Disasters Report 2010—Urban Risk.* International Federation of Red Cross and Red Crescent Societies Web site. http://www.ifrc.org/en/publications-and-reports/world-disasters-report/wdr2010. Accessed November 28, 2016.

4. Population Distribution, Urbanization, Internal Migration and Development. The United Nations Web site. http://www.un.org/en/development/desa/population/publications/urbanization/population-distribution.shtml. Accessed November 28, 2016.

5. The World's Fastest Growing Cities and Urban Areas from 2006 to 2020. City Mayors Web site. http://www.citymayors.com/statistics/urban_growth1.html. Accessed November 28, 2016.

6. The Largest Cities in the World and Their Mayors. City Mayors Web site. http://www.city-mayors.com/statistics/largest-cities-mayors-1.html. Accessed November 28, 2016.

7. Vlahov D, Galea S. Urban health: A new discipline. *The Lancet.* 2003; 362(9390): 1091-2.

8. Kaplan GA. What is the role of the social environment in understanding inequalities in health? *Annals of the New York Academy of Sciences.* 1999; 896: 116-9.

9. Neckerman KM, et al. Disparities in the food environments of New York City public schools. *American Journal of Preventive Medicine.* 2010; 39(3): 195-202. doi:10.1016/j.amepre.2010.05.004

10. de Sa E, Ardern CI. Neighbourhood walkability, leisure-time and transport-related physical activity in a mixed urban-rural area. *PeerJ.* 2014; 2: e440. doi:10.7717/peerj.440

11. Hille P. Ebola virus a serious threat to urban areas. *DW.* January 8, 2014. http://www.dw.com/en/ebola-virus-a-serious-threat-to-urban-areas/a-17826190. Accessed November 28, 2016.

12. Galea S, Vlahov D. Urban health: Evidence, challenges, and directions. *Annual Review of Public Health.* 2005; 26: 341-65.

13. Fleisch AF, et al. Air pollution exposure and abnormal glucose tolerance during pregnancy: The project Viva cohort. *Environmental Health Perspectives.* 2014; 122(4): 378-83. doi:10.1289/ehp.1307065

14. 7 Million Premature Deaths Annually Linked to Air Pollution. World Health Organization Web site. http://www.who.int/mediacentre/news/releases/2014/air-pollution/en/#.UzD4e3UCm-o.twitter. Accessed November 28, 2016.

15. Saelens BE, et al. Obesogenic neighborhood environments, child and parent obesity: The Neighborhood Impact on Kids study. *American Journal of Preventive Medicine.* 2012; 42(5): e57-64. doi:10.1016/j.amepre.2012.02.008

16. Mujahid MS, et al. Neighborhood characteristics and hypertension. *Epidemiology.* 2008; 19(4): 590-8. doi:10.1097/EDE.0b013e3181772cb2

17. Nandi A, et al. Access to and use of health services among undocumented Mexican immigrants in a US urban area. *American Journal of Public Health.* 2008; 98(11): 2011-20. doi:10.2105/AJPH.2006.096222

18. Solorio MR, Milburn NG, Andersen RM, Trifskin S, Rodríguez MA. Emotional distress and mental health service use among urban homeless adolescents. *The Journal of Behavioral Health Services & Research.* 2006; 33(4): 381-93.

19. Guerrero EG, Kao D. Racial/ethnic minority and low-income hotspots and their geographic proximity to integrated care providers. *Substance Abuse Treatment, Prevention, and Policy.* 2013; 8: 34. doi:10.1186/1747-597X-8-34

20. Built Environment and Health Research Group at Columbia University Web site. https://beh.columbia.edu. Accessed November 28, 2016.

21. NYC OpenData Web site. https://nycopendata.socrata.com. Accessed November 28, 2016.

22. Thomas SB, Quinn SC. Poverty and elimination of urban health disparities: Challenge and opportunity. *Annals of the New York Academy of Sciences.* 2008; 1136: 111-25. doi:10.1196/annals.1425.018

23. CAF–Development Bank of Latin America, UN-HABITAT. *Construction of More Equitable Cities.* Kenya: UN-Habitat, CAF–Development bank of Latin America, Avina; 2014.

24. Zimmerman E, Evans BF, Woolf SH, Haley AD. *Social Capital and Health Outcomes in Boston.* Richmond, VA: Virginia Commonwealth University Center on Human Needs; 2012.

25. Chen JT, et al. Mapping and measuring social disparities in premature mortality: The impact of Census tract poverty within and across Boston neighborhoods, 1999-2001. *Journal of Urban Health.* 2006; 83(6): 1063-84. doi:10.1007/s11524-006-9089-7

26. Duncan DT, Kawachi I, White K, Williams DR. The geography of recreational open space: Influence of neighborhood racial composition and neighborhood poverty. *Journal of Urban Health.* 2013; 90(4): 618-31. doi:10.1007/s11524-012-9770-y

27. Pabayo R, Molnar BE, Cradock A, Kawachi I. The relationship between neighborhood socioeconomic characteristics and physical inactivity among adolescents living in Boston, Massachusetts. *American Journal of Public Health.* 2014; 104(11): e142-e149. doi:10.2105/AJPH.2014.302109

28. *Health of Boston 2014-2015.* Boston, MA: Boston Public Health Commission Research and Evaluation Office; 2015.

29. Types of Healthy Settings: Healthy Cities. World Health Organization Web site. http://www.who.int/healthy_settings/types/cities/en. Accessed November 28, 2016.

30. Galea S, Uddin M, Koenen K. The urban environment and mental disorders: Epigenetic links. *Epigenetics.* 2011; 6(4): 400-404.

42

Toward an Activist Public Health[1]

THERE ARE MANY organizations that work toward improving the health of the public, including government, social service organizations, community-based organizations, public health agencies, and advocacy groups. Each has a key role to play in ensuring the well-being of populations. Academic public health also has a role as part of this broader public health enterprise. Our central function is knowledge generation and transmission. But we have an added responsibility. It is our job to influence culture, to advance a conversation toward creating positive change. For this reason, a forward-looking school of public health should closely tie an activist practice agenda to its central function of thinking and teaching. An *activist* role—that is, one that aims to bring about foundational change—is unavoidable if one aspires to promote population health [1].

An engaged school of public health must therefore stay true to its core mission—knowledge generation and transmission—while at the same time contributing to the daily work that improves health at the community level and beyond.

This unique combination of knowledge generation and activism will enrich the experience of students, even as it helps to meet the practical needs of the populations we serve. An activist school is able to turn theoretical concepts into reality, allowing students, faculty, and staff to truly understand, and get to know, vulnerable populations. Principally, there are four key areas around which an activist academic public health agenda can engage, contributing to both our core academic mission and our aspirations for further engagement with the wider world.

---

[1] This chapter was co-written by Professor Harold Cox, Associate Dean for Public Health Practice at the Boston University School of Public Health.

First, we have a responsibility to generate scholarship around issues that are of direct relevance to public health practice. This means applying the tools of science and scholarship to the work of practitioners who engage regularly with the issues of population health and disease. In its simplest form, schools must hold forums to broaden understanding of current issues, such as Ebola response, homelessness, and gun control. At a deeper level, we must seek answers to entrenched, complex questions, with the kind of sustained, scholarly focus only a university can provide. For example, in recent years, as the public health practice world has grappled with emergency preparedness as part of its sphere of influence, substantial public health scholarship has considered how health system capacity can best be built to inform public health preparedness efforts [2]. Going forward, schools of public health must continue to take a longer, broader view of such issues.

Second, an activist public health agenda elevates our ambition to provide academic support for our public health practice partners. This builds on the responsibility of academic public health to transmit knowledge beyond the university walls. Doing so means that we need to build the capacity to effectively educate students across a range of sectors and to ensure we have the modalities at hand to make our educational opportunities readily available, and useful, to our practice partners.

Third, academic public health must develop innovative approaches to public health practice that can serve as pilots, or models, for future adoption by partners in practice communities. A caveat here. I do not suggest that it is the role of an academic institution to take on the mantle of direct service or program delivery in the longer term. However, one of our core functions is to incubate ideas that can be carried forward by practice partners, informing programs and projects going forward. We must continue to capitalize on our assets to improve the way in which public health is practiced, aiming to positively influence the health of populations.

Finally, an activist public health must embrace the diversity of industries and fields that shape the health of populations and must work to nudge these sectors toward productive, positive change. We need to extend our agenda beyond what has been traditionally viewed as the remit of public health practice. In many ways, this approach is simply a reflection of our current reality. It is now clearly understood that most of the drivers of population health are not within the control of traditional health sectors. Urban planning, tax code structure, health care resource allocation, and packaging of calorie-dense, nutrient-poor food all shape the health of the public. Decisions on these areas are all well outside the scope of what has historically been viewed as public health practice, but we cannot afford to ignore them. An activist academic public health engages these areas to inform and influence decisions that, in turn, influence the health of populations. There is a rich academic scholarship that examines the centrality of non-health actors in influencing health [3]. An activist academic public health moves beyond merely recognizing these forces, seeking, rather, to leverage our intellectual and creative assets to effect meaningful change.

REFERENCES

1. Activism. Oxford Dictionaries Web site. https://en.oxforddictionaries.com/definition/us/activism. Accessed November 27, 2016.

2. Walsh L, Craddock H, Gulley K, Strauss-Riggs K, Schor KW. Building health care system capacity to respond to disasters: Successes and challenges of disaster preparedness health care coalitions. *Prehospital and Disaster Medicine.* 2015; 30(2): 112-22. doi:10.1017/S1049023X14001459

3. House JS, Schoeni RF, Kaplan GA, Pollack H, eds. *Making Americans Healthier: Social and Economic Policy as Health Policy.* New York, NY: Russell Sage Foundation; 2008.

43

Promoting Prevention

IN 2015, I HAD the privilege of co-organizing a meeting about prevention science under the auspices of the Rockefeller Foundation [1]. The attendees were a varied group and included academics, public health practitioners, and industry partners. The purpose of the meeting was to discuss the state of prevention science worldwide and to identify strategies for promoting a global primary prevention agenda. The meeting was informed by a key recognition, one that is frustrating yet inescapable: Although substantial improvements to population health can be achieved with the broad adoption of prevention efforts, the vast proportion of health spending worldwide is on curative care. Evidence from high-income countries, for example, demonstrates that health systems that rely exclusively on secondary prevention and curative care often fail to substantially reduce morbidity and mortality, notwithstanding the extreme expense of treatment. The United States is a particularly glaring example of this. In 2010, the United States ranked 24th out of the 30 Organization for Economic Cooperation and Development countries with respect to life expectancy. This was driven largely by higher burdens of a number of preventable diseases in the United States, including diabetes, cardiovascular disease, and chronic respiratory disease, compared to other similar countries. However, Americans already spend far more on health care than any other country in the world. Between 2011 and 2015, 17.1 percent of US gross domestic product (GDP) was spent on health care [2]. More important, health care costs have grown faster in the United States than in any other country in the world during the past 40 years, even while the United States spends 3 to 5 percent of its health expenditure on public health or preventive services. The Institute of Medicine stated succinctly, "It is no longer sufficient to expect that reforms in the medical care delivery system alone will improve the public's health. Large proportions of the US disease burden are preventable" [3].

Prevention has the potential to minimize morbidity and mortality worldwide. There is little question of this. In particular, a comprehensive prevention approach could help us mitigate the burden and cost of noncommunicable diseases (NCDs). The opportunity is particularly great in lower- and middle-income countries (LMICs), where upwards of 80 percent of the world's disease burden is concentrated. That burden is high indeed. Currently, nearly 8 million people die of NCDs before the age of 60 years in LMICs annually, and the burden of NCDs is expected to grow: Estimates suggest a potential increase in the burden of NCDs in LMICs of nearly 17 percent overall and up to 27 percent in regions such as sub-Saharan Africa [4].

This worrying trend lent urgency to the subject of our meeting, as we searched for ways to capitalize on a growing recognition of the importance of prevention. There is an increasing awareness that primary prevention, as a centerpiece to a functioning health system, has the capacity to both decrease morbidity and mortality over the long-term and afford health systems substantial cost savings, particularly in contexts that may have limited resources. During the course of the discussion, five key points emerged that have, I think, particular utility in understanding and promoting a prevention approach.

AN IMPERATIVE FOR PREVENTION: THE CONSEQUENCES OF INACTION

In a rapidly changing health and health care environment, the need for a prevention approach is critical. This is particularly true as we witness the emergence of newer blockbuster drugs. Consider Sovaldi, discussed in Chapter 18. Sovaldi, manufactured by Gilead, is a remarkable drug capable of curing hepatitis C, a disease that leads to the death of approximately 500,000 people annually [5]. Sovaldi is (unsurprisingly) expensive, resulting in several calls for revisiting its pricing [6]. Without returning to the issue of drug pricing, the impact of Sovaldi and other similar drugs on health care budgets clarifies the appeal of a prevention focus. Hepatitis C, transmitted principally through drug use, is largely preventable. We know this, yet we have spent far too little on known and effective harm-reduction efforts. As a consequence, we are now faced with a far more expensive prospect: a treatment that is effective but potentially ruinous for health systems locally and globally. This argues strongly for a prevention imperative.

THE CONSTRAINTS ON PREVENTION

Many barriers obstruct the implementation of a widespread prevention approach. These barriers are centrally financial, political, and empirical. Financially, work in this area is hindered by the fact that the costs of prevention are frequently borne by actors who do not reap their benefits. A hospital, health system, or health department that implements a preventive program may be accruing benefits for a health payer who sees costs decrease but who is not involved in the original outlay. This mismatch can be problematic, challenging any one actor's incentive to introduce preventive efforts and see commensurate return on the investment. Politically, the temporal lag between preventive efforts and the benefits that emerge from these efforts is too often a nonstarter. Political actors tend to work on a short timeline, dictated by elections and term limits. For this reason, they often desire to see yield from efforts they invest in during their time in office. Empirically, we have a remarkable paucity of good data about the efficacy of large-scale primary prevention efforts worldwide. This reflects the nature of many of these efforts, which are implemented by systems that are not accustomed to rigorous evaluation. Unfortunately, this has left us with a limited body of data that we can use to muster arguments in favor of prevention.

PREVENTION AS A LINK BETWEEN THE CLINICAL AND PUBLIC HEALTH WORLDS

Despite the obstacles prevention faces, there are also many opportunities. These opportunities often present as areas for collaboration—for example, preventive efforts can serve as bridges between the clinical and public health worlds. This is true for primary prevention, which frequently involves direct implementation of efforts that engage with patients within clinical systems. It is perhaps even more true for secondary and tertiary prevention efforts that involve working with patients who have already been exposed to disease. Extending the example of hepatitis C, we can see this synergy at work. Secondary prevention of attendant liver disease involves regular monitoring and the early use of antiviral drugs as appropriate. Similarly, and conversely, immunization against hepatitis A and B for persons infected with hepatitis C substantially minimizes hepatitis-related morbidity. These efforts blur the lines between clinical medicine and public health, improving understanding and effectiveness in both areas and providing a useful template for future work.

PRIVATE INITIATIVES AND INNOVATION AND TECHNOLOGY

Innovation in prevention is increasingly emerging from sectors that have not traditionally been linked to public health. This is happening even as we approach prevention as a core responsibility of public health scientists and professionals. Such innovation has had the effect of further broadening the scope of the field and the opportunity for partnership. For example, treatment as prevention brings the biotechnology and pharmaceutical industry into the fold. Elsewhere, the emergence of pre-exposure prophylaxis has revolutionized HIV prevention; emerging insights, such as the use of metformin in cancer prevention, will do much the same for other areas. More prosaic treatment efforts rest on the innovation in, and adoption of, new technologies. This extends as far back as innovations in bed nets to prevent malaria, but it also extends forward to the application of genomic approaches to infectious pathogen analysis, identification, and vaccine development. And the rate of change continues to accelerate. Rapid diagnostic methods depend on technological development and present opportunities for prevention that were outside our armamentarium not so long ago. This represents a strong argument for a multisectoral conception of public health—one that embraces industry, government, and nongovernmental actors as partners in the production of population health and the prevention of disease.

STRATEGIC APPLICATION OF HIDDEN GOVERNMENT POLICY LEVERS
AND RESTRUCTURING OF HEALTH SYSTEMS

The constraints on prevention are real. They reflect deep, system-level barriers to more widespread dissemination of prevention efforts. However, just as prevention can spur innovation in technology, it can also inspire innovations in approach, helping us to better navigate the barriers our efforts face. Much as these obstacles exist, they depend on system incentives and structures; those same incentives and structures can be leveraged to optimize the likelihood of prevention efforts being implemented and succeeding. For example, at the domestic federal level, the Office of Management and Budget (OMB) is responsible for budgetary projections for new policy implementation. However, OMB time horizons are time-constrained, limiting the analysis of potential benefits of longer term initiatives such as preventive efforts. This limitation presents opportunities for seemingly unrelated policy lever re-engineering (i.e., lengthening the OMB review window) that can have substantial import for prevention efforts. Similar levers exist within health systems. With this in mind, the architecture of health systems can and should be engineered to maximize preventive approaches. This can range from payment and reimbursement systems to individual physician incentives. Given the size and expense of our health care system, failure to take these steps represents an enormous opportunity cost and an entrenchment in the curative status quo, with attendant poor health indicators.

REFERENCES

1. The Rockefeller Foundation Web site. https://www.rockefellerfoundation.org. Accessed November 27, 2016.

2. Health Expenditure, Total (% of GDP). The World Bank Group Web site. http://data.worldbank.org/indicator/SH.XPD.TOTL.ZS. Accessed November 27, 2016.

3. Institute of Medicine. *For the Public's Health: Investing in a Healthier Future*. Washington, DC: The National Academies Press; 2012.

4. Islam SM, et al. Non-communicable diseases (NCDs) in developing countries: A symposium report. *Globalization and Health*. 2014; 10: 81. doi:10.1186/s12992-014-0081-9

5. Hepatitis C. World Health Organization Web site. http://www.who.int/mediacentre/factsheets/fs164/en. Updated July 2016. Accessed November 27, 2016.

6. Pollack A. High cost of Sovaldi hepatitis C drug prompts a call to void its patents. *The New York Times*. May 19, 2015. http://www.nytimes.com/2015/05/20/business/high-cost-of-hepatitis-c-drug-prompts-a-call-to-void-its-patents.html. Accessed November 27, 2016.

44

Innovating for a Healthier Public

"INNOVATION," WROTE ROBERTA Ness, "is the engine of scientific progress" [1]. I agree, and I argue that we would be missing a tremendous opportunity if we did not actively consider how we may embrace innovative approaches in advancing the goals of public health. I briefly do so here, commenting on three fronts: first on the role of biological and pharmaceutical approaches, second on the role of less typical innovative technological approaches to the improvement of population health, and third on approaches to public health efforts that are not centered around drugs or technology at all but, rather, rest on novel attempts to improve the social, cultural, and economic conditions that shape health.

First, I comment on biological/pharmaceutical innovation. By way of example, let us consider the development of tenofovir disoproxil/emtricitabine (Truvada) [2]. Truvada is on the cutting edge of HIV prevention. In one study of all adult Kaiser Permanente San Francisco members evaluated for pre-exposure prophylaxis between July 2012 and February 2015, there were no new HIV infections among Truvada users [3]. This makes Truvada an exciting, potentially game-changing drug focused on prevention. Other pharmaceutical innovations involve using old drugs in new ways. Consider the adoption of metformin for possible use in cancer prevention [4]. Diabetic postmenopausal women aged 50 to 79 years have been shown to have a 45 percent greater risk of dying from invasive cancer compared to women without diabetes [5]. Research from the Women's Health Initiative has suggested, however, that over the long term, women managing their diabetes with metformin have a lower risk of getting cancer compared to other diabetic women [5]. Other studies have shown equally encouraging results, suggesting that metformin, designed for treatment, can be leveraged for disease prevention [6, 7].

The examples of metformin and Truvada are just two cases in which pharmaceutical innovations are creating the conditions for a healthier future in ways that are compatible with a prevention focus. And there is more to encourage us in this area. The use of biotechnology and genomics in vaccine development and the continued refinement of rapid diagnostic tests (RDTs) are helping to advance both primary and secondary prevention, including the potential of RDTs to make a tremendous difference, if broadly utilized, in the fight against malaria [8, 9, 10, 11].

We now move on to other, more diverse technologies. Let us start small. One of the most useful developments in the history of health technology is also one of the most basic—the mosquito net [12]. The use of mosquito netting has dramatically lowered the prevalence of malaria in Africa; the disease was once the number one killer of refugees on the continent; it now ranks fifth [13]. The mosquito net, simple but effective, is in many ways the perfect marriage of innovation and disease prevention.

Now let us jump ahead and consider contemporary innovations in a host of industries, beyond just the pharmaceutical or biological world, that contribute to improving population health. On the environmental front, the construction of ever-larger offshore wind turbines means cleaner air and all the attendant health benefits of a less polluted world, including longer life expectancy [14, 15, 16]. In architecture and urban design, we see schools being built with an eye toward improving the physical and mental health of students, and the lay-out of cities being modified to improve pedestrian well-being [17, 18]. Automobiles have also been upgraded and improved in the interest of safeguarding health. The widespread use of seat belts, a triumph of public health, is now one safety measure among many. More recent vehicular innovations include blind spot sensors, collision warning systems, and automatic breaking [19, 20]. Just as technological innovation has lessened the danger of driving, it also stands to make a difference in preventing gun deaths. The introduction of fingerprint-locking "smart guns" suggests a way that technology can mitigate the lethality of firearms, creating, amid the contentiousness of the gun debate, an area of possible compromise [21]. A recent study found that close to 60 percent of Americans would be open to buying a smart or childproof gun [22].

Finally, a note about how innovation may shape the conditions that make people healthy. There is little question that changing these conditions has to be at the core of the mission of public health. We have recently witnessed several spectacular efforts to this end that have failed—for example, attempts to change soda packaging norms in New York [23]. But for every such frustration, we have seen other highly successful efforts. When New York City successfully banned trans fats, it substantially reduced satu-rated fat content in meals consumed in the city [24, 25]. Elsewhere, in 2016, the city of Philadelphia enacted a soda tax; although this measure was not cast as a public health effort, its net effect will be the reduction of sugary soda consumption and, by conse-quence, an improvement in population health [26]. The Vision Zero program is another example of this type of macro-level innovation [27]. The program aimed to reduce urban traffic injuries, leading to a reduction in New York City pedestrian fatalities in its first 2 years of existence [28]. These programs are indeed innovations, and they are templates for future success. They take something that we thought could not be done (can trans fats be banned? Will consumers not just leave New York City and go eat in New Jersey?) and show that it can be.

Innovative approaches stand to improve population health in a variety of ways, rang-ing from what we may typically think of as innovative—the discovery of new molecular or genetic targeting techniques—to creative approaches that shape our social, economic, and political context and, consequently, our health. Importantly, many innovative approaches that may promote health do not necessarily arise from the pursuit of a population health goal but, rather, can equally well lend themselves to the improvement of population health. This, to my mind, suggests a need for public health's active engagement in partnerships across different sectors and an openness to an "any-means-necessary" approach to creating a healthier world.

REFERENCES

1. Ness RB. Tools for innovative thinking in epidemiology. *American Journal of Epidemiology.* 2012; 175(8): 733-8. doi:10.1093/aje/kwr412

2. How Is Truvada Used to Treat HIV-1 Infection? Truvada Web site. http://www.truvada.com/treatment-for-hiv. Published 2016. Accessed July 27, 2016.

3. Volk JE, et al. No new HIV infections with increasing use of HIV preexposure prophylaxis in a clinical practice setting. *Clinical Infectious Diseases.* 2015; 61: 1601-3. doi:10.1093/cid/civ778

4. Metformin. Drugs.com Web site. https://www.drugs.com/metformin.html. Accessed July 27, 2016.

5. Gong Z. Diabetes, metformin and incidence of and death from invasive cancer in postmenopausal women: Results from the Women's Health Initiative. *International Journal of Cancer.* 2016; 138(8): 1915-27. doi:10.1002/ijc.29944

6. DeCensi A, et al. Metformin and cancer risk in diabetic patients: A systematic review and meta-analysis. *Cancer Prevention Research.* 2010; 3: 1451–1461. doi:10.1158/1940-6207. CAPR-10-0157

7. Sakoda L, et al. Metformin use and lung cancer risk in patients with diabetes. *Cancer Prevention Research.* 2015; 8: 174–179.

8. Serruto D, et al. Biotechnology and vaccines: Application of functional genomics to *Neisseria meningitidis* and other bacterial pathogens. *Journal of Biotechnology.* 2004; 113(1-3): 15-32. doi:10.1016/j.jbiotec.2004.03.024

9. The National Academies Keck Futures Initiative. How can genomics facilitate vaccine development? In *The National Academies Keck Futures Initiative: The Genomic Revolution— Implications for Treatment and Control of Infectious Disease: Working Groups Summaries.* Washington DC: National Academies Press; 2005: 33-9.

10. Malaria: Rapid Diagnostic Tests. World Health Organization Web site. http://www.who.int/malaria/areas/diagnosis/rapid_diagnostic_tests/en. Updated March 14, 2016. Accessed July 27, 2016.

11. Wilson ML. Malaria rapid diagnostic tests. *Clinical Infectious Diseases.* 2012; 54: 1637–1641. doi:10.1093/cid/cis228

12. Insecticide-Treated Bed Nets. Centers for Disease Control and Prevention Web site. http://www.cdc.gov/malaria/malaria_worldwide/reduction/itn.html. Updated December 28, 2015. Accessed July 27, 2016.

13. Our Impact. Nothing But Nets Web site. http://www.nothingbutnets.net/new/saving-lives/our-impact.html. Accessed July 27, 2016.

14. Richard MG. 9 energy innovations that make the future brighter! Treehugger.com Web site. http://www.treehugger.com/renewable-energy/9-energy-innovations-make-future-brighter.html. Published August 2012. Accessed July 27, 2016.

15. Benefits and Costs of the Clean Air Act 1990-2020, the Second Prospective Study. US Environmental Protection Agency Web site. https://www.epa.gov/clean-air-act-overview/ benefits-and-costs-clean-air-act-1990-2020-second-prospective-study. Updated October 19, 2015. Accessed July 27, 2016.

16. Arden Pope C, Ezzati M, Dockery D. Fine-particulate air pollution and life expectancy in the United States. *The New England Journal of Medicine*. 2009; 360: 376-86. doi:10.1056/ NEJMsa0805646

17. Hunter's Point Campus. Center for Active Design Web site. https://centerforactivedesign. org/hunterspointcampus. Accessed July 27, 2016.

18. SPUR's Design for Walkability Initiative. Design for Walkability Web site. http://www. designforwalkability.com. Accessed July 27, 2016.

19. Achievements in public health, 1900-1999 motor-vehicle safety: A 20th century public health achievement. *Morbidity and Mortality Weekly Report (MMWR)*. 1999; 48(18): 369-74.

20. 5 Top Car Safety Innovations. Autotrader Web site. http://www.autotrader.com/car-tech/ 5-top-car-safety-innovations-212820. Published August 2013. Accessed July 27, 2016.

21. Fingerprint Guns. Smart Tech Foundation Web site. https://smarttechfoundation.org/ smart-firearms-technology/fingerprint-guns. Accessed 27, 2016.

22. Wolfson J, Teret S, Frattaroli S, Miller M, Azrael D. The US public's preference for safer guns. *American Journal of Public Health*. 2016; 106(3): 411-3. doi:10.2105/AJPH.2015.303041

23. Grynbaum M. New York's ban on big sodas is rejected by final court. *The New York Times*. June 26, 2014. http://www.nytimes.com/2014/06/27/nyregion/city-loses-final-appeal-on-limiting-sales-of-large-sodas.html?mtrref=undefined&gwh=CB015E9556FF8D01C3750592 67832E99&gwt=pay&assetType=nyt_now. Accessed July 27, 2016.

24. Ross GL. Determining the benefits of the New York City trans fat ban. *Annals of Internal Medicine*.2010;152(3):194;authorreply194-5.doi:10.7326/0003-4819-152-3-201002020-00016

25. MacMillan A. NYC's fat ban paying off. CNN Web site. http://www.cnn.com/2012/07/16/ health/nyc-fat-ban-paying-off. Published July 16, 2012. Accessed July 27, 2016.

26. Nadolny T. Soda tax passes; Philadelphia is first big city in nation to enact one. Philly.com Web site. http://articles.philly.com/2016-06-18/news/73844306_1_philadelphia-city-council-tax-credit-first-such-tax. Published June 18, 2016. Accessed July 28, 2016.

27. NYC Vision Zero Action Plan. NYC.gov Web site. http://www1.nyc.gov/nyc-resources/ser-vice/3860/nyc-vision-zero-action-plan Accessed July 27, 2016.

28. The City of New York. *Vision Zero: Year Two Report*. New York, NY: Author; 2016.

45

Who Should We Talk to, and How?

WHY DO WE COMMUNICATE? At core, our communications represent an attempt to find spaces—in a variety of media—where ideas can be heard and engaged with. Even if this engagement results in disagreement or debate, the process of coming together to share thoughts and opinions is, I think, a perennially enriching exercise. Ultimately, we aim to influence the broader conversation as part of our responsibility as a field, to arrive at the confluence of knowledge and values needed to promote population health. Through our media engagement and our advocacy, we seek to use the power of language to effect positive change.

For our words to have maximum resonance, they must above all be clear. Finding this clarity begins with knowing our audience. We must be clear about to whom we are speaking and choose what we say accordingly—a time-tested communication technique. More than 2,000 years ago, Cicero summarized the importance of being able to speak comfortably to multiple groups, saying "He, therefore, is the man of genuine Eloquence, who can adapt his language to what is most suitable to each. By doing this, he will be sure to say every thing as it ought to be said" [1].

Who, then, are our main audiences? I suggest that they are threefold.

First, there is our academic audience, our peers. As scholars, our engagement with the academic world is the backbone of our work. When we conduct our research and give voice to our findings, we do so to advance knowledge and establish a scientific basis for our arguments. There are, of course, limitations to this dialogue. The audience for academic writing is a comparatively small one. However, this can make for a robust transmission of ideas and feedback, as concepts quickly circulate among a tight-knit, connected community. There are many benefits to this. When we address our peers, our thought process is laid bare for their review. The scientific method, itself a kind of common tongue, gives us a shared framework through which we can evaluate one another, as we lay the foundations of our field [2]. From this interplay of empiricism and argument arose many of the cornerstones of public health. This is the process through which initially controversial ideas can slowly (or not so slowly) become tenets of public health theory and practice. As discussed in Chapter 11, the utility of handwashing was once hotly debated in the academy. As strange as it may be to think something so seemingly self-evident used to be an academic question, many now "obvious" truths about health developed the same way—from the uselessness of bloodletting to the germ theory of disease and the declassification of same-sex love as a mental illness [3, 4, 5]. The fates of what we now accept as truisms were once dependent on the clear and consistent expression of an argument, often over the course of years. In these cases, understanding progressed through a combination of methodological rigor and disciplined communication, with language playing a key role in changing minds and shaping paradigms.

Our second audience represents a slightly larger sampling of people: the influencers working across many sectors who are in a position to change the policies that affect health. Our engagement with this group allows us access to the kind of real-world leverage that gives public health solutions the broadest possible reach. This engagement may expose us to ways of behaving and communicating that seem unfamiliar. If so, all the better. By learning to "speak the language" of those who are in a position to make change happen, we are better able to find areas of confluence and opportunities for collaboration.

By way of illustration, let us return to a subject we have covered previously—economics. Economics is a field that, like public health, concerns itself with the distribution of well-being within and across populations. Yet, between disciplines, the words used to describe this common mission can be quite different. Where we say "health," the economist might say "utility"; where we say "minimizing disparities," she might refer to a "Rawlsian function." To collaborate with an economist, then, we must familiarize ourselves with how an economist talks. This has the added benefit of familiarizing us with how an economist *thinks*. By opening ourselves to the vocabulary of others, we open ourselves to different habits of mind, improving our ability to make connections and identify areas of overlap between the work of public health and the many less obviously health-related fields that nevertheless shape the well-being of populations [6].

Finally, there is our outreach to the general public. This communication is critical if we are to change the culture around matters of health. It also helps us to keep track of the progress we have already made. With the exception of certain watershed moments, such as 2015's marriage equality victory, it can be difficult to measure the progress of change in real time [7]. One key benchmark can be language—the public conversation about issues related to health. Consider our efforts to curb the gun violence epidemic. That the word "epidemic" is now used prominently in reference to this ongoing tragedy is itself a sign of progress. It suggests our success in nudging the conversation forward—in framing gun violence as a public health crisis rather than simply a matter of law and order [8, 9]. This shift demonstrates the power of words to both define a problem and create a context in which it might be solved.

We need to deepen and extend this influence. From education to income inequality, there are many other areas in which the language of public health may be brought to bear [10]. Just as our own speech must draw from the language of other disciplines, we must not be shy about applying the words and phrases of our field to sectors in which they might make a difference. As we work to shift perception and culture, we must likewise work to influence the way people talk about health, changing—literally—the terms of the debate, as we move toward the ultimate goal of changing minds and societies.

REFERENCES

1. Cicero MT, Jones E, trans. *Cicero's Brutus or History of Famous Orators; Also His Orator, or Accomplished Speaker*. Urbana, IL: Project Gutenberg; 2006. http://www.gutenberg.org/cache/epub/9776/pg9776-images.html. Accessed November 28, 2016.

2. Steps of the Scientific Method. Science Buddies Web site. http://www.sciencebuddies.org/science-fair-projects/project_scientific_method.shtml. Accessed November 28, 2016.

3. Anders EO. "A Plea for the Lancet": Bloodletting, therapeutic epistemology, and professional identity in late nineteenth-century American medicine. *Social History of Medicine*. 2016; 29(4): 781–801. doi:10.1093/shm/hkw026

4. Metzner R. The causes of disease: The great debate. Functional Medicine University Web site. http://www.functionalmedicineuniversity.com/public/937.cfm. Accessed November 28, 2016.

5. Drescher J. Out of DSM: Depathologizing homosexuality. *Behavioral Sciences*. 2015; 5(4): 565-75. doi:10.3390/bs5040565

6. Chomsky's Philosophy. Noam Chomsky—Language and Thought. Online video clip. YouTube Web site. https://www.youtube.com/watch?v=KEmpRtj34xg. Accessed November 28, 2016.

7. Chappell B. Supreme Court declares same-sex marriage legal in all 50 states. *NPR*. June 26, 2015. http://www.npr.org/sections/thetwo-way/2015/06/26/417717613/supreme-court-rules-all-states-must-allow-same-sex-marriages. Accessed November 28, 2016.

8. Freking K. Obama pledges to do more to stop the "epidemic of gun violence." *The Huffington Post*. January 1, 2016. http://www.huffingtonpost.com/entry/obama-gun-control_us_56869330e4b0b958f65bbb1b. Accessed November 28, 2016.

9. Leonard K. Should gun violence be treated like car accidents? *US News & World Report*. July 7, 2015. http://www.usnews.com/news/articles/2015/07/07/the-rise-of-gun-violence-as-a-public-health-issue. Accessed November 28, 2016.

10. Sanger-Katz M. Income inequality: It's also bad for your health. *The New York Times*. March 30, 2015. http://www.nytimes.com/2015/03/31/upshot/income-inequality-its-also-bad-for-your-health.html?_r=0. Accessed November 28, 2016.

46

On Engaging the Media

THE GOAL OF academic public health is, ultimately, to advance a conversation toward improving the health of populations. This means that our job does not stop with the generation of scholarship, or with the transmission of knowledge to our students. It must also include our commitment to translating that knowledge for the broader public, as we work to make sure that the thought we produce leaves the university's, or the academy's, walls. If it does not, it cannot inform and inflect the public conversation in a way that supports our agenda of improving the health of the public.

As I wrote in a previous chapter, the aspirations of public health "continue to be about the conditions that make people healthy, and thus must unstintingly engage the social, political, and economic foundations that determine population health." This inevitably argues for the engagement of the media, given the media's role in informing culture and shaping the values that, in turn, shape the foundations of health.

What are some of the challenges of engaging with the media? How can we turn these challenges into opportunities and contribute to the public conversation with an eye toward furthering the goals of public health? It strikes me that there are three central challenges to our engaging with the media in communicating our message. First, there is the challenge of making our voice heard amid multiple competing influences that aim to shape media messaging. Public health is only one, rather small, player in this larger game, and we often have limited resources with which to play it. In contrast, stakeholders whose interests may run counter to the interests of public health often hold a substantial advantage in resources, which can then be marshaled toward influencing media narratives and messages. The tobacco industry is a prominent example of this. In its heyday, the tobacco industry had the capital to produce high-quality advertisements that made smoking appear glamorous and ubiquitous. These advertisements have since been banned—one of the great triumphs of public health advocacy [1]. However, other industries continue to successfully market unhealthy behaviors. This includes the makers of soda, fast food, and sugary snacks, many of which even incorporate trendy words such as "healthy" and "fat free" into advertising where they are not appropriate [2, 3]. Thus, our messaging must inevitably compete for space with the messaging of well-funded organizations whose aims are often at odds with our own.

Second, there is the challenge of personalizing our work. Media narratives engage through the power of individual stories, appealing to the public's empathy to trigger interest in a given issue. This has been shown to be a very effective means of communicating—as the aphorism has it, "a single death is a tragedy; a million deaths is a statistic" [4]. However, it creates an uphill climb for those us who would advance the population-based, data-driven prevention efforts that are at the heart of public health. We see this perhaps most clearly in the recent focus on "lifestyle" diseases, a trend I decried in Chapter 37. Even when media communication focuses on the challenges presented, for example, by the obesity epidemic, messaging tends to elide a population focus, emphasizing the individual instead. Such messaging suggests that it is up to said individual to exercise, eat well, and maintain day-to-day well-being. This sells weight-loss programs and gym memberships, but it misses the larger, and far more important, role of the cultural, economic, and social factors that shape the conditions that encourage or discourage population healthy behaviors [5]. In many ways, therefore, the language of the medium works against the goals of public health, creating a challenging engagement for us indeed.

Third, there is a substantial gulf between the complexity of the real world and the simplification needed to convey messages compellingly through the media. This makes it difficult for the media to deliver complicated messages concisely, particularly in the case of rapidly emerging stories. Coverage of the Zika virus in 2015, for example, made this challenge quite clear [6]. The difficulties in covering Zika echoed another at-the-time current public health issue, as news outlets tried (and often failed) to deliver accurate and reliable information about the rapidly evolving Ebola epidemic [7]. We share much of the responsibility here, and it seems to me self-evident that academics need to be adept at communicating clearly, working closely with the press, both online and in print, to make sure that messages are indeed conveyed accurately and in a timely manner.

How can we best engage with the media to promote the health of the public? It seems to me that a clear awareness of the challenges we face is an important first step. We must also acknowledge, and capitalize on, opportunities. We are at a remarkable point in the history of communication, where the democratization of messaging as part of the digital revolution has created spaces for smaller players to communicate their messages directly. The growth of social media during the past decade represents a cost-effective way to get our message across via Twitter, Instagram, Facebook, and other outlets. We should engage, creatively, with these platforms, using our energy and savvy to truly take ownership of our messaging.

Public heath, although somewhat slow to the party, is increasingly engaging these methods, with one study showing that more than 60 percent of public health departments are using at least one social media application, the most common of which is Twitter [8]. These are not the only examples of public health's success in communicating its messages. It has also made use of online videos, to memorable effect. For example, in order to combat the soda industry's constant advertisements, the New York City Department of Health and Mental Hygiene released a vivid advertisement showing soda literally turn into fat [9]. This ad was viewed millions of times on YouTube and shared frequently. The water filter company Brita released similar ads for its own company using a parallel visual tactic [10]. These successes speak to the potential health-promoting power of active, energetic media engagement and to the kind of reach our messaging can achieve when public health "goes viral."

REFERENCES

1. Nixon Signs Legislation Banning Cigarette Ads on TV and Radio. The History Channel Web site. http://www.history.com/this-day-in-history/nixon-signs-legislation-banning-cigarette-ads-on-tv-and-radio. Accessed November 28, 2016.

2. The Impact of Food Advertising on Childhood Obesity. American Psychological Association Web site. http://www.apa.org/topics/kids-media/food.aspx. Accessed November 28, 2016.

3. Collins SPK. Parents sue fruit snack company for advertising its candy as a healthy choice. *ThinkProgress.* September 30, 2015. https://thinkprogress.org/parents-sue-fruit-snack-company-for-advertising-its-candy-as-a-healthy-choice-c27caad6affd#.bp5tiz3n9. Accessed November 28, 2016.

4. A Single Death Is a Tragedy; A Million Deaths Is a Statistic. Quote Investigator Web site. http://quoteinvestigator.com/2010/05/21/death-statistic. Accessed November 28, 2016.

5. NCHHSTP Social Determinants of Health, Frequently Asked Questions. Centers for Disease Control and Prevention Web site. http://www.cdc.gov/nchhstp/socialdeterminants/faq.html. Updated March 21, 2014. Accessed November 28, 2016.

6. Annas G, Galea S, Thea D. Zika virus is not Ebola. *The Boston Globe.* February 1, 2016. https://www.bostonglobe.com/opinion/2016/02/01/zika-virus-not-ebola/gbBZA18ILkLcLK2VN-M7XfM/story.html. Accessed November 28, 2016.

7. Mulholland Q. Be very afraid: How the media failed in covering Ebola. *Harvard Political Review.* November 26, 2014. http://harvardpolitics.com/covers/afraid-media-failed-coverage-ebola. Accessed November 28, 2016.

8. Thackeray R, Neiger BL, Smith AK, Van Wagenen SB. Adoption and use of social media among public health departments. *BMC Public Health.* 2012; 12: 242. doi:10.1186/1471-2458-12-242

9. Are You Pouring on the Pounds? Man Drinking Fat. NYC Health Anti-Soda Ad. Are You Pouring on the Pounds? Online video clip. YouTube Web site. https://www.youtube.com/watch?v=-F4t8zL6Foc. Accessed November 28, 2016.

10. Velvet Mediendesign. Brita—Sugar buildings. Online video clip. YouTube Web site. https://www.youtube.com/watch?v=ZScPGeoLz-w. Accessed November 28, 2016.

47

Making the Acceptable Unacceptable

PUBLIC HEALTH IS concerned with the health of populations, and it aims to improve all aspects of physical and mental health both locally and globally. This concern is informed by our ever-growing understanding of the challenges we face—of their stubbornness and their scope. We have relatively sophisticated methods of assessing the burden of disease—including mortality and disability-adjusted life years—as well as several ways of assessing morbidity [1, 2, 3]. This understanding has tangible effects, such as the establishment of funding and research priorities. The more we learn, however, the clearer it becomes that these priorities do not always match need. The mismatch between some aspects of burden of disease and health spending is well documented, with ample evidence that health concerns such as mental health are funded far less than physical health concerns [4]. Why is this? How are the goals of public health set in such a way as to motivate policy action that aims to mitigate the consequences of a particular disease? Perhaps most important, how can we nudge those goals toward greater health for all?

A useful framework for considering these questions derives from a 1958 paper published by Sir Geoffrey Vickers, a pioneering systems scientist and former president of the society that was the precursor to the International Society for the Systems Science [5, 6]. In his paper, "What Sets the Goals of Public Health?" he argues that we are motivated by the health challenges we consider to be intolerable and that action arises when a condition we considered a "given" becomes, indeed, "intolerable."

Let us consider Vickers' idea within the context of a few illustrations. In 1832, cholera epidemics were common throughout much of the world; in 2 months of that year, there were 3,500 deaths in New York City alone [7]. Today, however, the threat of cholera has greatly diminished, particularly in the United States. What changed? Through better understanding of germ theory, improvements in our capacity to deliver safe water and sanitation, political will to control cholera, and the economic means to implement cholera control measures, cholera has essentially been eradicated from the United States. Between 1995 and 2000, there was only one death in the entire country, and only 61 cases, the majority of which were acquired through international travel [8]. This represents a remarkable example of a health challenge once considered common and acceptable being dealt with through public health interventions spurred by the conviction that regular cholera outbreaks were not, in fact, acceptable after all.

Another key illustration of public health action concerns the dramatic reduction in motor vehicle accidents during the past half-century. In 1963, there were 41,723 motor vehicle deaths in the United States, with a fatality rate of 5.2 deaths per 100 million vehicle miles traveled [9]. In 2011, there were 33,561 deaths, with a fatality rate of 1.1 per 100 million vehicle miles traveled [9]. Despite a dramatic increase in the number of vehicle miles traveled, we reduced, in a single generation, the risk of motor vehicle fatality fivefold. This reduction came about in much the same way the decline of cholera occurred in the United States—through political will and attention to the broader context in which the threat was allowed to flourish. In reducing traffic deaths, this meant attending to road safety, advocating for safer driving, and creating legal disincentives for unsafe driving. All of these contributed to a rapidly growing unacceptability of the rates of motor vehicle fatalities and an adoption of measures geared toward positive change.

There are other examples in which making the acceptable unacceptable has created improvements in health. They include a drop in the US infant mortality rate from 55.7 per 1,000 live births in 1935 to 6.1 per 1,000 live births today—a nearly 10-fold decrease in 80 years—and a drop in the prevalence of elevated blood lead levels in children from 8.6 percent 20 years ago to 1.4 percent during the subsequent 10-year period [10, 11]. Changes in smoking habits (and attendant declines in related cancers) during the past 50 years provide another dramatic, and heartening, example [12].

All of these examples speak to the power of making the acceptable unacceptable and the good that can come of such a shift in attitudes. Vickers notes,

> The landmarks of political, economic, and social history are the moments when some condition passed from the category of the given into the category of the intolerable.
> . . . I believe that the history of public health might well be written as a record of successful redefinings of the unacceptable. [5]

Each of the previously discussed examples can serve as a case study for public action. They illustrate how particular conditions can reach tipping points, becoming unacceptable and triggering action. These tipping points were prompted by a confluence of circumstance—similar to the one characterized by Vickers more than 50 years ago—when society realized that a particular health hazard should no longer be tolerated. It then becomes possible to apply the technical (often therapeutic or preventive) know-how and economic capacity toward creating change. All these cases provide dramatic examples of what public health efforts can indeed achieve when the time is right—when a long-standing disease or danger finally prompts a society to collectively say "no more."

Encouraging as these examples are, there are also, unfortunately, many cases in which circumstances have not triggered action. This is particularly tragic in cases in which we have both the technical know-how and the economic resources to make a difference. For example, many of the health conditions that we have substantially improved in the United States remain at catastrophically high levels globally, particularly in low-income countries. The infant mortality rate in low-income countries is 76 per 1,000 live births; cholera continues to kill 2,102 annually; and 91 percent of the world's motor vehicle fatalities occur in low- and middle-income countries, despite those countries representing only half of the world's vehicles [13, 14, 15]. This begs the question: Why is cholera unacceptable in the United States but acceptable in Bangladesh? Why is it acceptable to have a 12-fold difference in the infant mortality rate between the United States and Cameroon? Yet we do not even have to leave the United States to find examples of needless, preventable death that we could easily stop but do not. Why is it acceptable, for example, that 33,636 Americans die annually from fire-arm deaths [16]? Or that 4,169 Americans die in motorcycle crashes in the absence of helmet laws [17]? We must continue to ask these questions until we can finally trigger meaningful action on these issues.

We must also work toward the "successful redefining" that can shape the goals of social action on public health. This is necessary if we are to both create positive change and avoid backsliding when hard-won successes, such as the dramatic decline in many early childhood diseases through vaccination, face opposition that has the potential to reintroduce long-eliminated health hazards. How might we best do this? Relatedly, how do we make sure that it is diseases that are viewed as unacceptable, rather than people, so that we may minimize stigma as we work to prevent future illness [18, 19]? Vickers suggests a way forward: "For public health has a unique opportunity, as well as a duty, to clarify our understanding of health and disease, and hence our attitude towards it" [5]. I agree.

However, this places a tremendous onus on academic public health to indeed "clarify our understanding of health and disease." It suggests that we need to make a particular effort to ask ourselves, in Vickers' formulation, "that critical and ubiquitous question: 'What matters most now?'" and work toward making it clear to the wider world exactly which determinants of heath matter most. This expression must be central to our work if we wish to create the social momentum necessary to implement public health solutions on the widest possible scale. It therefore does matter—very much so—if we articulate that the most common cause of death is heart disease, or being overweight, or lacking education, because the formulation of the causes of death contributes to changing how these causes are viewed by society and whether or not they are considered unacceptable and, ultimately, worth changing [20].

REFERENCES

1. Mathers C, Boerma T. Mortality measurement matters: Improving data collection and estimation methods for child and adult mortality. *PLoS Medicine*. 2010; 7(4): e1000265.

2. Metrics: Disability-Adjusted Life Year (DALY). World Health Organization Web site. http://www.who.int/healthinfo/global_burden_disease/metrics_daly/en. Accessed November 29, 2016.

3. International Classification of Functioning, Disability and Health (ICF). World Health Organization Web site. http://www.who.int/classifications/icf/en. Accessed November 29, 2016.

4. Gillum LA, et al. NIH disease funding levels and burden of disease. *PLoS One*. 2011; 6(2): e16837. doi:10.1371/journal.pone.0016837

5. Vickers G. What sets the goals of public health? *The New England Journal of Medicine*. 1958; 258(12): 589-96. doi:10.1056/NEJM195803202581205

6. International Society for the Systems Sciences Web site. http://www.isss.org/world. Accessed November 29, 2016.

7. Cholera in 1832. Virtual New York City Web site. http://www.virtualny.cuny.edu/cholera/ 1832/cholera_1832_set.html. Accessed November 29, 2016.

8. Steinberg EB, et al. Cholera in the United States, 1995-2000: Trends at the end of the twentieth century. *Journal of Infectious Diseases*. 2001; 184(6): 799-802.

9. Data. National Highway Traffic Safety Administration Web site. http://www.nhtsa.gov/ Data. Accessed November 29, 2016.

10. MacDorman MF, Hoyert DL, Mathews TJ. *Recent Declines in Infant Mortality in the United States, 2005-2011*. NCHS data brief No. 120. Hyattsville, MD: National Center for Health Statistics; 2013.

11. Jones RL, et al. Trends in blood lead levels and blood lead testing among US children aged 1 to 5 years, 1988-2004. *Pediatrics*. 2009; 123(3): e376–85. doi:10.1542/peds.2007-3608

12. Saad L. One in five US adults smoke, tied for all-time low. Gallup, Inc. Web site. http:// www.gallup.com/poll/156833/one-five-adults-smoke-tied-time-low.aspx. Published August 22, 2012. Accessed November 29, 2016.

13. Under-Five Mortality. World Health Organization Web site. http://www.who.int/gho/ child_health/mortality/mortality_under_five_text/en. Accessed November 29, 2016.

14. Number of Reported Deaths Due to Cholera. World Health Organization Web site. http:// www.who.int/gho/epidemic_diseases/cholera/deaths/en. Accessed November 29, 2016.

15. Road Traffic Injuries. World Health Organization Web site. http://www.who.int/mediacentre/factsheets/fs358/en. Accessed November 29, 2016.

16. National Center for Health Statistics: All Injuries. Centers for Disease Control and Prevention Web site. http://www.cdc.gov/nchs/fastats/injury.htm. Updated October 7, 2016. Accessed November 29, 2016.

17. National Center for Health Statistics: Accidents or Unintentional Injuries. Centers for Disease Control and Prevention Web site. http://www.cdc.gov/nchs/fastats/accidental-injury.htm. Updated September 15, 2016. Accessed November 29, 2016.

18. Stuber J, Galea S, Link BG. Smoking and the emergence of a stigmatized social status. *Social Science & Medicine*. 2008; 67(3): 420-30. doi:10.1016/j.socscimed.2008.03.010

19. Ahern J, Stuber J, Galea S. Stigma, discrimination and the health of illicit drug users. *Drug and Alcohol Dependence*. 2007; 88(2-3): 188-96.

20. Galea S, Tracy M, Hoggatt KJ, Dimaggio C, Karpati A. Estimated deaths attributable to social factors in the United States. *American Journal of Public Health*. 2011; 101(8): 1456-65. doi:10.2105/AJPH.2010.300086

48

Social Movements and the Conditions of Health

THERE IS LITTLE question that a consideration of public health would be incomplete without a consideration of the social movements that influence the attitudes and actions of the populations we serve. This point is well made in the report on "population health movement," part of an Institute of Medicine Population Health Improvement Roundtable [1]. Nancy Adler and colleagues point out that "some of the challenges to establishing population health derive from political and social concerns . . . [and] one of the hallmarks of the field is its attention to the social causes of disease and health" [1]. This observation speaks to the importance of social causes and, by extension, social movements—the roots of public health. The report argues that research and action must go hand in hand in order to facilitate change and that new technological developments such as electronic medical records, or "big data," in the form of social media, have the potential to integrate economic or social information into both research and policy change. These developments represent an exciting new chapter in the ongoing story of social movements and public health. With this possible future in mind, a look back at the history of social movements and public health and how each has at various points shaped, and been shaped by, the other.

Perhaps the most iconic public health-inspired social movement is the push to limit tobacco consumption that began in the 1950s and continued for the next several decades. This effort provides useful insights into the often incremental phases that lead to broad social change. Constance Nathanson argued in 1999 that compared to many other movements, the relative success of tobacco control efforts had much to do with the dissemination of information about the health risks of smoking, as well as grassroots mobilization geared toward protecting the right of nonsmokers to be healthy [2]. Nathanson breaks down the movement into three main phases. In the first phase, the health connection was made between tobacco and lung cancer, primarily in the medical press. This included the famous Doll and Hill reports, as well as the 1964 "Surgeon General's Report on Smoking and Health." The second phase entailed the "struggle for regulation," in which Congress excluded tobacco from being regulated under several acts, and loopholes were used to create milder warning labels. The third phase involved the "discovery of innocent victims." This gave birth to the nonsmokers' rights movement; in 1971, the Surgeon General urged the addition of a bill of rights for the nonsmoker to include a ban on smoking in all public spaces [3, 4]. Nathanson argued that restaurant smoking bans may have been due to nonsmokers' rights activism in conjunction with greater consumer sensitivity to health risks and media hyperbole. Particularly on point was Nathanson's reflection that "in a society increasingly skeptical of experts and expert knowledge, it is critically important to develop agile institutional mechanisms that link population health science and practice . . . [because] research alone will not produce change" [2]. This agitates for academic engagement in generating content that is accessible and aims to inflect such institutional mechanisms toward broader social ends. Of course, the work is not done, even on smoking—arguably public health's greatest achievement during the past century—with many groups suffering a high prevalence of smoking even today; however, we have seen great strides during the past half-century, due in large part to social movements [5, 6].

The story of change around motor vehicle safety is another example of progress being made due to the patient work of informing social movements. As with tobacco, we return to the theme of making the acceptable unacceptable. Indeed, progress on road safety would not have been possible without the denormalization of previously accepted behavior [7]. This case study provides some perhaps generalizable lessons about the elements of social norm transformation that can be leveraged toward change. Lawrence Green and Andrea Gielen suggest, in a book they co-edited, that three key elements emerged to contribute to changing norms around seat belt use [7]. First, public health initiatives provoke less controversy when they involve children compared to when similar restraints are advocated for adults. To this point, child car seat use was an aspect of vehicle safety that was easier to adopt compared to other measures. Second, there was the confluence of many sectors that came together to create safer roads. This was the case in the late 1980s, when transportation and law enforcement collaborated with community advocates to support legislation and education on car seats. Third, media and social marketing were paramount in promoting vehicle safety; the National Highway Traffic Safety Administration conducted large public education programs that helped to shape public opinion and garner support for policy change. One of the most successful campaigns that we all recognize is the "Click It or Ticket" slogan [8]. Taken together, the success of these efforts has been dramatic. In 1984, seat belt use was only approximately 15 percent in the United States; by 2007, it had increased to 82 percent—an extraordinary feat [9].

How might we apply these historical examples to two topics of contemporary relevance? As discussed in previous chapters, the evidence around the health consequences of racism and the unconscionable and persistent health inequalities in the United States is incontrovertible. The Black Lives Matter (BLM) movement has helped to bring the racial injustice at the heart of these issues to the forefront of the public debate, infusing this conversation with the weight of moral urgency [10]. BLM arose as a consequence of long-standing racial inequities and has been compared to the civil rights movement [11]. Both movements are arguably predicated on opposing the same core injustice, although the civil rights movement was catalyzed primarily by voting rights, and the BLM movement focuses more on institutionalized racism and the treatment of black individuals by the justice system. Speaking to these goals, a group of BLM activists published a set of specific policy recommendations called Campaign Zero, which proposed policing changes and compared the 2016 presidential candidates' positions on issues central to the concerns of the movement [12]. This approach aims to mobilize a diverse organizational constituency and bring about a convergence of political opportunities with target vulnerabilities. In a more up-to-date twist, social media and technology have played a key role in shaping BLM thus far, helping the group mobilize and spread awareness and news of events [13].

There is little doubt that moral urgency also rings true with the issue of climate change [14]. As the global temperature on the surface of the earth continues to rise, millions of people are expected to be pushed into poverty in the next 15 years [15]. Despite this threat, and recent moves by the Trump administration to roll back climate protections, there are encouraging signs of potential progress. For example, there is widespread consensus about the need to safeguard our planet—82 percent of Americans now believe it is their "moral duty" to protect the environment for future generations [16]. The climate change movement has especially gained momentum in the United States in recent years, as former President Obama rejected the Keystone XL pipeline, and the United Nations, in its 21st Conference of the Parties, urged action on climate change [17, 18]. Many have argued that the climate change movement has finally succeeded in convincing the public of global warming's dangers, and that the next step is government action [19, 20]. This would then conform to the three phases noted by Nathanson in her analysis of the anti-tobacco movement, as the initial establishment of a problem's health effects morphs into a struggle for regulation. It would be heartening if success on climate change did not need to wait until stage three—the discovery of "innocent victims"—but, rather, achieves the needed changes in time to ward off adverse health consequences.

In summary, the successful anti-smoking and car safety movements provide some lessons that can, it is hoped, have utility for future efforts. Going forward, success around the issues of climate change and racial inequities would do much to both improve our world and demonstrate, once again, the centrality of social movements to the business of creating healthier populations.

REFERENCES

1. Activity: Roundtable on Population Health Improvement. The National Academies of Sciences, Engineering, and Medicine Web site. http://www.nationalacademies.org/hmd/Activities/PublicHealth/PopulationHealthImprovementRT.aspx. Accessed November 29, 2016.
2. Nathanson CA. Social movements as catalysts for policy change: The case of smoking and guns. *Journal of Health Politics, Policy and Law.* 1999; 24(3): 421-88.
3. Doll R, Hill AB. The mortality of doctors in relation to their smoking habits. *British Medical Journal.* 1954; 1(4877): 1451-5.
4. Public Health Service. *Smoking and Health: Report of the Advisory Committee to the Surgeon General of the Public Health Service.* Washington, DC: Author; 1964.
5. Jacobson PD, Banerjee A. Social movements and human rights rhetoric in tobacco control. *Tobacco Control.* 2005; 14: ii45-ii49. doi:10.1136/tc.2004.008029

6. Brown DW. Smoking prevalence among US veterans. *Journal of General Internal Medicine.* 2010; 25(2): 147-9. doi:10.1007/s11606-009-1160-0

7. Kahan S, Gielen AC, Fagan PJ, Green LW, eds. *Health Behavior Change in Populations.* Baltimore, MD: Johns Hopkins University Press; 2014.

8. National Highway Traffic Safety Administration Web site. https://www.nhtsa.gov/risky-driving/seat-belts. Accessed November 29, 2016.

9. Accessible text file for GAO report No. GAO-08-477 titled "Traffic Safety: Improved Reporting and Performance Measures Would Enhance Evaluation of High-Visibility Campaigns." US Government Accountability Office Web site. http://www.gao.gov/assets/280/274733.html. Published April 25, 2008. Accessed November 29, 2016.

10. Eligon J, Pérez-Peña R. University of Missouri protests spur a day of change. *The New York Times.* November 9, 2015. http://www.nytimes.com/2015/11/10/us/university-of-missouri-system-president-resigns.html. Accessed November 29, 2016.

11. Harris FC. The next civil rights movement? *Dissent.* Summer 2015. https://www.dissentmagazine.org/article/black-lives-matter-new-civil-rights-movement-fredrick-harris. Accessed November 29, 2016.

12. Campaign Zero Web site. http://www.joincampaignzero.org/solutions/#solutionsoverview. Accessed November 29, 2016.

13. Stephen B. How Black Lives Matter uses social media to fight the power. *Wired.* November 2015. https://www.wired.com/2015/10/how-black-lives-matter-uses-social-media-to-fight-the-power. Accessed November 29, 2016.

14. Bieber M. Marshall Ganz, Obama's 2008 organizer-in-chief, on the moral urgency of Occupy Wall Street. *The Huffington Post.* November 14, 2011. http://www.huffingtonpost.com/matt-bieber/marshall-ganz-occupy-wall-street_b_1083078.html. Updated January 14, 2012. Accessed November 29, 2016.

15. Rapid, Climate-Informed Development Needed to Keep Climate Change from Pushing More than 100 Million People into Poverty by 2030. The World Bank Group Web site. http://www.worldbank.org/en/news/feature/2015/11/08/rapid-climate-informed-development-needed-to-keep-climate-change-from-pushing-more-than-100-million-people-into-poverty-by-2030. Published November 8, 2015. Accessed November 29, 2016.

16. Moore P. Poll results: Religion & climate change. YouGov Web site. https://today.yougov.com/news/2015/05/27/poll-results-religion-climate-change. Accessed November 29, 2016.

17. Davenport C. Citing climate change, Obama rejects construction of Keystone XL oil pipeline. *The New York Times.* November 6, 2015. http://www.nytimes.com/2015/11/07/us/obama-expected-to-reject-construction-of-keystone-xl-oil-pipeline.html. Accessed November 29, 2016.

18. COP 21 United Nations Conference on Climate Change Web site. http://www.cop21.gouv.fr/en. Accessed November 29, 2016.

19. Aronoff K. The climate-change movement is winning the argument—Now it must force the government to act. *In These Times.* July 20, 2015. http://inthesetimes.com/article/18186/turning-up-the-heat-on-washington. Accessed November 29, 2016.

20. Gitlin T. The climate change movement is not wishful thinking anymore. *Mother Jones.* October 6, 2014. http://www.motherjones.com/environment/2014/10/climate-change-movement-peoples-march-wishful. Accessed November 29, 2016.

49

Public Health as Public Good

∽——————————————————————————————

IN ECONOMICS, THE classic understanding of a public good is as follows: a good that is non-excludable and non-rivalrous—that is, where no one can be excluded from the good's use and where the use by one does not diminish the availability of the good to others [1]. Examples of public goods include such commonly available assets as air, water, parks, and national security. This original definition posits public goods as a "product (i.e., a good or service) of which anyone can consume as much as desired without reducing the amount available for others" [2]. A public good could then be characterized as the opposite of a private good, which is "any product for which consumption by one person reduces the amount available for others, at least until more is produced" [2]. By these definitions, a public good is not necessarily connected to the public sector, nor is a private good necessarily connected to the private sector.

This early conception of a public good has been much discussed and modified over time. In *The Affluent Society*, John Kenneth Galbraith describes public goods as "things [that] do not lend themselves to [market] production, purchase and sale. They must be provided for everyone if they are to be provided for anyone, and they must be paid for collectively or they cannot be had at all" [3]. Challenging established definitions, June Sekera offers a definition of public goods with three distinct elements: "Public goods are goods and services that are supplied through non-market, public production. I.e., they are: a. created through collective choice, b. paid for collectively, and c. supplied without charge (or below cost) to recipients" [4]. For his part, Marc Wuyts concluded that "public goods are socially defined and constructed according to what is perceived as a 'public need' rather than containing certain inherent characteristics of non-excludability and non-rivalry" [5].

What are some challenges associated with the provision of public goods, and how can we best mitigate them? From a classic economic perspective, the production of public goods can lead to a market failure, an imbalance that manifests when a free market economy does not achieve results efficient for the whole economy [6]. Such failure is mainly attributed to what is known as the "free rider" problem [7]. This arises as a consequence of when individuals choose to receive the benefits of a public good without helping to pay the costs of producing said benefits [7]. For this reason, public goods are frequently supplied by governments rather than private companies, and the bill is paid for collectively. In her book, *Why Democracy Needs Public Goods*, Angela Kallhoff argues that public goods contribute to the generation of civil society by creating conditions that assist citizens in identifying with a larger community of equal citizenship [8]. Moreover, she argues that social justice, engendered by fairness implicit in the availability of public goods, contributes to robust democracies. It is worth noting that Kallhoff does not argue that the state should provide public goods; she does, however, suggest that groups (e.g., nongovernmental organizations or actors with private resources) can provide public goods if they ensure open access.

Health is not generally considered a public good because nonpaying individuals (i.e., nonpaying for health insurance, healthy food, etc.) may not be able to achieve good health. However, health may be moving closer to this status as countries attempt to implement universal health coverage to ensure that all citizens are cared for [9]. Further steps include the adoption of social insurance systems or other publicly financed health insurance so that all citizens are insured and can utilize health care services, regardless of whether they can afford them or not; such measures suggest that insured health services might eventually become non-excludable and non-rivalrous, better approximating a public good [10].

Where does public health fit into our conception of public goods? I argue that public health is a prime example of public goods and that, viewed through this lens, we can better understand the true contribution of public health to society. There are three principle reasons for this.

First, building on the classical definition of public goods, public health is a collective property that depends principally on the economic, social, and political forces that create health rather than on any individual action. These conditions are features of social structures that are not owned, or purchasable, by individuals. Salutogenic urban environments, for example, are both non-excludable and non-rivalrous. So are policies that incentivize healthier foods and environmentally conscious efforts to minimize pollution. As was well-articulated in *Global Public Goods for Health*, the provision of public health is inextricably linked to government action and other classic public goods [11]. It follows, then, that the conditions that promote the health of the public are also classic public goods, even if our increasingly assertive ownership society may occasionally seem at odds with this characterization. Knowledge (e.g., knowledge of health risks), technology, policy, and health systems have many properties of considered public goods, but as Richard Smith argues, modern health technologies are "increasingly patented and thus made artificially excludable" [12, 13]. This is also the case with health systems, which, absent public financing, are not affordable to many.

Second, public health—which is to say, the health of the collective—is a clear example of shared gain resulting from a shared good. As David Woodward and Richard Smith argue, whereas a person (or group of people) may be the primary beneficiary of his or her (or the entity's) health, public health represents a collective benefit, from which no one is excluded; this is amply illustrated by examples of herd immunity or the protection from adverse health behaviors provided by salutogenic group behavior [12, 14]. For example, no one can be excluded from the benefit of infectious disease reduction, and one person benefiting certainly does not prevent others from benefiting as well.

Third, as the world rapidly globalizes, the quality of our health increasingly depends on that of the people living in other countries. This relationship—indeed, symbiosis—was well illustrated by the Ebola and SARS epidemics. The reality of this interconnectedness suggests that notions of nation-specific public goods are becoming outmoded and that the provision of public health is dependent on global public goods. This speaks to a need for universal solutions, defined as reaching more than one country or generation [12]. For example, no country can be excluded from benefitting from reduction in carbon dioxide emissions, which benefits the health of all.

Fourth, a core element of public health has always been, and should continue to be, the promotion of greater equity. Equity, in the context of health, means the opportunity for all to live in conditions that promote health and the minimization of intergroup health differences. This is synchronous with a conception of public goods whereby access to a positive resource is not limited by individual circumstance. Public health is then both a good in itself and a chance to access other goods and apply them toward the goal of creating a more "level playing field" [15].

Why does all of this matter? To answer that question, I refer to the suggestion, more than 20 years old, that public goods are socially defined and a matter of perceived public need [16]. We must make it clear that the core elements of public health are indeed public goods that manifest collectively, benefitting us all. We must further emphasize that these goods are interdependent with other public goods and essential for a healthy workforce and healthy consumers—thereby linking public goods to the production and consumption of private goods. This gives us the basis to agitate for collectively investing in policies that create and sustain health. It also implies that this investment should be cross-sectoral, opening the door for multiple actors to invest resources in the social, physical, and economic circumstances that shape the health of populations, for everyone's good.

REFERENCES

1. Cowen T. Public goods (from *The Concise Encyclopedia of Economics*). Library of Economics and Liberty Web site. http://www.econlib.org/library/Enc/PublicGoods.html#abouttheauthor. Accessed November 29, 2016.

2. Public Goods: A Brief Introduction. The Linux Information Project Web site. http://www.linfo.org/public_good.html. Accessed November 29, 2016.

3. Galbraith JK. *The Affluent Society, 40th Anniversary Edition*. New York, NY: Houghton Mifflin; 1998.

4. Sekera J. Re-thinking the definition of "public goods." Real-World Economics Review Blog Web site. https://rwer.wordpress.com/2014/07/09/re-thinking-the-definition-of-public-goods. Accessed November 29, 2016.

5. Deneulin S, Townsend N. Public goods, global public goods and the common good. *International Journal of Social Economics*. 2007; 34 (1-2): 19-36.

6. Market Failures, Public Goods, and Externalities. Library of Economics and Liberty Web site. http://www.econlib.org/library/Topics/College/marketfailures.html. Accessed November 29, 2016.

7. A Glossary of Political Economy Terms: Free Rider. Web page of Dr. Paul M. Johnson. Auburn University Web site. https://www.auburn.edu/~johnspm/gloss/free_rider. Accessed November 29, 2016.

8. Kallhoff A. *Why Democracy Needs Public Goods*. Lanham, MD: Lexington Books (Rowman & Littlefield); 2011.

9. What Is Universal Health Coverage? World Health Organization Web site. http://www. who.int/features/qa/universal_health_coverage/en. Accessed November 29, 2016.

10. Five Capitalist Democracies & How They Do It (from *Frontline: Sick Around the World*). Public Broadcasting Service Web site. http://www.pbs.org/wgbh/pages/frontline/sick-aroundtheworld/countries. Accessed November 29, 2016.

11. Smith R, Beaglehole R, Woodward D, Drager N, eds. *Global Public Goods for Health: Health Economics and Public Health Perspectives*. Oxford, UK: Oxford University Press; 2003.

12. Woodward D, Smith RD. Global public goods and health: Concepts and issues. World Health Organization Web site. http://www.who.int/trade/distance_learning/gpgh/gpgh1/en/index10.html. Accessed November 29, 2016.

13. Smith RD. Global public goods and health. *Bulletin of the World Health Organization*. 2003; 81(7): 475.

14. Smith KP, Christakis NA. Social networks and health. *Annual Review of Sociology*. 2008; 34(1): 405-29. doi:10.1146/annurev.soc.34.040507.134601

15. Stiglitz JE. Equal opportunity, our national myth. *The New York Times*. February 16, 2013. http://opinionator.blogs.nytimes.com/2013/02/16/equal-opportunity-our-national-myth. Accessed November 29, 2016.

16. Wuyts M, Mackintosh M, Hewitt T. *Development Policy and Public Action*. Oxford, UK: Oxford University Press; 1992.

50

A World Without Public Health

THIS BOOK ARGUES that improving the health of populations is the core goal of the academic health enterprise. Sometimes that goal seems frustratingly difficult to reach. I have commented on this frustration in previous chapters, commenting on the lives that could be saved by action on various areas, including firearms, or through better vaccination of populations.

However, it is important to acknowledge that during the past century, public health has also realized tremendous successes. We have much to learn, and perhaps celebrate, from these achievements. To that end, this chapter examines four of the great triumphs of public health and considers their implications. These four are drawn from the Centers for Disease Control and Prevention's "Ten Great Public Health Achievements in the 20th Century" list, highlighting advances related to tobacco, control of infectious disease, motor vehicle safety, and cardiovascular disease (CVD) [1]. For a fuller understanding of the significance of these achievements, we ask, in the case of each, the question: What would the world have looked like if we did not have success in these areas?

We start, perhaps inevitably, with the success of tobacco control in the United States in the 20th century [2]. This success can be attributed to a number of factors, including a successful campaign to educate the public about the health risks associated with smoking, public health efforts to reduce consumption, shifting public norms about smoking, and increased cigarette taxation. To illustrate the sweep of these measures, the rate of per capita cigarette consumption in the United States in the 20th century is presented in Figure 50.1A, annotated with relevant events that contributed to this success [2].

Figure 50.1A makes it clear that the doubling of the federal cigarette tax, the Fairness Doctrine, and the Master Settlement Agreement were all key inflection points in the larger effort to reduce tobacco consumption [2]. Attention to these textbook examples of macro-social determinants was instrumental in improving population health [3].

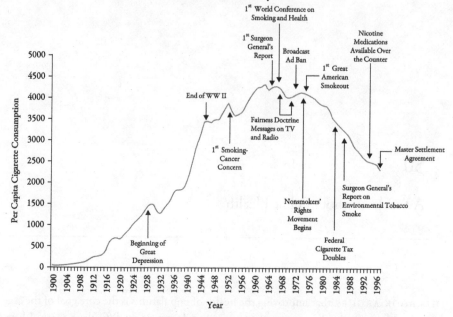

(A) **Annual adult per capita cigarette consumption and major smoking and health events in the United States: 20th Century**

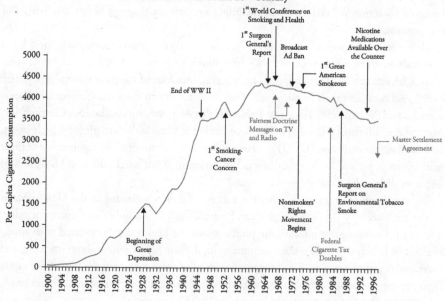

(B) **Annual adult per capita cigarette consumption and major smoking and health events in the United States: an alternate 20th Century**

FIGURE 50.1 (A) Tobacco consumption in the 20th century. (B) Tobacco consumption in an alternate 20th century. Created from Figure 1 of Created Created from Figure 1 of Achievements in Public Health, 1900–1999: Tobacco Use—United States, 1900–1999. *Morbidity and Mortality Weekly Report (MMWR)*. 1999; 48(43): 986–993 [2].

But what if these efforts had not been implemented? Or what if they had failed? For example, what if the federal cigarette tax had not doubled and the Fairness Doctrine and the Master Settlement Agreement had not been passed? One version of this alternate reality is presented in Figure 50.1B [2].

Figure 50.1B extends the preexisting trajectory while removing some of the key public health efforts that inflected the shape of the tobacco consumption curve. What would this alternate reality have looked like? We would estimate that the difference between the original and the revised curve represents an annual 451 cigarettes per capita on average between 1968 and 1997. At an ecologic level, we know that consumption of 3 million cigarettes is associated with one lung cancer death and that the time lag between consumption and death is 35 years on average [4]. Performing an area under the curve calculation, this would then mean an excess of 1,005,778 deaths from lung cancer between 2003 and 2032.

Now we move on to another major advance of the 20th century—control of infectious diseases. This achievement is due to a number of salutary factors, including a combination of sanitation and hygiene improvements, the advent of antibiotics, and universal vaccination programs [5]. The crude annual death rate attributable to infectious disease deaths in the United States is presented in Figure 50.2A, annotated with key events of import [5].

In this case, we do not ask what would have happened if key public health actions had never occurred; we simply imagine the effect of their delayed application. Figure 50.2B presents an alternate version, in which the initiation of widespread state health departments and the continuous use of chlorine were delayed by 10 to 20 years [5].

The might-have-been costs of this delay are dramatic. We estimate, based on the difference between the two curves, that between 1900 and 1995, this difference would translate into an excess of 21,651,243 infectious disease deaths.

Now we discuss the decline in CVD, a hallmark health improvement of the 20th century [6]. As with previous examples, success in this area can be traced to many factors, including societal changes in diet and smoking habits and advances in medical care. Particularly important were the Surgeon General's reports on smoking and environmental smoke, as well as the advent of statins. Figure 50.3A presents the death rate due to total CVD from 1900 to 2010 [7].

Again, we ask what this curve might have looked like if those societal advances had not occurred. This alternate reality is presented in Figure 50.3B, which supposes that the identification of CVD risk factors and the Surgeon General's reports on smoking and secondhand smoke did not happen [7]. According to our calculations, the consequence would have been 19,948,307 excess deaths between 1960 and 2010.

Finally, motor vehicle safety represents another signature public health achievement of the 20th century—it is also my favorite example of how structural change can improve health on a grand scale [8]. The core drivers of improved motor vehicle safety were federal regulatory efforts that improved the safety of vehicles and roads, changes in driving behavior and enforcement of driving laws, and public health communication efforts. The steep downward progression shown in Figure 50.4A illustrates the diminished rate of death per million vehicle miles traveled during the 20th century [8].

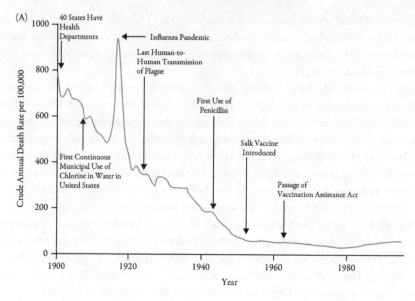

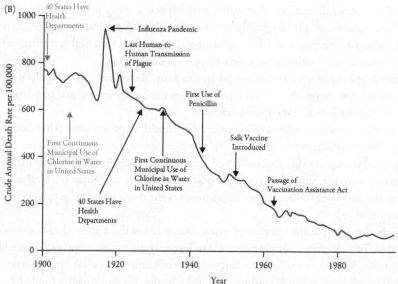

FIGURE 50.2 (A) Infectious Disease Control in the 20th century. (B) Infectious Disease Control in an alternate 20th century. Created from Figure 1 of Achievements in Public Health, 1900–1999: Control of Infectious Diseases. *Morbidity and Mortality Weekly Report (MMWR)*. 1999; 48(29): 621–629 [5].

Figure 50.4B shows an alternate version of this success story, providing a potential answer to the question: What if regulation of motor vehicle safety and enforcement of motor vehicle laws had never been instituted? Taking into account the difference between the two curves, we estimate that this would have meant an excess of 1,218,915 deaths in the United States between 1967 and 1999.

(A)

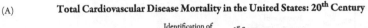

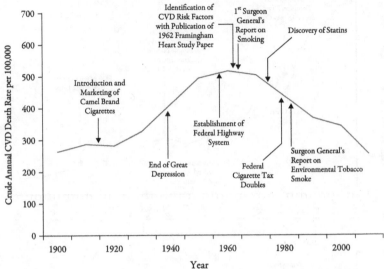

(B)

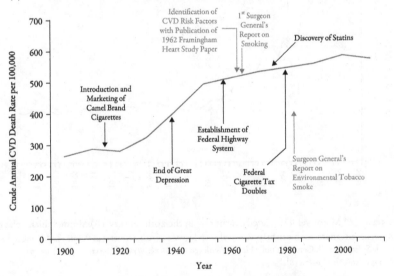

FIGURE 50.3 (A) Cardiovascular disease in the 20th century. (B) Cardiovascular disease in an alternate 20th century. Created from Disease Statistics Data Points for Graphics. National Heart, Lung, and Blood Institute Web site [7].

It is true that we can all ask, in dark moments, whither public health? But a fresh look at the achievements of public health suggests that if key public health interventions did not happen or were delayed, we would see about 50 million excess deaths from four major causes of death in the United States between 1901 and 2032. These figures, I think, speak for themselves, providing ample justification for the work we are engaged in and an inspiring preview of the world we could create through the broader application of our methods.

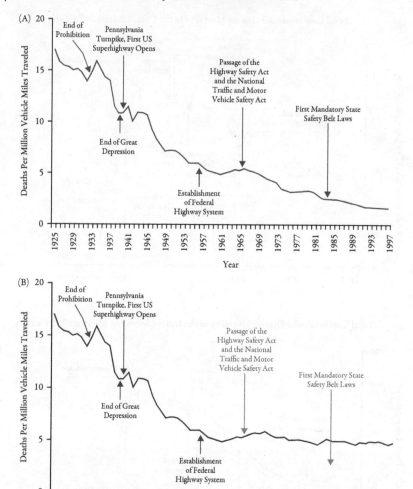

FIGURE 50.4 (A) Motor vehicle related deaths rate in the 20th century. (B) Motor vehicle related death rate in an alternate 20th century. Created from Figure 1 of Achievements in Public Health, 1900–1999 Motor-Vehicle Safety: A 20th Century Public Health Achievement. *Morbidity and Mortality Weekly Report* (*MMWR*). 1999; 48(18): 369–374 [8].

TECHNICAL NOTE

The estimates in this chapter were calculated with the assistance of Gregory Cohen, MSW. To derive the estimates, we extended the best-fit line beyond the date of the key public health action that we "deleted" and then calculated the new area under the curve to obtain excess mortality:

$$\sum \Big[\big(\text{Hypothetical rate}_i - \text{True rate}_i\big) * \big(\text{Population at risk}_i\big)\Big]$$

where i = year.

The equation for motor vehicle-related deaths is the same, with the exception that "Millions of vehicle miles traveled$_i$," is substituted for "Population at risk$_i$".

In the case of cigarette smoking, assuming that consumption of 3 million cigarettes is associated with one lung cancer death and 90 percent of lung cancer in the United States is caused by tobacco, we obtained an estimate of excess tobacco-related lung cancer deaths associated with cigarettes consumed between 1968 and 1997 using the following formula [4]:

$$\sum \frac{\left[\left(\text{Hypothetical consumption}_i - \text{True consumption}_i\right) * \left(\text{Population at risk}_i\right) * (0.90)\right]}{3,000,000}$$

where i = year.

REFERENCES

1. Ten Great Public Health Achievements in the 20th Century. Centers for Disease Control and Prevention Web site. http://www.cdc.gov/about/history/tengpha.htm. Updated April 26, 2013. Accessed November 29, 2016.

2. Achievements in public health, 1900-1999: Tobacco use—United States, 1900-1999. *Morbidity and Mortality Weekly Report (MMWR)*. 1999; 48(43): 986-93.

3. Galea S, ed. *Macrosocial Determinants of Population Health*. New York, NY: Springer; 2007.

4. Proctor RN. Tobacco and the global lung cancer epidemic. *Nature Reviews Cancer*. 2001; 1(1): 82-6.

5. Achievements in public health, 1900-1999: Control of infectious diseases. *Morbidity and Mortality Weekly Report (MMWR)*. 1999; 48(29): 621-9.

6. Achievements in public health, 1900-1999: Decline in deaths from heart disease and stroke—United States, 1900-1999. *Morbidity and Mortality Weekly Report (MMWR)*. 1999; 48(30): 649-56.

7. Disease Statistics Data Points for Graphics. National Heart, Lung, and Blood Institute Web site. https://www.nhlbi.nih.gov/about/documents/factbook/2012/chapter4data#gr6. Accessed November 29, 2016.

8. Achievements in public health, 1900-1999: Motor-vehicle safety: A 20th century public health achievement. *Morbidity and Mortality Weekly Report (MMWR)*. 1999; 48(18): 369-74.

INDEX

Note: Page numbers followed by *f* and *t* indicate figures and tables, respectively.